Hormone Optimization
In Preventive/Regenerative Medicine – Second Edition

A "Nuts and Bolts" Approach to Management

Ron Rothenberg MD
Kris Hart MN, RN-C, FNP
Roger Rothenberg BA

Hormone Optimization in Preventive/Regenerative Medicine- Second Edition

A "Nuts and Bolts" Approach to Management

By

Ron Rothenberg, MD
Kris Hart, MN, FNP, RN-C
Roger Rothenberg BA

California HealthSpan Institute
320 Santa Fe Drive, Suite 211
Encinitas, CA 92024
1-800-943-3331
1-760-635-1996
1-760-635-1994 (fax)
eHealthSpan.com

The information contained in this book is based on scientific research and the professional experiences of the authors over the past fifteen years. The information is not intended to be a substitute for consulting with your physician or other health care providers. The publisher and the authors are not responsible for any possible adverse effects resulting from the suggestions contained in this book.

Published by:
Panda Press
Encinitas, CA

Printed in the United States of America

AUTHORS' NOTE

Hormone Optimization in Preventive/ Regenerative Medicine- a "Nuts and Bolts" Approach to Management was written to educate physicians about hormone optimization and to be a reference and a companion guide. We realize that there is a large amount of information to absorb in this book. Practicing good medicine requires state of the art scientific information, clinical experience and judgment. What we hope to provide here is showing you our approach to managing our patients and providing you with peer review literature to support our management style. There are many aspects of this field of medicine that are controversial and even lead to emotional arguments. "Conventional wisdom" is often supported by myths not evidence. Because of these controversies we have provided the full abstracts of the medical literature we cite. In this way the reader can get a deeper understanding of the scientific information that is the basis of hormone optimization.

Note to Patients- This is not a guide to self-treatment. Please discuss this with your physician and hand her the book if you wish.

TABLE OF CONTENTS

FOREWORD

Hormones control information flow between cells, organs, tissues and even between individual organisms. As we age, adult hormone deficiencies become clinically relevant. Replacing adult hormone deficiencies is a major factor in maintaining health and fitness and can help to prevent the decline of physical and cognitive function that usually begins around the age of 40.

Hormonal optimization cannot be done in a vacuum. Optimal lifestyle including nutrition, exercise and stress reduction is an essential simultaneous treatment modality.

CHAPTER 1

The Neuroendocrine Theory:

The causes of aging, physiologic deterioration, and increased chance of death with time are multifactorial. Multiple explanatory theories exist including telomere loss, oxidative stress, "wear and tear" and glycation. The neuroendocrine theory proposes that a major cause of aging is the deterioration of optimal neuroendocrine controls that typically manifests in adult endocrine hormone deficiencies, but may also involve endocrine hormone excesses. This concept leads to the paradigm shift: "We age because our hormones decline, our hormones do not decline because we age." This is one of the paradigm shifts that anti-aging medicine explores, analyzes, and acts upon with balanced hormone replacement therapy. Important concepts to understand include what the difference is between "normal" hormone levels and desirable or ideal levels. We can discard the old concept that "normal for age" is really normal and acceptable. We can discard the concept that simply being in the "reference range' produces optimal health. For example, if a 75-year-old woman's estrogen level is zero, this might be "normal for age". But this absence of estrogen, which her body needs to function properly, may have grave consequences by causing decline in brain, bone, and cardiovascular and sexual function.

Endocrine hormones are the chemical messengers produced in one area of the body that travel to other areas to regulate cellular function. Autocrine hormones are made by all of our 60-90 trillion cells and report information back to the cell by interacting with the receptors on the surface and nucleus. These hormones are evolutionarily preserved from our one-celled ancestors. Paracrine hormones such as dopamine or serotonin transmit information across the synapse to adjacent neurons as well as neurons in the nearby area. This chapter details optimization of endocrine hormones, but simultaneous attention should be paid towards the optimization of autocrine and paracrine hormones through lifestyle and nutraceuticals. We now know that hormones have multiple roles that are just being discovered and the old idea of a limited and specific role for most hormones is obsolete. For example, testosterone is more than a male hormone and more than a sex hormone--androgen receptors are found throughout male and female tissues.

One of the most exciting aspects of the neuroendocrine theory of aging and hormones is that we can directly treat the loss of our hormones with balanced bio-identical hormone replacement therapy. Testing can assess hormone levels and hormone deficiencies can be replaced to the 20-30 year old level indefinitely.

Hormone replacement therapy has been studied in depth, and robust supportive data is present in the medical literature for the benefits of bio-identical hormone replacement therapy. A bioidentical hormone is simply a hormone that is identical to a hormone endogenously produced in the human body, atom for atom. This term should not be necessary since "bio-identical" is already within the definition of a hormone. However, since nonendogenous molecules have been used for "hormone replacement therapy" (with multiple adverse consequences) this distinction is unfortunately essential. Since this area is so controversial and emotional reactions to this paradigm shift are frequent among physicians, we have provided an extensive reference list, from peer reviewed medical literature, to back up the management plans in this chapter. Conclusions from studies of non-bioidentical hormones that are not part of human physiology do not apply to bioidentical hormones.

Stem Cells:

The next step to maintain health and fitness after hormone optimization will be via stem cell treatments. Optimization of each hormone improves our endogenous stem cell function. This is a major factor in improving and maintaining our natural repair mechanism. Hormone optimization improves endothelial progenitor cell function to maintain the cardiovascular system. Progesterone metabolites turn on neural stem cells in the brain. Testosterone activates satellite cells in muscle. In optimizing hormones we have taken the first step in stem cell therapies.

Inflammation:

Current theories of health and disease are centered on limiting chronic inflammation. As we will demonstrate from the literature, optimization of each hormone is anti-inflammatory. Even though the focus of this text is hormone replacement, do not forget other lifestyle interventions such as low glycemic diet, exercise (incorporating interval training, resistance and flexibility), stress reduction and elimination of infections as methods of inflammation reduction. Key nutraceuticals such as optimal vitamin D, Resveratrol, Omega 3 fatty acids and the synergism of all vitamins, minerals and other supplements, based on individual needs, are anti-inflammatory as well.

CHAPTER 2

Laboratory Testing:

It is useful to have baseline lab tests prior to evaluating and treating patients. A traditional medical lab evaluation is required to rule out disease and to assess hormone levels for deficiencies. Since this is a clinical specialty, lab tests should be used to confirm diagnosis, not to make the diagnosis. An engineering approach where we try to achieve a specific numerical value in a tightly controlled range is not part of the clinical model of hormone optimization. The reference range values are based on population statistics, but the optimal range is individualized for each patient.

Although there is controversy over the ideal type of testing (including serum, saliva and urine), serum testing has been the standard in endocrinology and is clinically useful. 24 hour urine testing, although more difficult to obtain patient compliance, is useful clinically and offers a more detailed evaluation of individual metabolic breakdown products. Salivary cortisol testing provides data points throughout the day and information regarding the diurnal pattern of cortisol release. Salivary assessment of other hormones has theoretical advantages but results have not been that useful for practical patient management in our experience. There are unlimited possibilities for testing, but the initial evaluation needs to be cost effective and easy to obtain. Further detailed testing can be done on an individual basis after the evaluation.

The suggested baseline tests that we order are:

- Complete Blood Count
- Comprehensive Metabolic Panel
- VAP panel or other expanded lipid profile
- Hemoglobin A1C
- Fasting Insulin
- Homocysteine
- Cardio C-Reactive Protein – high sensitivity
- Salivary Cortisol – 4 points
- DHEA-Sulfate
- Free and Total Testosterone and SHBG
- Estradiol and Estrone
- Progesterone
- IGF-1
- IGF-BP3
- LH
- FSH
- DHT
- TSH
- Free T4
- Free T3
- Reverse T3
- Thyroid peroxidase
- PSA
- CA-125
- Urine N-Telopeptides
- Urinalysis with culture if indicated
- 25 OH Vitamin D3

Although there are many options for vitamin and antioxidant levels a baseline assessment could include:

- Antioxidant Screen
- Fatty Acid Profile: Arachidonic Acid: Eicosapentanoic Acid (AA:EPA) ratio
- B 12 and folate serum levels
- CoEnzymeQ10
- Telomere analysis with attention to % critically short
- Comprehensive Stool Analysis to evaluate for concurrent leaky gut or parasitic infections.
- Heavy metal panels

It is important to mention that on the day of testing, these tests be done fasting, which includes not taking any supplements or medications the morning of the blood draw. This includes the application of the hormone creams. On occasion, patients have had to recheck their levels because the cream was applied to the same arm used to draw the blood, making levels supraphysiologic. If this is the standard, you will be able to compare future draws with consistency. The urine N-Telopeptides is a second morning random urine test, which makes it convenient when done with fasting lab testing. Hormone testing for women who are still cycling should be done during the mid-luteal phase (days 19-21). If weekly testosterone injections are being used, awareness of peak level at 48 hours and trough levels is necessary.

Additional testing should be done as baseline screening for patients prior to starting on hormone management. This includes the basic preventive medicine screens such as Pap smears and mammography or thermography for women. Colonoscopy, either direct or virtual, for men and women over 40 is recommended. Dental exams to evaluate for underlying infection and eye exams for visual changes that can occur with aging are also part of health management. Cardiac evaluation should be done, including Coronary Calcium Score, stress test and echocardiogram, if indicated by history. Annual dermatological evaluation is recommended. The basics of preventive medicine should not be neglected while advanced treatments are performed.

CHAPTER 3

Thyroid Hormones

Thyroid physiology:

The thyroid gland impacts every function in the body because it controls metabolism. Having thyroid levels in an optimal range is critical for good health and well-being. Approximately 80% of the thyroid hormone produced in the body is thyroxine (T4) and 20% is triiodothyronine (T3). Trace amounts of T1 and T2 are also synthesized in the thyroid, but have limited and poorly defined function. T3 is the active hormone and T4 is a prohormone; we do not have any T4 receptors in the body, only receptors for T3. Clinically, T3 is approximately 4 times more powerful than T4. Thyroid hormone synthesis involves putting two tyrosine rings together and adding four iodine molecules to comprise T4. We produce about 100 mcg per day of T4, synthesized by the thyroid gland. 30 mcg of T3 is also produced per day, though the majority by deiodination of T4. Deiodination (via selenodeiodinases) consists of removing an iodine molecule and thereby converting T4 to T3. The selenodeiodinases D1 and D2 catalyze conversion of T4 to T3. D3 (another selenodeiodinase) catalyzes conversion of T4 to Reverse T3, the stereoisomer of T3, which is inactive and may block receptor sites, effectively turning off thyroid function. D1 and D2 attenuate the effects of reverse T3 by converting it to T2, whereas D3 turns of T3 and converts it to T2. Hence D1 and D2 promote thyroid function on the front and back end, while D3 inhibits thyroid. Feedback controls of the thyroid hormones require hypothalamic secretion of Thyroid

Releasing Hormone (TRH) and pituitary secretion of the Thyroid Stimulating Hormone (TSH) to maintain balance.

Many factors decrease the conversion of T4 to T3, decreasing the active hormone and its effects. Beta-blockers, lithium, anticonvulsants, amiodarone and others can decrease conversion. Note, however, that a syndrome of amiodarone-induced hyperthyroidism also exists. Other factors affecting conversion include inflammation and infections, smoking, mental and physical stress, dieting, radiation and cancer. Selenium and iodine deficiencies (being required for selenodeiodinase and the construction of thyroid, respectively) can result in less available thyroid activity.

Thyroid Activation and Inactivation
Catalyzed by seleno deiodinases (D1-3)

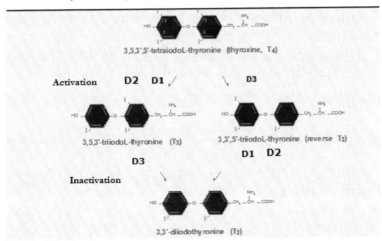

Thyroid lab:

Traditionally we are taught that the diagnosis of hypothyroidism should be made by evidence of elevated TSH and low T4. However, free T4 (the prohormone) and TSH often can be normal in hypothyroidism. The free T3, if low, is a much better indicator of suboptimal thyroid function, especially if paired with clinical symptoms. In contrast to the typical diagnostic black or white of hypo/hyperthyroidism, there is a continuum between euthyroid and hypothyroid, as there is between normal and elevated TSH. The mean TSH in America is about 1.4 without known thyroid disease. The thyroid peroxidase antibody (TPO), if elevated, screens for Hashimoto's thyroiditis or other autoimmune thyroid disorders. Hashimoto's disease is present in 13% of the U.S. population. African-Americans have the lowest incidence of Hashimoto's with an average TSH of 1.18. That is close to the "true", or optimal normal—in our clinical experience, patients feel best with a TSH of around 1.0. Low thyroid levels can also cause increased cortisol levels, which can eventually lead to adrenal fatigue. Patients with TSH levels greater than 2.0 are often clinically hypothyroid. Thyroid resistance, like insulin resistance, can occur even when TSH levels appear normal.

Thyroid Symptoms:

The most common symptoms of hypothyroidism are cold intolerance and cold hands and feet. The symptoms of hypothyroidism can vary widely, and can be counterintuitive, such as heat intolerance. The Hertoghe sign of lateral eyebrow thinning is a useful physical diagnostic clue. Hypothyroid patients cannot lose fat with exercise. To burn fat in the mitochondria beta 2 and thyroid nuclear receptor stimulation is required. For example, without thyroid you can't lose weight and you're too tired to exercise. The tiredness could have an adrenal component, which needs to be evaluated simultaneously. Fluid retention with the classic pretibial ankle edema, periorbital edema, and hypertension can also be present as well as depression, cognitive dysfunction, anxiety, arthralgias, dry skin and hair. Patients may only have a few symptoms from the list below to be clinically hypothyroid.

Thyroid Deficiency Symptoms:

- Cold Intolerance, cold hands and feet
- Handshake test
- Hertogue's sign (lateral eyebrow thinning)
- Fatigue
- Dry Skin
- Constipation
- Difficulty losing weight
- Depression
- Memory loss – Cognitive dysfunction
- Anxiety, Insomnia
- Arthralgias, muscle aches, headache
- Dry rough skin, thinning hair
- Hoarseness
- Too tired to exercise
- Lowered body temperature
- May have heat intolerance as well as cold intolerance
- Fluid Retention
- Periorbital or ankle edema
- Hypertension
- Brain Fog
- Muscle aches

Literature Review:

El-Shaikh in June 2006 looked at thyroid and the immune system. You need thyroid for immune system on various levels. As thyroid function declines the immune system deteriorates. Wartofsky in August 2006 evaluated thyroid in women. Thyroid disease is common in women. The incidence of Hashimoto's thyroiditis has risen to 15%. It is important to treat mild hypothyroidism in women and just like the other medical problems in women it is often overlooked. Danzi and Klein in 2004 studied thyroid and the cardiovascular system. In patients with low T3 syndrome and cardiovascular disease, T3 increased cardiac contractility and decreased systemic vascular resistance and improved the clinical outcome in cardiac disease. Patients with CHF may benefit from T3 replacement. Symptoms and signs of low T3 in cardiovascular disease include bradycardia, narrowed pulse pressure, diastolic hypertension, elevated CRP, inflammation markers and homocysteine. T3 has a role in the treatment of CHF and shows a synergistic effect with standard management. T3 treatment is antiarrhythmic because it shortens the QT interval and makes lethal arrhythmias less likely. It also improves cognitive and neuropsychiatric parameters. Decreased systemic vascular resistance results in decreased diastolic blood pressure, leading to decreased afterload and increased cardiac output. T3 also increases thermogenesis, burning fat and improving lipids. Christ-Crain et al. reviewed thyroid and CRP. Hypothyroidism is associated with premature atherosclerosis, cardiovascular disease and elevated CRP. Treatment of hypothyroidism improves elevated CRP. Nedrobo et al in 1998 demonstrated that hypothyroidism is associated with elevated homocysteine, which improves with treatment. Hak et al demonstrated that mild (subclinical) hypothyroidism is associated with aortic atherosclerosis and increased frequency of acute MI. Hamilton (1996) found that low T3 predicted mortality in CHF. More specifically, a low ratio of T3 to Reverse T3 was the strongest predictor of mortality. He (1998) also studied the use of IV T3 in advanced heart failure. There was no change in heart rate or metabolic rate, it was well tolerated, and there was increased cardiac output and decreased systemic vascular resistance. Danzi in 2005 found that 30 percent of patients with CHF have low T3 syndrome. Yoneda, in 1998, found that T3 dilated the coronary arteries, and that there was no effect from reverse T3. Shimoyama et al. in 1993, published in the Journal of Cardiology, studied thyroid and chronic CHF. The incidence of ventricular tachycardia was associated with low T3 and a high reverse T3. Cerrillo et al, 2003, reviewed patients post coronary artery bypass graft (CABG) and found that the strongest predictor of atrial fibrillation post operatively was low free T3 at P= 0.001. Iervase in Circulation, 2003, found that low T3 predicts death in cardiac patients. It is the strongest independent predictor of death, more than lipids or ejection fraction. Friberg et al. in 2001 looked at the association between reverse T3 and AMI mortality. They found that with elevated reverse T3, there was three times the mortality. Fernandez–Real, in 2006 looked at healthy euthyroid subjects and found that optimal thyroid function is needed for insulin sensitivity, HDL and for endothelial function. Asvold, in March 2007, 30,000 individuals without previously known thyroid disease were evaluated regarding thyroid function and blood pressure. Inclusion criteria were TSH within the reference range: 0.5 to 3.5. There was a linear increase in blood pressure with increasing

19

TSH. Just within that normal range, having thyroid optimal lowered blood pressure. Asvold in 2007 studied the same group of individuals and found the lower the TSH, the higher the HDL, and the lower the LDL and triglycerides. Schulte et al in 1998 found that a low T3, high reverse T3 predicts mortality in ICU patients. Berger et al. in 2001 looked at selenium and post trauma thyroid changes. 500 mcg of selenium in selenium deficient patients was needed to normalize thyroid function.

Thyroid Management:

The traditional method of thyroid replacement therapy is to replace T4 (thyroxine) rather than a combination of T4 and T3 (thyroxine, liothyronine). Some patients may be adequately treated with this therapy, however multiple studies reflect that patients may feel better and actually prefer the combination therapy. Since many patients poorly convert T4 to T3, optimal treatment should include a combination of treatment with both T4 and T3. Best clinical results for thyroid replacement are achieved with desiccated porcine thyroid. Desiccated thyroid is a natural substance derived from the thyroid glands of pigs. Each grain (60 mg) of desiccated porcine contains 38 mcg T4 and 9 mcg T 3, as well as trace amounts of T1 and T2. This combination can also be prepared by a compounding pharmacy utilizing either porcine or non-porcine ingredients. The dose prescribed for thyroid replacement is dependent upon the clinical presentation, the TSH and free T3 levels. The question arises that if T3 is the active hormone why prescribe a combination treatment? The half-life of T 4 is about 6 days and the half-life of T3 is about 18 hours. Combination treatment has the advantages of maintaining levels as the T3 wears off.

Even if the patient is a poor converter there will be some conversion and the patient will not be at risk of "crashing" if a dose is forgotten.

Based on lab and clinical symptoms we initially recommend desiccated Thyroid 1 grain (60mg) one tab daily in the morning on an empty stomach and titrate as needed. It would be more physiologic to divide the dose with a second dose around 2 pm, but for patient compliance, it is better to start with a single morning dose. We educate our patients on the signs and symptoms of hyperthyroidism like palpitations, sweating etc. We make sure that they have incorporated adequate selenium and iodine in their diet and that the other hormones are also being replaced if deficient. Follow up lab testing in 8 weeks with ultimate clinical goals of improved energy and focus, warmer hands and lab goals of Free T3 in upper quartile of the reference range. If results suboptimal, continued titration up or down by ½ grain, until desired results are obtained. Monitor N-telopeptide urines for evidence of bone stability and EKG for heart rhythm if indicated. Bone density scans can be obtained but they take years to show the effect of treatment.

Thyroid Troubleshooting:

1. Patient with symptoms of thyroid excess- palpitations, shakiness-
    - Decrease the dosages by ½ grain; if still symptomatic hold it for a 5-7 days and restart at half the original dosage.
    - Evaluate for atrial fibrillation or other arrhythmia if palpitations are present.

2.   Patient notices no change-
   - If early in the treatment, patience, as it can take 3-4 weeks to notice clinical improvement, even if serum testing adequate.

3.   Reverse T3 remains high and T3/T4 treatment not clinically adequate-
   - Consider treating with time release T3 exclusively since reverse T3 is produced from T4 and by not adding exogenous T4, the substrate for reverse T3 is decreased.

THYROID ALGORITHM

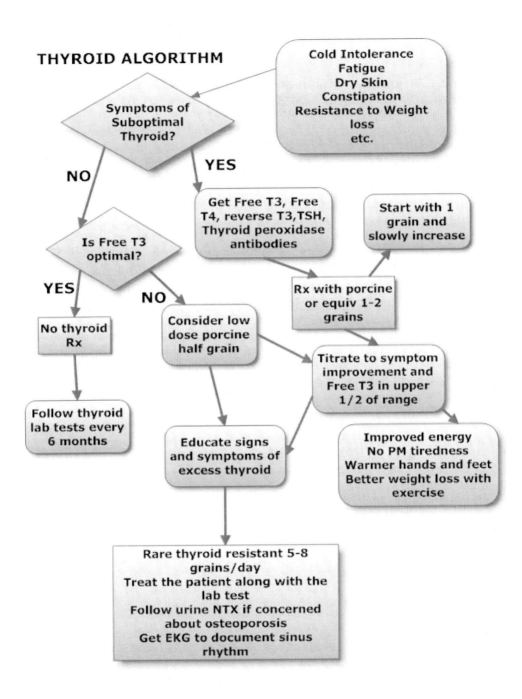

Cold Intolerance
Fatigue
Dry Skin
Constipation
Resistance to Weight loss
etc.

Symptoms of Suboptimal Thyroid?

NO

YES

Get Free T3, Free T4, reverse T3,TSH, Thyroid peroxidase antibodies

Start with 1 grain and slowly increase

Is Free T3 optimal?

YES

NO

No thyroid Rx

Rx with porcine or equiv 1-2 grains

Consider low dose porcine half grain

Titrate to symptom improvement and Free T3 in upper 1/2 of range

Follow thyroid lab tests every 6 months

Educate signs and symptoms of excess thyroid

Improved energy
No PM tiredness
Warmer hands and feet
Better weight loss with exercise

Rare thyroid resistant 5-8 grains/day
Treat the patient along with the lab test
Follow urine NTX if concerned about osteoporosis
Get EKG to document sinus rhythm

THYROID ABSTRACTS

Agid O. Triiodothyronine augmentation of selective serotonin reuptake inhibitors in posttraumatic stress disorder. J Clin Psychiatry 2001 Mar; 62(3):169-73 BACKGROUND: There is considerable comorbidity of major depression and posttraumatic stress disorder (PTSD), and antidepressants have been reported to be effective in treating PTSD. Addition of triiodothyronine (T3) to ongoing antidepressant treatment is considered an effective augmentation strategy in refractory depression. We report the effect of T3 augmentation of antidepressants in patients with PTSD. METHOD: T3 (25 microg/day) was added to treatment with a selective serotonin reuptake inhibitor (SSRI) (paroxetine or fluoxetine, 20 mg/day for at least 4 weeks and 40 mg/day for a further 4 weeks) of 5 patients who fulfilled DSM-IV criteria for PTSD but not for major depressive disorder (although all patients had significant depressive symptoms). The Clinician-Administered PTSD Scale, the 21-item Hamilton Rating Scale for Depression, and the Clinical Global Impressions-Severity of Illness scale were administered every 2 weeks, and self-assessments were performed with a 100 mm visual analog mood scale. RESULTS: In 4 of the 5 patients, partial clinical improvement was observed with SSRI treatment at a daily dose of 20 mg with little further improvement when the dose was raised to 40 mg/day. This improvement was substantially enhanced by the addition of T3. Improvement was most striking on the Hamilton Rating Scale for Depression. CONCLUSION: T3 augmentation of SSRI treatment may be of therapeutic benefit in patients with PTSD, particularly those with depressive symptoms. Larger samples and controlled studies are needed in order to confirm this observation.

Asakura H. et al. Severity of Hyperemesis gravidarum correlates with serum levels of reverse T3. Arch Gyn Obs 2000, 264 257-262 To investigate the possible physiological relevance of extra-thyroidal production of reverse T3 (rT3) in hyperemesis gravidarum, measurements of serum rT3, free T3 (FT3), free T4, (FT4), and nonesterified fatty acids (NEFA) were correlated with weight loss of hyperemetic women. All the thyroid hormones, NEFAs and weight loss were significantly higher in hyperemesis gravidarum than in control subjects, and also higher than in those with milder symptoms of morning sickness ($p < 0.05$). Elevations of FT3, FT4 and NEFAs correlated with the extent of weight loss, the latter taken as the index of the severity of hyperemesis gravidarum ($p < 0.05$). Only rT3 correlated with both weight loss and the rate of lipolysis, as reflected by elevations of NEFAs ($p < 0.05$). The data are consistent with a shift from T3 to rT3 as products of 5'-monodeiodination of thyroxine in hyperemesis gravidarum. Because reverse T3 is physiologically inactive a control mechanism may be postulated wherein T3 production is minimized, thereby reducing weight loss and lipolysis in patients with hyperemesis gravidarum.

Baldini M et al. Treatment of benign nodular goitre with mildly suppressive doses of L-thyroxine: effects on bone mineral density and on nodule size. J Intern Med. 2002 May; 251(5):407-14. OBJECTIVES: To evaluate (i) the demineralizing effect of L-thyroxine (LT4) therapy at doses mildly inhibiting serum thyroid stimulating hormone (TSH) in patients with benign nodular goitre; (ii) the efficacy of treatment on nodule size. DESIGN: Cross-sectional study comparing euthyroid women with nodular goitre treated with LT4 for > or = 2 years (52 +/- 32 months, range 24-138, median 42) and a matched group with untreated goitre. SUBJECTS: A total of 89 female outpatients (53.3 +/- 9 years; 36 pre- and 53 postmenopausal), 43 treated and 46 untreated. MAIN OUTCOME MEASURES: Bone mineralization was measured with total body and regional mineralometry [dual energy X-ray absorptiometry (DEXA)], and indirectly evaluated with biochemical parameters (alkaline phosphatase, osteocalcin). Efficacy of LT4 therapy was assessed by measuring the nodule size during ultrasonography. The adequacy of the treatment was evaluated on the basis of serum TSH levels. RESULTS: No significant differences were found at DEXA for total body and regional mineralization (P > 0.05 for all comparisons) in treated and untreated patients, both in pre- and postmenopausal states. Evaluation of the nodule size during the ultrasound scan showed a reduction of > or = 30% in 11 of 43 treated patients (26%) versus none of the untreated, an unchanged size in 29 treated patients (67%) versus 18 untreated, an increase of nodules and/or new nodule development in three treated patients (7%) versus 28 untreated (61%). CONCLUSIONS: L-thyroxine (LT4) treatment at doses slightly suppressing TSH does not significantly affect bone mineralization, nor does it represent a risk factor for osteoporosis, even in postmenopausal patients. The efficacy of this therapeutic schedule on goitre size is comparable with the effects previously reported with suppressive doses.

Berger MM et al. Influence of selenium supplements on the post-traumatic alterations of the thyroid axis: a placebo-controlled trial. Intensive Care Med 2001 Jan;27(1):91-100 OBJECTIVE: To investigate whether early selenium (Se) supplementation can modify the post-traumatic alterations of thyroid hormone metabolism, since the first week after trauma is characterised by low plasma Se and negative Se balances. DESIGN: Prospective, placebo-controlled randomised supplementation trial. SETTING: Surgical ICU in a tertiary university hospital. PATIENTS: Thirty-one critically ill trauma patients aged 42 +/- 16 years (mean +/- SD), with severe multiple injury (Injury Severity Score 30 +/- 7). INTERVENTION: Supplementation during the first 5 days after injury with either Se or placebo. The selenium group was further randomised to receive daily 500 microg Se, with or without 150 mg alpha-tocopherol (AT) and 13 mg zinc supplements. The placebo group received the vehicle. Circulating Se, AT, zinc, and thyroid hormones were determined on D0 (= day 0, admission), D1, D2, D5, D10, and D20. RESULTS: Plasma Se, low on D0, normalised from D1 in the selenium group; total T4 and T3 increased more and faster after D2 (P

= 0.04 and 0.08), reverse T3 rising less between D0 and D2 (P = 0.05). CONCLUSIONS: Selenium supplements increased the circulating Se levels. Supplementation was associated with modest changes in thyroid hormones, with an earlier normalisation of T4 and reverse T3 plasma levels. The addition of AT and zinc did not produce any additional change.

Bianco et al. Biochemistry, Cellular and Molecular Biology and Physiological Roles of the Iodothyroine Selenodeiodinases. Endocrine Reviews, 2002

The goal of this review is to place the exciting advances that have occurred in our understanding of the molecular biology of the types 1, 2, and 3 (D1, D2, and D3, respectively) iodothyronine deiodinases into a biochemical and physiological context. We review new data regarding the mechanism of selenoprotein synthesis, the molecular and cellular biological properties of the individual deiodinases, including gene structure, mRNA and protein characteristics, tissue distribution, subcellular localization and topology, enzymatic properties, structure-activity relationships, and regulation of synthesis, inactivation, and degradation. These provide the background for a discussion of their role in thyroid physiology in humans and other vertebrates, including evidence that D2 plays a significant role in human plasma T(3) production. We discuss the pathological role of D3 overexpression causing "consumptive hypothyroidism" as well as our current understanding of the pathophysiology of iodothyronine deiodination during illness and amiodarone therapy. Finally, we review the new insights from analysis of mice with targeted disruption of the Dio2 gene and overexpression of D2 in the myocardium.

Biondi, B et al. Combination replacement of T4 and T3: toward personalized replacement in hypothyroidism.   JCEM 2012 Jul;97(7):2256-71

Context: Levothyroxine therapy is the traditional lifelong replacement therapy for hypothyroid patients. Over the last several years, new evidence has led clinicians to evaluate the option of combined T(3) and T(4) treatment to improve the quality of life, cognition, and peripheral parameters of thyroidhormone action in hypothyroidism. The aim of this review is to assess the physiological basis and the results of current studies on this topic. Evidence Acquisition: We searched Medline for reports published with the following search terms: hypothyroidism, levothyroxine, triiodothyronine,thyroid, guidelines, treatment, deiodinases, clinical symptoms, quality of life, cognition, mood, depression, body weight, heart rate, cholesterol, bone markers, SHBG, and patient preference for combined therapy. The search was restricted to reports published in English since 1970, but some reports published before 1970 were also incorporated. We supplemented the search with records from personal files and references of relevant articles and textbooks. Parameters analyzed included the rationale for combination treatment, the type of patients to be selected, the optimal T(4)/T(3) ratio, and the potential benefits of this therapy on symptoms of hypothyroidism, quality of life, mood, cognition, and peripheral parameters of thyroid hormone action. Evidence Synthesis: The outcome of our analysis suggests that it may be time to consider a personalized regimen of thyroid hormone replacement therapy in hypothyroid patients. Conclusions: Further prospective randomized controlled studies are needed to clarify this important issue. Innovative formulations of the thyroid hormones will be required to mimic a more perfect thyroid hormone replacement therapy than is currently available

Bunevicius R et al. Effects of thyroxine as compared with thyroxine plus triiodothyronine in patients with hypothyroidism. N Engl J Med 1999 Feb 11; 340(6):424-9
BACKGROUND: Patients with hypothyroidism are usually treated with thyroxine (levothyroxine) only, although both thyroxine and triiodothyronine are secreted by the normal thyroid gland. Whether thyroid secretion of triiodothyronine is physiologically important is unknown. METHODS: We compared the effects of thyroxine alone with those of thyroxine plus triiodothyronine (liothyronine) in 33 patients with hypothyroidism. Each patient was studied for two five-week periods. During one period, the patient received his or her usual dose of thyroxine. During the other, the patient received a regimen in which 50 microg of the usual dose of thyroxine was replaced by 12.5 microg of triiodothyronine. The order in which each patient received the two treatments was randomized. Biochemical, physiologic, and psychological tests were performed at the end of each treatment period. RESULTS: The patients had lower serum free and total thyroxine concentrations and higher serum total triiodothyronine concentrations after treatment with thyroxine plus triiodothyronine than after thyroxine alone, whereas the serum thyrotropin concentrations were similar after both treatments. Among 17 scores on tests of cognitive performance and assessments of mood, 6 were better or closer to normal after treatment with thyroxine plus triiodothyronine. Similarly, among 15 visual-analogue scales used to indicate mood and physical status, the results for 10 were significantly better after treatment with thyroxine plus triiodothyronine. The pulse rate and serum sex hormone-binding globulin concentrations were slightly higher after treatment with thyroxine plus triiodothyronine, but blood pressure, serum lipid concentrations, and the results of neurophysiologic tests were similar after the two treatments. CONCLUSIONS: In patients with hypothyroidism, partial substitution of triiodothyronine for thyroxine may improve mood and neuropsychological function; this finding suggests a specific effect of the triiodothyronine normally secreted by the thyroid gland.

Canaris GJ, et al. The Colorado thyroid disease prevalence study. Arch Intern Med. 2000; 160:526-534. CONTEXT: The prevalence of abnormal thyroid function in the United States and the significance of thyroid dysfunction remain controversial. Systemic effects of abnormal thyroid function have not been fully delineated, particularly in cases of mild thyroid failure. Also, the relationship between traditional hypothyroid symptoms and biochemical thyroid function is unclear. OBJECTIVE: To determine the prevalence of abnormal thyroid function and the relationship between (1) abnormal thyroid function and lipid levels and (2) abnormal thyroid function and symptoms using modern and sensitive thyroid tests. DESIGN: Cross-sectional study. PARTICIPANTS: Participants in a statewide health fair in Colorado, 1995 (N = 25 862). MAIN OUTCOME MEASURES: Serum thyrotropin (thyroid-stimulating hormone [TSH]) and total thyroxine (T4) concentrations, serum lipid levels, and responses to a hypothyroid symptoms questionnaire. RESULTS: The prevalence of elevated TSH levels (normal range, 0.3-5.1 mIU/L) in this population was 9.5%, and the prevalence of decreased TSH levels was 2.2%. Forty percent of patients taking thyroid medications had abnormal TSH levels. Lipid levels increased in a graded fashion as thyroid function declined. Also, the mean total cholesterol and low-density lipoprotein cholesterol levels of subjects with TSH values between 5.1 and 10 mIU/L were significantly greater than the corresponding mean lipid levels in euthyroid subjects. Symptoms were reported more often in hypothyroid vs euthyroid individuals, but individual symptom sensitivities were low. CONCLUSIONS: The prevalence of abnormal biochemical thyroid function reported here is substantial and confirms previous reports in smaller populations. Among patients taking thyroid medication, only 60% were within the normal range of TSH. Modest elevations of TSH corresponded to changes in lipid levels that may affect cardiovascular health. Individual symptoms were not very sensitive, but patients who report multiple thyroid symptoms warrant serum thyroid testing. These results confirm that thyroid dysfunction is common, may often go undetected, and may be associated with adverse health outcomes that can be avoided by serum TSH measurement.

Cerillo AG et al. Free Triiodothyronine: a novel predictor of postoperative atrial fibrillation. Eur J. Cardiothorac Surg 2003 Oct, 24(4) 487-92. OBJECTIVE: Despite improved perioperative management, atrial fibrillation (AF) after coronary artery bypass grafting (CABG) remains a relevant clinical problem, whose pathogenetic mechanisms remain incompletely explained. A reduced incidence of postoperative AF has been described in CABG patients receiving IV tri-iodothyronine (T3). This study was designed to define the role of thyroid metabolism on the genesis of postoperative AF. METHODS AND RESULTS: Free T3 (fT3), free thyroxine (fT4), and thyroid stimulating hormone were assayed at admission in 107 consecutive patients undergoing isolated CABG surgery. Patients with thyroid disease or taking drugs known to interfere with thyroid function were excluded. A preoperative rhythm other than sinus rhythm was considered an exclusion criterion. Thirty-three patients (30.8%) had postoperative AF. An older age (P=0.03), no therapy with beta-blockers (P=0.08), chronic obstructive pulmonary disease (P=0.08), lower left ventricle ejection fraction (P=0.09) and lower fT3 concentration (P=0.001), were univariate predictors of postoperative AF. On multivariate analysis, low fT3 concentration and lack of beta-blocking therapy were independently related with the development of postoperative AF (odds ratio, OR, 4.425; 95% confidence interval, CI, 1.745-

11.235; P=0.001 and OR 3.107; 95% CI 1.087-8.875; P=0.03, respectively). Postoperative AF significantly prolonged postoperative hospital stay (P=0.002). CONCLUSIONS: Low basal fT3 concentration can reliably predict the occurrence of postoperative AF in CABG patients.

Christ-Crain M et al. Elevated C-reactive protein and homocysteine values: cardiovascular risk factors in hypothyroidism? A cross-sectional and a double-blind, placebo-controlled trial. Atherosclerosis 2003 Feb; 166(2): 379-86
Hypothyroidism is associated with premature atherosclerosis and cardiovascular disease. Recently, total homocysteine (tHcy) and C-reactive protein (CRP) emerged as additional cardiovascular risk factors. We first investigated CRP and tHcy in different severities of primary hypothyroidism and in a second study we evaluated the effect of L-thyroxine treatment in patients with subclinical hypothyroidism (SCH) in a double-blind, placebo-controlled trial. One hundred and twenty-four hypothyroid patients (63 with subclinical, 61 with overt hypothyroidism, OH) and 40 euthyroid controls were evaluated. CRP was measured using a latex-based high sensitivity immunoassay; tHcy was determined by a fluorescence polarization immunoassay. tHcy values were significantly elevated in OH (P=0.01). In SCH tHcy levels were not augmented as compared to controls. CRP values were significantly increased in OH (P=0.016) and SCH (P=0.022) as compared to controls. In a univariate analysis tHcy correlated significantly with fT4, vitamin B12, folic acid and creatinine levels. In multiple regression analysis only fT4 (beta=0.33) had a significant effect on tHcy. CRP did not correlate with thyroid hormones. In SCH, L-T4 replacement had no significant effect on either tHcy or CRP levels. This is the first paper to show that CRP values increase with progressive thyroid failure and may count as an additional risk factor for the development of coronary heart disease in hypothyroid patients. In contrast to overt disease, only CRP, but not tHcy values, are affected in SCH, yet without significant improvement after L-thyroxine therapy.

Clyde PW et al. Combined levothyroxine plus liothyronine compared with levothyroxine alone in primary hypothyroidism: a randomized controlled trial. JAMA. 2003 Dec 10; 290(22):2952-8. CONTEXT: Standard therapy for patients with primary hypothyroidism is replacement with synthetic thyroxine, which undergoes peripheral conversion to triiodothyronine, the active form of thyroid hormone. Within the lay population and in some medical communities, there is a perception that adding synthetic triiodothyronine, or liothyronine, to levothyroxine improves the symptoms of hypothyroidism despite insufficient evidence to support this practice. OBJECTIVE: To evaluate the benefits of treating primary hypothyroidism with levothyroxine plus liothyronine combination therapy vs levothyroxine monotherapy. DESIGN, SETTING, AND PATIENTS: Randomized, double-blind, placebo-controlled trial conducted from May 2000 to February 2002 at a military treatment facility that serves active duty and retired military personnel and their family members. The trial included a total of 46 patients aged 24 to 65 years with at least a 6-month history of treatment with levothyroxine for primary hypothyroidism. INTERVENTION: Patients received either their usual dose of levothyroxine (n = 23) or combination therapy (n = 23), in which their usual levothyroxine dose was reduced by 50 micro g/d and substituted with liothyronine, 7.5 micro g, taken twice daily for 4 months. MAIN OUTCOME MEASURES: Scores on a hypothyroid-specific health-related quality-of-life (HRQL) questionnaire, body weight, serum lipid levels, and 13 neuropsychological tests measured before and after treatment. RESULTS: Serum thyrotropin levels remained similar and within the normal range in both treatment groups from baseline to 4 months. Body weight and serum lipid levels did not change. The HRQL questionnaire scores improved significantly in both the control group (23%; P<.001) and the combination therapy group (12%; P =.02), but these changes were statistically similar (P =.54). In 12 of 13 neuropsychological tests, outcomes between groups were not significantly different; the 1 remaining test (Grooved Peg Board) showed better performance in the control group. CONCLUSION: Compared with levothyroxine alone, treatment of primary hypothyroidism with combination levothyroxine plus liothyronine demonstrated no beneficial changes in body weight, serum lipid levels, hypothyroid symptoms as measured by a HRQL questionnaire, and standard measures of cognitive performance.

Danzi S et al. Potential uses of T3 in the treatment of human disease.Clin Cornerstone. 2005; 7 Suppl 2:S9-15. Treatments for hypothyroidism have been available since the late 19th century, and have been continually improved by advancing our understanding of thyroid hormone pharmacology. Thyroxine (T4) monotherapy is currently the standard of care, but may leave some hypothyroid symptoms unaddressed. Triiodothyronine (T3), formed by the monodeiodination of T4, is the biologically active form of thyroid hormone based upon its ability to regulate gene expression at the nuclear level. A variety of human and animal studies have raised the question of whether T4 monotherapy is sufficient to restore tissue and organ intracellular T3 levels to normal. Furthermore, some evidence, albeit controversial, suggests that the addition of T3 (Cytomel) to T4 replacement therapy may improve patients' quality of life, psychometric performance and mood. Further developmental work is needed to refine T3 therapy in a way to enhance efficacy and lower the potential for unwanted effects.

Danzi S and Klein I Thyroid hormone and the cardiovascular system. Minerva Endocrinol. 2004 Sep; 29(3):139-50Thyroid hormone is an important regulator of cardiac function and cardiovascular hemodynamics. Triiodothyronine, (T(3)), the physiologically active form of thyroid hormone, binds to nuclear receptor proteins and mediates the expression of several important cardiac genes, inducing transcription of the positively regulated genes including alpha-myosin heavy chain (MHC) and the sarcoplasmic reticulum calcium ATPase. Negatively regulated genes include beta-MHC and phospholamban, which are down regulated in the presence of normal serum levels of thyroid hormone. T (3) mediated effects on the systemic vasculature include relaxation of vascular smooth muscle resulting in decreased arterial resistance and diastolic blood pressure. In hyperthyroidism, cardiac contractility and cardiac output are enhanced and systemic vascular resistance is decreased, while in hypothyroidism, the opposite is true. Patients with subclinical hypothyroidism manifest many of the same cardiovascular changes, but to a lesser degree than that which occurs in overt hypothyroidism. Cardiac disease states are sometimes associated with the low T (3) syndrome. The phenotype of the failing heart resembles that of the hypothyroid heart, both in cardiac physiology and in gene expression. Changes in serum T(3) levels in patients with chronic congestive heart failure are caused by alterations in thyroid hormone metabolism suggesting that patients may benefit from T(3) replacement in this setting.

El-Shaikh KA Recovery of age-dependent immunological deterioration in old mice by thyroxine treatment. J Anim Physiol Anim Nutr (Berl). 2006 Jun; 90(5-6):244-54. On the basis that multiple interactions exist between thyroid hormones and immune system, and ageing is accompanied by changes in thyroid hormone secretion, it seems possible that thyroid hormones may be involved in the age-related immune dysfunction. The present study was conducted to evaluate in vivo and in vitro effects of thyroxine (T (4)) treatment on both cell-mediated and humoral immune responses of aged mice. In a trial to improve age-associated immune dysfunction, T (4) (0.2, 1.0 and 5.0 microg) was subcutaneously supplemented to BALB/c mice (over 18 months old) for 30 consecutive days. The present results showed that exogenous treatment of aged mice with T(4) was associated with a marked increase in serum T(4) level, and the total number of peripheral blood leukocytes as well as the total cellularity of thymus, spleen, peripheral lymph nodes (PLNs), mesenteric lymph nodes (MLNs) and bone marrow (BM). T(4) treatment also caused a significant increase in the total and differential numbers of peritoneal exudate cells (PECs), while it caused a slight increase in macrophages' phagocytic activity of PEC. Moreover, T (4) treatment elicited a statistically significant increase in both plaque-forming cell and rosette-forming cell responses. In vitro results showed that the addition of T (4) at concentrations of 0.001, 0.005 and 0.025 microg/well substantially potentiated the ability of splenocytes from aged mice to proliferate in the presence of concanavalin-A mitogen. Histological examination of thymuses from T (4)-treated aged mice revealed that the cortex was preferentially enlarged and repopulated with immature thymocytes. The present study postulates that thyroid hormones may be involved in the observed decrease in the immune responsiveness during ageing, and that T(4) treatment to aged mice is able to restore the age-related decline of the immune efficiency.

Escobar-Morreale HF et al. Thyroid hormone replacement therapy in primary hypothyroidism: a randomized trial

comparing L-thyroxine plus liothyronine with L-thyroxine alone. Ann Intern Med. 2005 Mar 15; 142(6):412-24

BACKGROUND: Substituting part of the dose of l-thyroxine with small but supraphysiologic doses of liothyronine in hypothyroid patients has yielded conflicting results. OBJECTIVE: To evaluate combinations of L-thyroxine plus liothyronine in hypothyroid patients that match the proportions present in normal secretions of the human thyroid gland. DESIGN: Randomized, double-blind, crossover trial. SETTING: Academic research hospital. PARTICIPANTS: 28 women with overt primary hypothyroidism. INTERVENTION: Crossover trial comparing treatment with l-thyroxine, 100 microg/d (standard treatment), versus treatment with L-thyroxine, 75 microg/d, plus liothyronine, 5 microg/d (combination treatment), for 8-week periods. All patients also received L-thyroxine, 87.5 microg/d, plus liothyronine, 7.5 microg/d (add-on combination treatment), for a final 8-week add-on period. MEASUREMENTS: Primary outcomes included serum thyroid hormone levels, results of quality-of-life and psychometric tests, and patients' preference. Multiple biological thyroid hormone end points were studied as secondary outcomes. RESULTS: Compared with standard treatment, combination treatment led to lower free thyroxine levels (decrease, 3.9 pmol/L [95% CI, 2.5 to 5.3 pmol/L]), slightly higher serum levels of thyroid-stimulating hormone (increase, 0.62 mU/L [CI, 0.01 to 1.23 mU/L]), and unchanged free triiodothyronine levels. No improvement was observed in the other primary and secondary end points after combination treatment, with the exception of the Digit Span Test, in which the mean backward score and the mean total score increased slightly (0.6 digit [CI, 0.1 to 1.0 digit] and 0.8 digit [CI, 0.2 to 1.4 digits], respectively). The add-on combination treatment resulted in overreplacement. Levels of thyroid-stimulating hormone decreased by 0.85 mU/L (CI, 0.27 to 1.43 mU/L) and serum free triiodothyronine levels increased by 0.8 pmol/L (CI, 0.1 to 1.5 pmol/L) compared with standard treatment; 10 patients had levels of thyroid-stimulating hormone that were below the normal range. Twelve patients preferred combination treatment, 6 patients preferred the add-on combination treatment, 2 patients preferred standard treatment, and 6 patients had no preference (P = 0.015). LIMITATIONS: Treatment with L-thyroxine, 87.5 microg/d, plus liothyronine, 7.5 microg/d, was an add-on regimen and was not randomized. CONCLUSIONS: Physiologic combinations of L-thyroxine plus liothyronine do not offer any objective advantage over l-thyroxine alone, yet patients prefer combination treatment.

Faber J et al. Changes in bone mass during prolonged subclinical hyperthyroidism due to L-thyroxine treatment: a meta-analysis.Eur J Endocrinol 1994 Apr; 130(4):350-6 L-Thyroxine (L-T4) in the treatment of thyroid disease resulting in reduced serum thyrotropin (TSH) has been associated with reduced bone mass and thus the potential risk of premature development of osteoporosis. However, several recent studies have failed to show such a detrimental effect. These disagreements are probably due to only a small number of patients taking part in each study, decreasing the change of finding significant differences and increasing the risk of missing a real difference (type 1 and 2 errors, respectively). We therefore performed a meta-analysis on the available papers (N = 13), in which bone mass was measured in the distal forearm, femoral neck or lumbar spine in a cross-sectional manner in women with suppressed serum TSH due to L-T4 treatment and in a control group. The women were divided according to their pre- and postmenopausal state, because preserved estrogen production plays a protective role against irreversible bone loss. Based on the number of measurements performed on the different sites of the skeleton, a theoretical bone composed of 30.4% distal forearm, 28.8% femoral neck and 40.8% lumbar spine could be constructed in premenopausal women (441 measurements). A premenopausal woman at an average age of 39.6 years and treated with 164 micrograms L-T4/day for 8.5 years, leading to suppressed serum TSH, had 2.67% less bone mass than controls (NS), corresponding to an excess annual bone loss of 0.31% after 8.5 years of treatment (NS). The risk of not detecting an excess bone loss of at least 1% per year (type 2 error) was $p < 0.15$.

Fernandez-Real JM et al. Thyroid function is intrinsically linked to insulin sensitivity and endothelium-dependent vasodilation in healthy euthyroid subjects. J Clin Endocrinol Metab. 2006 Jun 27 CONTEXT: Levels of TSH respond to fluctuations in serum free T (4) (fT (4)) but remain in a very narrow individual range. There exists current controversy regarding the upper limit of normal serum TSH values above which treatment should be indicated. OBJECTIVE: We aimed to study whether the individually determined fT (4)-TSH relationship was associated with plasma lipids, insulin sensitivity, and endothelial dysfunction in healthy subjects with strictly normal thyroid function according to recent recommendations (0.3-3.0 mU/liter). DESIGN: This was a cross-sectional study. SETTING: The study consisted of a cohort of healthy men from the general population (n = 221). MAIN OUTCOME MEASURES: Oral glucose tolerance, insulin sensitivity (S (I), minimal model), endothelium-dependent vasodilation (high-resolution ultrasound), and plasma lipids were measured in relation to thyroid function tests. RESULTS: Both serum TSH and fT (4).TSH product were positively associated with fasting and postload insulin concentration and negatively with S (I). After body mass index stratification, these associations were especially significant among lean subjects. Serum TSH and fT (4).TSH product also correlated positively with fasting triglycerides and negatively with high-density lipoprotein cholesterol. In a multiple linear regression analysis, age (P = 0.007) and S(I) (P = 0.02) but not body mass index, fasting triglycerides, or serum high-density lipoprotein concentration contributed independently to 3.7 and 3.3%, respectively, of the variance in fT(4).TSH. Those subjects over the median of fT (4).TSH showed reduced endothelium-dependent vasodilation. CONCLUSIONS: Thyroid function tests are intrinsically linked to variables of insulin resistance and endothelial function. It is possible that underlying factors lead simultaneously to increased serum TSH, insulin resistance, ensuing dyslipidemia, and altered endothelial function even within current normal TSH levels.

Friberg L et al. Association between increased levels of reverse triiodothyronine and mortality after acute myocardial infarction. Am J Med. 2001 Dec 15; 111(9):699-703 PURPOSE: The thyroid hormone system may be downregulated temporarily in patients who are severely ill. This "euthyroid sick syndrome" may be an adaptive response to conserve energy. However, thyroid hormone also has beneficial effects on the cardiovascular system, such as improving cardiac function, reducing systemic vascular resistance, and lowering serum cholesterol levels. We investigated whether thyroid hormone levels obtained at the time of myocardial infarction are associated with subsequent mortality. PATIENTS AND METHODS: Serum levels of thyroid hormones (triiodothyronine [T3], reverse T3, free thyroxine [T4], and thyroid-stimulating hormone) were measured in 331 consecutive patients with acute myocardial infarction (mean age [+/- SD], 68 +/- 12 years), from samples obtained at the time of admission. RESULTS: Fifty-three patients (16%) died within 1 year. Ten percent (16 of 165) of patients with reverse T3 levels (an inactive metabolite) >0.41 nmol/L (the median value) died within the first week after myocardial infarction, compared with none of the 166 patients with lower levels (P <0.0004). After 1 year, the corresponding figures were 24% (40 of 165) versus 7.8% (13 of 166; P <0.0001). Reverse T3 levels >0.41 nmol/L were associated with an increased risk of 1-year mortality (hazard ratio = 3.0; 95% confidence interval: 1.4 to 6.3; P = 0.005), independent of age, previous myocardial infarction, prior angina, heart failure, serum creatinine level, and peak serum creatine kinase-MB fraction levels. CONCLUSION: Determination of reverse T3 levels may be a valuable and simple aid to improve identification of patients with myocardial infarction who are at high risk of subsequent mortality.

Gorres G et al. Bone mineral density in patients receiving suppressive doses of thyroxine for differentiated thyroid carcinoma Eur J Nucl Med 1996 Jun; 23(6):690-2 To determine bone mineral density in patients with differentiated thyroid carcinoma receiving thyroxine replacement therapy in suppressive doses, we studied 65 patients (47 women and 18 men; age 25-83 years, mean+/-SD 52.5+/-15.4 years). Patients were free of thyroid cancer in clinical and laboratory examinations at the time of the study. Bone mineral density of the lumbar spine and both hips was measured by dual-energy X-ray absorptiometry. There was no decrease in bone density in either 32 postmenopausal or 15 premenopausal women compared with an age- and sex-matched control group, nor was any decrease in bone density found in men. Our data suggest that thyroxine treatment in suppressive doses in patients with differentiated thyroid carcinoma is not a risk factor for the development of osteoporosis.

Guo TW et al. Positive association of the DIO2 (deiodinase type 2) gene with mental retardation in the iodine-deficient areas of China. J Med Genet. 2004 Aug; 41(8):585-90. BACKGROUND: Iodine deficiency is the commonest cause of preventable mental retardation (MR) worldwide. However, in iodine-deficient areas not everyone is affected and familial aggregation is common. This suggests that genetic factors may also contribute. Thyroid hormone (TH) plays an important role in fetal and early postnatal brain development. The pro-hormone T4 (3, 3', 5, 5'-triiodothyronine) is converted in the brain to its active form, T3, or its inactive metabolite, reverse T3, mainly by the action of deiodinase type 2 (DIO2). METHODS: To investigate the potential genetic contribution of the DIO2 gene, we performed a case-control association study using three common SNPs in the gene (rs225014, rs225012, and rs225010) that were in strong linkage disequilibrium with each other. RESULTS: Single marker analysis showed a positive association of MR with rs225012 and rs225010. Particularly with rs255012 [corrected], CC [corrected] genotype frequency was significantly higher in MR cases than in controls (chi squared [corrected] = 9.18, p = 0.00246). When we compared the distributions of common haplotypes, we also found significant differences between mental retardation and controls in the haplotype combination of rs225012 and rs225010 (chi2 = 15.04, df 2, global p = 0.000549). This association remained significant after Bonferroni correction (p = 0.0016470). CONCLUSION: We conclude that allelic variation in the DIO2 gene may affect the amount of T3 available and in an iodine-deficient environment may partly determine overall risk of MR.

Hak AE et al. Subclinical hypothyroidism is an independent risk factor for atherosclerosis and myocardial infarction in elderly women: the Rotterdam Study Ann Intern Med 2000 Feb 15; 132(4):270-8 BACKGROUND: Overt hypothyroidism has been found to be associated with cardiovascular disease. Whether subclinical hypothyroidism and thyroid autoimmunity are also risk factors for cardiovascular disease is controversial. OBJECTIVE: To investigate whether subclinical hypothyroidism and thyroid autoimmunity are associated with aortic atherosclerosis and myocardial infarction in postmenopausal women. DESIGN: Population-based cross-sectional study. SETTING: A district of Rotterdam, The Netherlands. PARTICIPANTS: Random sample of 1149 women (mean age +/- SD, 69.0 +/- 7.5 years) participating in the Rotterdam Study. MEASUREMENTS: Data on thyroid status, aortic atherosclerosis, and history of myocardial infarction were obtained at baseline. Subclinical hypothyroidism was defined as an elevated thyroid-stimulating hormone level (>4.0 mU/L) and a normal serum free thyroxine level (11 to 25 pmol/L [0.9 to 1.9 ng/dL]). In tests for antibodies to thyroid peroxidase, a serum level greater than 10 IU/mL was considered a positive result. RESULTS: Subclinical hypothyroidism was present in 10.8% of participants and was associated with a greater age-adjusted prevalence of aortic atherosclerosis (odds ratio, 1.7 [95% CI, 1.1 to 2.6]) and myocardial infarction (odds ratio, 2.3 [CI, 1.3 to 4.0]). Additional adjustment for body mass index, total and high-density lipoprotein cholesterol level, blood pressure, and smoking status, as well as exclusion of women, who took beta-blockers, did not affect these estimates. Associations were slightly stronger in women who had subclinical hypothyroidism and antibodies to thyroid peroxidase (odds ratio for aortic atherosclerosis, 1.9 [CI, 1.1 to 3.6]; odds ratio for myocardial infarction, 3.1 [CI, 1.5 to 6.3]). No association was found between thyroid autoimmunity itself and cardiovascular disease. The population attributable risk percentage for subclinical hypothyroidism associated with myocardial infarction was within the range of that for known major risk factors for cardiovascular disease. CONCLUSION: Subclinical hypothyroidism is a strong indicator of risk for atherosclerosis and myocardial infarction in elderly women.

Haluzik M et al. Effects of hypo- and hyperthyroidism on noradrenergic activity and glycerol concentrations in human subcutaneous abdominal adipose tissue assessed with microdialysis. J Clin Endocrinol Metab. 2003 Dec; 88(12):5605-8 Thyroid hormones play a major role in lipid metabolism. However, whether they directly affect lipolysis locally in the adipose tissue remains unknown. Therefore, we measured abdominal sc adipose tissue norepinephrine (NE), basal, and isoprenaline-stimulated lipolysis in 12 hypothyroid patients (HYPO), six hyperthyroid patients (HYPER), and 12 healthy controls by in vivo microdialysis. Adipose tissue NE was decreased in HYPO and increased in HYPER compared with controls (90.4 +/- 2.9 and 458.0 +/- 69.1 vs. 294.9 +/- 19.5 pmol/liter, P < 0.01). Similarly, basal lipolysis, assessed by glycerol assay, was lower in HYPO and higher in HYPER than in controls (88.2 +/- 9.9 and 566.0 +/- 42.0 vs. 214.3 +/- 5.1 micromol/liter P < 0.01). The relative magnitude of isoprenaline-induced glycerol increase was smaller in HYPO (39 +/- 19.4%, P < 0.05 vs. basal) and higher in HYPER (277 +/- 30.4%, P < 0.01) than in controls (117 +/- 5.6%, P < 0.01). The corresponding changes in NE after isoprenaline stimulation were as follows: 120 +/- 9.2% (P < 0.05), 503 +/- 113% (P < 0.01), and 267 +/- 17.2 (P < 0.01). In summary, by affecting local NE levels and adrenergic postreceptor signaling, thyroid hormones may influence the lipolysis rate in the abdominal sc adipose tissue.

Hamilton MA Safety and hemodynamic effects of intravenous triiodothyronine in advanced congestive heart failure. Am J Cardiol 1998 Feb 15; 81(4):443-7 Most patients with advanced congestive heart failure have altered thyroid hormone metabolism. A low triiodothyronine level is associated with impaired hemodynamics and is an independent predictor of poor survival. This study sought to evaluate safety and hemodynamic effects of short-term intravenous administration of triiodothyronine in patients with advanced heart failure. An intravenous bolus dose of triiodothyronine, with or without a 6- to 12-hour infusion (cumulative dose 0. 1 5 to 2.7 microg/kg), was administered to 23 patients with advanced heart failure (mean left ventricular ejection fraction 0.22 +/- 0.01). Cardiac rhythm and hemodynamic status were monitored for 12 hours, and basal metabolic rate by indirect calorimetry, echocardiographic parameters of systolic function and valvular regurgitation, thyroid hormone, and catecholamine levels were measured at baseline and at 4 to 6 hours. Triiodothyronine was well tolerated without episodes of ischemia or clinical arrhythmia. There was no significant change in heart rate or metabolic rate and there was minimal increase in core temperature. Cardiac output increased with a reduction in systemic vascular resistance in patients receiving the largest dose, consistent with a peripheral vasodilatory effect. Acute intravenous administration of triiodothyronine is well tolerated in patients with advanced heart failure, establishing the basis for further investigation into the safety and potential hemodynamic benefits of longer infusions, combined infusion with inotropic agents, oral triiodothyronine replacement therapy, and new triiodothyronine analogs.

Hamilton MA Thyroid hormone abnormalities in heart failure: possibilities for therapy Thyroid 1996 Oct;6(5):527-9 Though thyroid hormone abnormalities have been identified in many cardiac conditions, the role of thyroid hormones in congestive heart failure has not been well defined. In a population of patients with advanced heart failure, a reduction in triiodothyronine (T3) with an increase in reverse T3 was identified in many patients, with an abnormally low ratio of T3/reverse T3 being the strongest predictor of mortality. Normalization of thyroid indices appeared to be necessary for prolonged survival to occur. To address the concern of T3 administration possibility exacerbating a hypermetabolic state, basal metabolic rate was measured in a group of advanced heart failure patients and was found to be generally within the normal range. A preliminary safety study of short-term intravenous T3 administration (bolus +/- 6 h infusion, total dose 0.15-2.7 micrograms/kg) was then performed in 23 patients under hemodynamic and electrocardiographic monitoring. There were neither adverse events nor substantial hemodynamic changes, but some patients had an increase in cardiac output, consistent with a peripheral vasodilatory effect. With this foundation, further investigation into the possible role of T3 and its analogs in congestive heart failure therapy may be pursued.

Hollowell JG, Serum TSH, T(4), and thyroid antibodies in the United States population (1988 to 1994): National Health and Nutrition Examination Survey (NHANES III).J Clin Endocrinol Metab. 2002 Feb;87(2):489-99.NHANES III measured serum TSH, total serum T(4), antithyroperoxidase (TPOAb), and antithyroglobulin (TgAb) antibodies from a sample of 17,353 people aged > or =12 yr representing the geographic and ethnic distribution of the U.S. population. These data provide a reference for other studies of these analytes in the U.S. For the 16,533 people who did not report thyroid disease, goiter, or taking thyroid medications (disease-free population), we determined mean concentrations of TSH, T (4), TgAb, and TPOAb. A reference population of 13,344 people was selected from the disease-free population by excluding, in addition, those who were pregnant, taking androgens or estrogens, who had thyroid antibodies, or biochemical hypothyroidism or hyperthyroidism. The influence of demographics on TSH, T (4), and antibodies was examined. Hypothyroidism was found in 4.6% of the U.S. population (0.3% clinical and 4.3% subclinical) and hyperthyroidism in 1.3% (0.5% clinical and 0.7% subclinical). (Subclinical hypothyroidism is used in this paper to mean mild hypothyroidism, the term now preferred by the American Thyroid Association for the laboratory findings described.) For the disease-free population, mean serum TSH was 1.50 (95% confidence interval, 1.46-1.54) mIU/liter, was higher in females than males, and higher in white non-Hispanics (whites) [1.57 (1.52-1.62) mIU/liter] than black non-Hispanics (blacks) [1.18 (1.14-1.21) mIU/liter] (P < 0.001) or Mexican Americans [1.43 (1.40-1.46) mIU/liter] (P < 0.001). TgAb were positive in 10.4 +/- 0.5% and TPOAb, in 11.3 +/- 0.4%; positive antibodies were more prevalent in women than men, increased with age, and TPOAb were less prevalent in blacks (4.5 +/- 0.3%) than in whites (12.3 +/- 0.5%) (P < 0.001). TPOAb were significantly associated with hypo or hyperthyroidism, but TgAb were not. Using the reference population, geometric mean TSH was 1.40 +/- 0.02 mIU/liter and increased with age, and was significantly lower in blacks (1.18 +/- 0.02 mIU/liter) than whites (1.45 +/- 0.02 mIU/liter) (P < 0.001) and Mexican Americans (1.37 +/- 0.02 mIU/liter) (P < 0.001). Arithmetic mean total T (4) was 112.3 +/- 0.7 nmol/liter in the disease-free population and was consistently higher among Mexican Americans in all populations. In the reference population, mean total T (4) in Mexican Americans was (116.3 +/- 0.7 nmol/liter), significantly higher than whites (110.0 +/- 0.8 nmol/liter) or blacks (109.4 +/- 0.8 nmol/liter) (P < 0.0001). The difference persisted in all age groups. In summary, TSH and the prevalence of antithyroid antibodies are greater in females, increase with age, and are greater in whites and Mexican Americans than in blacks. TgAb alone in the absence of TPOAb is not significantly associated with thyroid disease. The lower prevalence of thyroid antibodies and lower TSH concentrations in blacks need more research to relate these findings to clinical status. A large proportion of the U.S. population unknowingly have laboratory evidence of thyroid disease, which supports the usefulness of screening for early detection.

Iervasi, G et al. Low-T3 Syndrome, A Strong Prognostic Predictor of Death in Patients With Heart Disease Circulation. 2003; 107:708 BACKGROUND: Clinical and experimental data have suggested a potential negative impact of low-T3 state on the prognosis of cardiac diseases. The aim of the present prospective study was to assess the role of thyroid hormones in the prognosis of patient population with heart disease. METHODS AND RESULTS: A total of 573 consecutive cardiac patients underwent thyroid function profile evaluation. They were divided in two subgroups: group I, 173 patients with low T3, ie, with free T3 (fT3) <3.1 pmol/L, and group II, 400 patients with normal fT3 (>or=3.1 pmol/L). We considered cumulative and cardiac death events. During the 1-year follow-up, there were 25 cumulative deaths in group I and 12 in group II (14.4% versus

3%, P<0.0001); cardiac deaths were 13 in group I and 6 in group II (7.5% versus 1.5%, P=0.0006). According to the Cox model, fT3 was the most important predictor of cumulative death (hazard ratio [HR] 3.582, P<0.0001), followed by dyslipidemia (HR 2.955, P=0.023), age (HR 1.051, P<0.005), and left ventricular ejection fraction (HR 1.037, P=0.006). At the logistic multivariate analysis, fT3 was the highest independent predictor of death (HR 0.395, P=0.003). A prevalence of low fT3 levels was found in patients with NYHA class III-IV illness compared with patients with NYHA class I-II (chi(2) 5.65, P=0.019). CONCLUSIONS: Low-T3 syndrome is a strong predictor of death in cardiac patients and might be directly implicated in the poor prognosis of cardiac patients.

Jakobs TC et al. Proinflammatory cytokines inhibit the expression and function of human type I 5'-deiodinase in HepG2 hepatocarcinoma cells.Eur J Endocrinol. 2002 Apr; 146(4):559-66. OBJECTIVE: The sick euthyroid syndrome in critically ill patients without primary disease of the thyroid gland is characterised by low serum total triiodothyronine (T3), normal to elevated thyroxine (T4), elevated reverse T3 (rT3) and normal TSH levels. The aim of this work was to clarify if impaired T4 and rT3 5'-deiodination is an underlying mechanism. DESIGN AND METHODS: We analysed the effect of the human recombinant proinflammatory cytokines interleukin (IL)-6 and IL-1beta, tumour necrosis factor-alpha (TNF-alpha) and interferon-gamma (IFN-gamma) on human type I 5'-iodothyronine deiodinase (5'DI) enzyme activity in the human hepatocarcinoma cell line HepG2, i.e. in a homologous human system. Furthermore, we analysed transcriptional effects of the cytokines by transient transfection assays using the luciferase or chloramphenicol acetyltransferase (CAT) reporter genes under the control of 1480 nucleotides of the human 5'DI promoter. RESULTS: IL-6 at 500 pg/ml and TNF-alpha at 25 ng/ml had no significant effect, whereas 100 ng/ml IFN-gamma or 10 ng/ml IL-1beta reduced 5'DI enzyme activity to 77.9 and 59.5% of control values. IFN-gamma did not alter, IL-6 and TNF-alpha moderately decreased (in the case of IL-6 only in the CAT system), and IL-1beta (0.01-10 ng/ml) dose-dependently inhibited 5'DI promoter activity to a minimum of 38.1%. CONCLUSION: IL-1beta inhibited both 5'DI enzyme and promoter activity and, thus, may exert its effect on thyroid hormone metabolism at least partially through direct inhibition of hepatic 5'DI gene transcription.

Knudsen N et al. Small differences in thyroid function may be important for body mass index and the occurrence of obesity in the population.J Clin Endocrinol Metab. 2005 Jul; 90(7):4019-24 CONTEXT: Increasing prevalence of overweight in the population is a major concern globally; and in the United States, nearly one third of adults were classified as obese at the end of the 20th century. Few data have been presented regarding an association between variations in thyroid function seen in the general population and body weight. OBJECTIVE: The aim of this study was to investigate the association between thyroid function and body mass index (BMI) or obesity in a normal population. DESIGN: A cross-sectional population study (The DanThyr Study) was conducted. PARTICIPANTS: In all, 4649 participants were investigated, and 4082 were eligible for these analyses after exclusion of subjects with previous or present overt thyroid dysfunction. MAIN OUTCOME MEASURES: The study examined the association between category of serum TSH or serum thyroid hormones and BMI or obesity in multivariate models, adjusting for possible confounding. RESULTS: We found a positive association between BMI and category of serum TSH (P < 0.001) and a negative association between BMI and category of serum free T (4) (P < 0.001). No association was found between BMI and serum free T (3) levels. The difference in BMI between the groups with the highest and lowest serum TSH levels was 1.9 kg/m (2), corresponding to a difference in body weight of 5.5 kg among women. Similarly, the category of serum TSH correlated positively with weight gain during 5 yr (P = 0.04), but no statistically significant association was found with weight gain during 6 months (P = 0.17). There was an association between obesity (BMI > 30 kg/m (2)) and serum TSH levels (P = 0.001). CONCLUSIONS: Our results suggest that thyroid function (also within the normal range) could be one of several factors acting in concert to determine body weight in a population. Even slightly elevated serum TSH levels are associated with an increase in the occurrence of obesity.

Krotkiewski M Thyroid hormones in the pathogenesis and treatment of obesity.Eur J Pharmacol. 2002 Apr 12; 440(2-3):85-98. Thyroid hormones (TH) are potent modulators of adaptive thermogenesis and can potentially contribute to development of obesity. The decrease of T (3) in association with reduction of calorie intake is centrally regulated via decreases in leptin and melanocortin concentrations and peripherally via a decrease in deiodinase activity, all aimed at protein and energy sparing. The use of TH in the treatment of obesity is hardly justified except in cases of elevated thyrotropin (TSH) with low/normal T(3) and T(4) and/or a low T(3) or T'(3)/T(4) or a high TSH/T(3) ratio. TH treatment with small doses of T(3) can also be exceptionally applied in obese patients resistant to dietary therapy who are taking beta-adrenergic blockers or with obesity developed after cessation of cigarette smoking and with hyperlipidemia and a concomitant high thryrotropin/T(3) ratio. Supplementation with Se (2+) and Zn (2+) may be tried along with more severe calorie restriction to prevent decline of T (3).

Lange U et al. Thyroid disorders in female patients with ankylosing spondylitis.Eur J Med Res 1999 Nov 22;4(11):468-74 The association between rheumatological and thyroid disorders has long been known, the most common being the association of rheumatoid arthritis and autoimmune thyroiditis. Little is known as to possible thyroid involvement in ankylosing spondylitis (AS). In 22 female patients with AS and 22 healthy age-matched control subjects parameters of thyroid gland function, rheumatic activity, as well as a subtle drug anamnesis of the rheumatic medication, and an ultrasonographic examination of the thyroid gland were determined. Thyroid function was tested by intravenous injection of 400 microg thyrotropin-releasing hormone (TRH). In parallel basal levels of reverse-T3 (rT3), calcium and anti-thyroid antibodies were estimated. In the AS-group an enlarged thyroid volume was seen in 10 cases, basal FT4, FT3 and TT3 were significantly lower, TSH and TT4 were found to be in the normal range and rT3 was significantly increased. The prevalence of anti-thyroid antibodies was significantly higher in the AS-group. The AS-patients responded as well as the controls with thyroid hormone secretion to TRH, within an observation period of 2 hours. No differences were observed in TSH response. Free serum calcium showed in both groups no significant difference.

Medina-Gomez G et al. Potent thermogenic action of triiodothyroacetic acid in brown adipocytes. Cell Mol Life Sci. 2003 Sep; 60(9):1957-67 Triiodothyroacetic acid (TRIAC) is a triiodothyronine (T3) metabolite with high affinity for T3 nuclear receptors. We compared the thermogenic action of TRIAC versus T3 in brown adipocytes, by studying target genes known to mediate thermogenic action: uncoupling protein 1 (UCP-1), a marker of brown adipocytes, and type II-5'deiodinase (D2), which provides the T3 required for thermogenesis. TRIAC is 10-50 times more potent than T3 at increasing the adrenergic induction of UCP-1 mRNA and D2 activities. TRIAC action on UCP-1 is exerted at the transcriptional level. In the presence of an adrenergic stimulus, TRIAC is also more potent than T3, inducing lipoprotein lipase mRNA and 5 deiodinase (D3) activity and mRNA. Maximal effects occur at very low concentrations (0.2 nM). The greater potency of TRIAC is not due to preferential cellular or nuclear uptake. Therefore, TRIAC is a potent thermogenic agent that might increase energy expenditure and regulate T3 production in brown adipocytes.

Nedrebo BG et al. Plasma total homocysteine levels in hyperthyroid and hypothyroid patients. Metabolism. 1998 Jan;47(1):89-93 We found a higher plasma concentration of total homocysteine (tHcy), an independent risk factor for cardiovascular disease, in patients with hypothyroidism (mean, 16.3 micromol/L; 95% confidence interval [CI], 14.7 to 17.9 micromol/L) than in healthy controls (mean, 10.5 micromol/L; 95% CI, 10.1 to 10.9 micromol/L). The tHcy level of hyperthyroid patients did not differ significantly from that of the controls. Serum creatinine was higher in hypothyroid patients and lower in hyperthyroid patients than in controls, whereas serum folate was higher in hyperthyroid patients compared with the two other groups. In multivariate analysis, these differences did not explain the higher tHcy concentration in hypothyroidism. We confirmed the observation of elevated serum cholesterol in hypothyroidism, which together with the hyperhomocysteinemia may contribute to an accelerated atherogenesis in these patients.

Neeck G Neuroendocrine perturbations in fibromyalgia and chronic fatigue syndrome. Rheum Dis Clin North Am 2000 Nov; 26(4):989-1002 A large body of data from a number of different laboratories worldwide has demonstrated a general tendency for reduced adrenocortical responsiveness in CFS. It is still not clear if this is secondary to CNS abnormalities leading to decreased activity of CRH- or AVP-producing hypothalamic neurons. Primary hypofunction of the CRH neurons has been described on the basis of genetic and environmental influences. Other pathways could secondarily influence HPA axis activity, however. For example, serotonergic and noradrenergic input acts to stimulate HPA axis activity. Deficient serotonergic activity in CFS has been suggested by some of the studies as reviewed here. In addition, hypofunction of sympathetic nervous system function has been described and could contribute to abnormalities of central components of the HPA axis. One could interpret the clinical trial of glucocorticoid replacement in patients with CFS as confirmation of adrenal insufficiency if one were convinced of a positive therapeutic effect. If patient symptoms were related to impaired activation of central components of the axis, replacing glucocorticoids would merely exacerbate symptoms caused by enhanced negative feedback. Further study of specific components of the HPA axis should ultimately clarify the reproducible abnormalities associated with a clinical picture of CFS. In contrast to CFS, the results of the different hormonal axes in FMS support the assumption that the distortion of the hormonal pattern observed can be attributed to hyperactivity of CRH neurons. This hyperactivity may be driven and sustained by stress exerted by chronic pain originating in the musculoskeletal system or by an alteration of the CNS mechanism of nociception. The elevated activity of CRH neurons also seems to cause alteration of the set point of other hormonal axes. In addition to its control of the adrenal hormones, CRH stimulates somatostatin secretion at the hypothalamic level, which, in turn, causes inhibition of growth hormone and thyroid-stimulating hormone at the pituitary level. The suppression of gonadal function may also be attributed to elevated CRH because of its ability to inhibit hypothalamic luteinizing hormone-releasing hormone release; however, a remote effect on the ovary by the inhibition of follicle-stimulating hormone-stimulated estrogen production must also be considered. Serotonin (5-HT) precursors such as tryptophan (5-HTP), drugs that release 5-HT, or drugs that act directly on 5-HT receptors stimulate the HPA axis, indicating a stimulatory effect of serotonergic input on HPA axis function. Hyperfunction of the HPA axis could also reflect an elevated serotonergic tonus in the CNS of FMS patients. The authors conclude that the observed pattern of hormonal deviations in patients with FMS is a CNS adjustment to chronic pain and stress, constitutes a specific entity of FMS, and is primarily evoked by activated CRH neurons.

Nuzzo V et al. Bone mineral density in premenopausal women receiving levothyroxine suppressive therapy. Gynecol Endocrinol 1998 Oct; 12(5): 333-7 Osteoporosis is a well-known complication of thyrotoxicosis. Prolonged subclinical hyperthyroidism due to L-thyroxine treatment has been associated with reduced bone mass and thus with the potential risk of premature development of osteoporosis. The aim of this study was to assess the effect of a chronic L-thyroxine suppressive treatment on bone mineral density (BMD) in a group of premenopausal women. Forty consecutive patients (mean age +/- SE = 40.95 +/- 1.56 years) affected by non-toxic goiter underwent bone mineral densitometry (dual energy X-ray absorptiometry; DEXA) of the lumbar spine (L1-L4) and right femoral neck. At the time of the study the patients had been under thyroid stimulating hormone (TSH) suppressive therapy for 74.95 +/- 10.34 months (range 17-168 months). Baseline levels of free thyroxine (fT4), free triiodothyronine (fT3), TSH, calcium and phosphorus were measured and correlated with BMD. The age of starting, duration of treatment, main daily dose, cumulative dose of treatment and body mass index (BMI) were also correlated with BMD. Statistical analysis was performed by multiple linear regression. BMD among female patients was not significantly different from that of the general population matched for age and sex. With the use of the regression model, no significant correlation was found between BMD and the variables considered. In conclusion, our data suggest that L-thyroxine suppressive therapy, if carefully carried out and monitored has no significant effect on bone mass.

Okamoto R et al. Adverse effects of reverse triiodothyronine on cellular metabolism as assessed by 1H and 31P NMR spectroscopy. Res Exp Med (Berl) 1997;197(4):211-7 Effects of 3,3',5'-triiodothyronine (rT3) in connection with 3,3',5-triiodothyronine (T3) on 3T3 cells were studied in vitro by means of 1H and 31P NMR spectroscopy. In the cells incubated with 5 nM T3 for 3 h at pH 7.4, the ATP/ADP ratio was elevated from 6.9 to 8.4, whereas it was reduced to 6.1 in cells incubated with rT3. When the cells were incubated at pH 6.7, the ATP/ADP ratio was reduced to 6.6 and 5.2 at 1 and 2 h, respectively. In the presence of 5 nM of T3, however, the ratio was maintained above the control level. A 1-h preincubation with rT3 dramatically augmented the reductions caused by elevated acidity. These reductions were completely reversed when the cells were incubated with T3.

Peeters RP et al. Reduced Activation and Increased Inactivation of Thyroid Hormone in Tissues of Critically Ill Patients The Journal of Clinical Endocrinology & Metabolism Vol. 88, No. 7 3202-3211, 2003 Critical illness is often associated with reduced TSH and thyroid hormone secretion as well as marked changes in peripheral thyroid hormone metabolism, resulting in low serum T (3) and high rT (3) levels. To study the mechanism(s) of the latter changes, we determined serum thyroid hormone levels and the expression of the type 1, 2, and 3 iodothyronine deiodinases (D1, D2, and D3) in liver and skeletal muscle from deceased intensive care patients. To study mechanisms underlying these changes, 65 blood samples, 65 liver, and 66 skeletal muscle biopsies were obtained within minutes after death from 80 intensive care unit patients randomized for intensive or conventional insulin treatment. Serum thyroid parameters and the expression of tissue D1-D3 were determined. Serum TSH, T (4), T (3), and the T (3)/rT (3) ratio were lower, whereas serum rT (3) was higher than in normal subjects (P < 0.0001). Liver D1 activity was down-regulated and D3 activity was induced in liver and skeletal muscle. Serum T (3)/rT (3) ratio correlated positively with liver D1 activity (P < 0.001) and negatively with liver D3 activity (ns). These parameters were independent of the type of insulin treatment. Liver D1 and serum T(3)/rT(3) were highest in patients who died from severe brain damage, intermediate in those who died from sepsis or excessive inflammation, and lowest in patients who died from cardiovascular collapse (P < 0.01). Liver D3 showed an opposite relationship. Acute renal failure requiring dialysis and need of inotropes were associated with low liver D1 activity (P < 0.01 and P = 0.06) and high liver D3 (P < 0.01) and skeletal muscle D3 (P < 0.05) activity. Liver D1 activity was negatively correlated with plasma urea (P = 0.002), creatinine (P = 0.06), and bilirubin (P < 0.0001). D1 and D3 mRNA levels corresponded with enzyme activities (both P < 0.001), suggesting regulation of the expression of both deiodinases at the pretranslational level. This is the first study relating tissue deiodinase activities with serum thyroid hormone levels and clinical parameters in a large group of critically ill patients. Liver D1 is down-regulated and D3 (which is not present in liver and skeletal muscle of healthy individuals) is induced, particularly in disease states associated with poor tissue perfusion. These observed changes, in correlation with a low T (3)/rT (3) ratio, may represent tissue-specific ways to reduce thyroid hormone bioactivity during cellular hypoxia and contribute to the low T (3) syndrome of severe illness.

Riedel W Secretory pattern of GH, TSH, thyroid hormones, ACTH, cortisol, FSH, and LH in patients with fibromyalgia syndrome following systemic injection of the relevant hypothalamic-releasing hormones Z Rheumatol 1998;57 Suppl 2:81-7 To study the hormonal perturbations in FMS patients we injected sixteen FMS patients and seventeen controls a cocktail of the hypothalamic releasing hormones: Corticotropin-releasing hormone (CRH), Thyrotropin-releasing hormone (TRH), Growth hormone-releasing hormone (GHRH), and Luteinizing hormone-releasing hormone (LHRH) and observed the hormonal secretion pattern of the pituitary together with the hormones of the peripheral endocrine glands. We found in FMS patients elevated basal values of ACTH and cortisol, lowered basal values of insulin-like growth factor I (IGF-I) and of triiodothyronine (T3), elevated basal values of follicle-stimulating hormone (FSH) and lowered basal values of estrogen. Following injection of the four releasing-hormones, we found in FMS patients an augmented response of ACTH, a blunted response of TSH, while the prolactin response was exaggerated. The effects of LHRH stimulation were investigated in six FMS patients and six controls and disclosed a significantly blunted response of LH in FMS. We explain the deviations of hormonal secretion in FMS patients as being

44

caused by chronic stress, which, after being perceived and processed by the central nervous system (CNS), activates hypothalamic CRH neurons. CRH, on the one hand, activates the pituitary-adrenal axis, but also stimulates at the hypothalamic level somatostatin secretion which, in turn, causes inhibition of GH and TSH at the pituitary level. The suppression of gonadal function may also be attributed to elevated CRH by its ability to inhibit hypothalamic LHRH release, although it could act also directly on the ovary by inhibiting FSH-stimulated estrogen production. We conclude that the observed pattern of hormonal deviations in FMS patients is a CNS adjustment to chronic pain and stress, constitutes a specific entity of FMS, and is primarily evoked by activated CRH neurons.

Sawka AM et al. 2003 Does a combination regimen of thyroxine (T4) and 3, 5, 3'-triiodothyronine improve depressive symptoms better than T4 alone in patients with hypothyroidism? Results of a double-blind, randomized, controlled trial. J Clin Endocrinol Metab 88:4551–4555 Some hypothyroid patients receiving levothyroxine replacement therapy complain of depressive symptoms despite normal TSH measurements. It is not known whether adding T (3) can reverse such symptoms. We randomized 40 individuals with depressive symptoms who were taking a stable dose of levothyroxine for treatment of hypothyroidism (excluding those who underwent thyroidectomy or radioactive iodine ablation of the thyroid) to receive T(4) plus placebo or the combination of T(4) plus T(3) in a double-blind manner for 15 wk. Participants receiving combination therapy had their prestudy dose of T(4) dropped by 50%, and T(3) was started at a dose of 12.5 micro g, twice daily. T (4) and T (3) doses were adjusted to keep goal TSH concentrations within the normal range. Compared with the group taking T(4) alone, the group taking both T(4) plus T(3) did not report any improvement in self-rated mood and well-being scores that included all subscales of the Symptom Check-List-90, the Comprehensive Epidemiological Screen for Depression, and the Multiple Outcome Study (P > 0.05 for all indexes). In conclusion, the current data do not support the routine use of combined T (3) and T (4) therapy in hypothyroid patients with depressive symptoms.

Schulte C et al. Low T3-syndrome and nutritional status as prognostic factors in patients undergoing bone marrow transplantation. Bone Marrow Transplant 1998 Dec;22(12):1171-8 Bone marrow transplantation is known to be associated with considerable morbidity and mortality. The aim of this study was to determine the influence of nutritional status and development of sick euthyroid syndrome as prognostic factors for outcome after BMT. In 100 patients who underwent transplantation the following parameters were assessed before and at day 14 and 28 after transplantation: anthropometric data (body weight, body mass index, body composition, grip strength), rapid turnover proteins transferrin and prealbumin, T4, T3, free T4, reverse T3, thyroid-stimulating hormone and thyroglobulin. Following bone marrow transplantation, 22 patients died in the short-term follow-up (group A) before day 140 after BMT, 21 patients died during further follow-up between days 140 and 365 (group B) and 57 patients survived longer than 365 days (group C). All patients experienced a significant decrease of transferrin and T3, accompanied by an increase of rT3 and rT3/T3 ratio at day 14 after BMT. At day 28 after BMT, patients in group C showed recovery from these changes with an increase of transferrin and a fall in rT3 and the rT3/T3-ratio, which was not seen in patients who died during further follow-up (groups A and B). The observed changes were independent of other prognostically relevant factors (type of disease, HLA-match, immunosuppression). Impaired nutritional status and development of a sick euthyroid syndrome, without tendency to recovery, are associated with a higher probability of fatal outcome after bone marrow transplantation and have prognostic relevance in this group of patients.

Shimoyama N et al. Serum thyroid hormone levels correlate with cardiac function and ventricular tachyarrhythmia in patients with chronic heart failure. J Cardiol 1993; 23(2):205-13

The relationship between cardiac function and serum thyroid hormone levels was investigated in 41 patients with chronic heart failure (25 men and 16 women, mean age 63.7 +/- 11.1 years) and 15 normal subjects (5 men and 10 women, mean age 55.5 +/- 12.2 years). Patients with apparent thyroid disease were excluded from the study. All patients were evaluated according to the New York Heart Association (NYHA) classification using echocardiography, cardiothoracic ratios, mean daily heart rates calculated from ambulatory electrocardiograms (ECG), and ventricular tachyarrhythmias greater than triplets based on either Holter or ECG monitoring. The serum free triiodothyronine (FT3), free thyroxine (FT4), and reverse triiodothyronine (rT3) levels were measured. Decreased FT3 levels and FT3/FT4 ratios, and increased rT3 levels were associated with worse NYHA class. FT3/FT4 was positively and rT3 was negatively correlated with echocardiographical fractional shortening. FT3 and rT3 were negatively and positively correlated with mean daily heart rates, in contrast to known hypothyroid patients. Patients with ventricular tachycardia demonstrated significantly lower serum values of FT3 and FT3/FT4, and significantly higher values of rT3. Serum thyroid hormone levels can provide a quantitative index for evaluating the severity of chronic heart failure and predicting ventricular tachycardia.

Surks MI et al. The thyrotropin reference range should remain unchanged. J Clin Endocrinol Metab. 2005 Sep; 90(9):5489-96.

CONTEXT: Recent recommendations to decrease the upper limit of the TSH reference range from 4.5 to 2.5 mIU/liter, based on the high proportion of normal people whose serum TSH is less than 2.5 mIU/liter and the observation that those with TSH between 2.5 and 4.5 mIU/liter [upper reference range (URR)] have increased risk of progression to overt hypothyroidism (Whickham, 20-yr data), have not been subjected to critical analysis. STUDY SUBJECTS:

The study subjects were from the Reference Group of NHANES III, 14,333 people more than 12 yr old, without known thyroid disease or antithyroid antibodies; 85% had TSH levels below 2.5 mIU/liter, and 2.3% had subclinical hypothyroidism (SCH). An additional 9.7% had URR TSH, representing 20.6 million Americans, who would also be identified as SCH if the upper TSH limit were decreased. Many with URR TSH do not have thyroid disease. INTERVENTION: The time of phlebotomy is important, because the TSH level varies throughout the day, with early morning values greater than later ones, and is accentuated by sleep deprivation, strenuous exercise, or working during the night or evening shifts. Repeated measurements in the same individual vary considerably over months. RESULTS: About half of those with URR TSH probably have thyroid disease, but most with thyroid disease, antithyroid peroxidase antibodies, have TSH below 2.5 mIU/liter. Those with URR TSH with thyroid disease probably have minimal thyroid deficiency, without any reported adverse health consequences or benefit of treatments with levothyroxine. CONCLUSION: Because routine levothyroxine treatment is not recommended for SCH, it is certainly not warranted in individuals with URR TSH. For all patients with URR TSH, it is reasonable to determine serum TSH every 1-2 yr.

Ursella S, Testa A, Mazzone M, Gentiloni Silveri Amiodarone-induced thyroid dysfunction in clinical practice. N.Eur Rev Med Pharmacol Sci. 2006 Sep-Oct;10(5):269-78. Amiodarone is a potent class III anti-arrhythmic drug used in clinical practice for the prophylaxis and treatment of many cardiac rhythm disturbances, ranging from paroxismal atrial fibrillation to life threatening ventricular tachyarrhythmias. Amiodarone often causes changes in thyroid function tests mainly related to the inhibition of 5'-deiodinase activity resulting in a decrease in the generation of T3 from T4 with a consequent increase in rT3 production and a decrease in its clearance. In a group of amiodarone-treated patients there is overt thyroid dysfunction, either amiodarone-induced thyrotoxicosis (AIT) or amiodarone-induced hypothyroidism (AIH). AIT is primarily related to excess iodine-induced thyroid hormone synthesis in an abnormal thyroid gland (type I AIT) or to amiodarone-related destructive thyroiditis (type II AIT). The pathogenesis of AIH is related to a failure to escape from the acute Wolff-Chaikoff effect due to defects in thyroid hormonogenesis, or, in patients with positive thyroid autoantibody test, to concomitant Hashimoto's thyroiditis. Both AIT and AIH may develop either in apparently normal thyroid glands or in glands with preexisting, clinically silent abnormalities. AIT is more common in iodine-deficient regions of the world, whereas AIH is usually seen in iodine-sufficient areas. In contrast to AIH, AIT is a difficult condition to diagnose and treat, and discontinuation of amiodarone is usually recommended. In this review we analyse, according to data from current literature, the alterations in thyroid laboratory tests seen in euthyroid patients under treatment with amiodarone and the epidemiology and treatment options available of amiodarone-induced thyroid dysfunctions (AIT and AIH).

Van Den Eeden SK et al. Thyroid hormone use and the risk of hip fracture in women > or = 65 years: a case-control study.J Womens Health (Larchmt). 2003 Jan-Feb; 12(1):27-31. BACKGROUND: There is controversy about whether thyroid hormone therapy may lead to osteoporosis, and less is known about the clinically more important end point of whether its use increases fracture risk. METHODS: We used a case-control study to examine the association between thyroid hormone use and hip fractures among older women in a large managed care organization in Northern California. The subjects were 501 women > or =65 years of age who were hospitalized for hip fractures and 533 age-matched controls without hip fractures. RESULTS: No difference in the ever use or duration of use of exogenous thyroid hormone was found between cases and controls (odds ratio [OR] 1.1, 95% confidence interval [CI] 0.8, 1.6). Hip fracture was associated with evidence of visual impairment, prior use of steroids, and number of falls. CONCLUSIONS: In women > or =65 years, an independent effect of thyroid hormone use on the risk of hip fracture was not found. This finding is reassuring, given the large number of women on thyroid hormone therapy today.

Walsh JP et al. Small changes in thyroxine dosage do not produce measurable changes in hypothyroid symptoms, well-being or quality of life: results of a double blind randomized clinical trial. J Clin Endocrinol Metab. 2006 May 2 CONTEXT: In patients with primary hypothyroidism, anecdotal evidence suggests that well-being is optimized by fine adjustment of T (4) dosage, aiming for a serum TSH concentration in the lower reference range. This has not been tested in a clinical trial. OBJECTIVE: Our objective was to test whether adjustment of T (4) dosage aiming for a serum TSH concentration less than 2 mU/liter improves well-being compared with a serum TSH concentration in the upper reference range. DESIGN: We conducted a double-blind, randomized clinical trial with a crossover design. PARTICIPANTS: Fifty-six subjects (52 females) with primary hypothyroidism taking T (4) (>/=100 microg/d) with baseline serum TSH 0.1-4.8 mU/liter participated. INTERVENTIONS: Each subject received three T (4) doses (low, middle, and high in 25-microg increments) in random order. OUTCOME MEASURES: Outcome measures included visual analog scales assessing well-being (the primary endpoint) and hypothyroid symptoms, quality of life instruments (General Health Questionnaire 28, Short Form 36, and Thyroid Symptom Questionnaire), cognitive function tests, and treatment preference. RESULTS: Mean (+/- sem) serum TSH concentrations were 2.8 +/- 0.4, 1.0 +/- 0.2, and 0.3 +/- 0.1 mU/liter for the three treatments. There were no significant treatment effects on any of the instruments assessing well-being, symptoms, quality of life, or cognitive function and no significant treatment preference. CONCLUSIONS: Small changes in T(4) dosage do not produce measurable changes in hypothyroid symptoms, well-being, or quality of life, despite the expected changes in serum TSH and markers of thyroid hormone action. These data do not support the suggestion that the target TSH range for the treatment of primary hypothyroidism should differ from the general laboratory range.

Walsh JP et al. 2003 Combined thyroxine/liothyronine treatment does not improve well-being, quality of life, or cognitive function compared to thyroxine alone: a randomized controlled trial in patients with primary hypothyroidism. J Clin Endocrinol Metab 88:4543–4550 T (4) is standard treatment for hypothyroidism. A recent study reported that combined T (4)/liothyronine (T (3)) treatment improved well-being and cognitive function compared with T (4) alone. We conducted a double-blind, randomized, controlled trial with a crossover design in 110 patients (101 completers) with primary hypothyroidism in which liothyronine 10 micro g was substituted for 50 micro g of the patients' usual T(4) dose. No significant (P < 0.05) difference between T(4) and combined T(4)/T(3) treatment was demonstrated on cognitive function, quality of life scores, Thyroid Symptom Questionnaire scores, subjective satisfaction with treatment, or eight of 10 visual analog scales assessing symptoms. For the General Health Questionnaire-28 and visual analog scales assessing anxiety and nausea, scores were significantly (P < 0.05) worse for combined treatment than for T(4) alone. Serum TSH was lower during T(4) treatment than during combined T(4)/T(3) treatment (mean +/- SEM, 1.5 +/- 0.2 vs. 3.1 +/- 0.2 mU/liter; P < 0.001), a potentially confounding factor; however, subgroup analysis of subjects with comparable serum TSH concentrations during each treatment showed no benefit from combined treatment compared with T(4) alone. We conclude that in the doses used in this study, combined T (4)/T (3) treatment does not improve well-being, cognitive function, or quality of life compared with T (4) alone

Wartofsky L et al. Overt and 'subclinical' hypothyroidism in women. Obstet Gynecol Surv. 2006 Aug; 61(8):535-42. Thyroid disease in general and hypothyroidism in particular, are very common in women. In the USA, the most common cause of primary thyroid deficiency is on an autoimmune basis due to lymphocytic (Hashimoto) thyroiditis. Because there are thyroid hormone receptors in virtually every tissue of the body, the manifestations of hypothyroidism are varied, but problems with abnormal menses, conception, fertility, and pregnancy can be especially troubling in young women. The single most important diagnostic test is measurement of serum thyrotropin (TSH). The overwhelming majority of patients with hypothyroidism are treated with a single daily dose of synthetic levothyroxine with the goal of therapy being restoration of a normal metabolic state with return of the TSH level down to the range of 0.5 to 1.5 mIU/L. "Subclinical" hypothyroidism refers to those patients with early or mild thyroid hypofunction manifested as slight elevations of thyrotropin (approximately 4-10 mIU/L) although serum thyroxine (T4) and triiodothyronine (T3) levels are within their reference ranges. The entity is somewhat controversial in regard to its consequences if left untreated, and whether or not we should be screening patients, at least susceptible populations, for the condition. Reports indicate an association between subclinical hypothyroidism and poor outcomes of pregnancy, as well as dyslipidemias, atherogenesis, and increased mortality in the long term. We believe these consequences are sufficiently compelling to warrant screening and treatment with levothyroxine when found to halt progression to overt hypothyroidism, and improve symptoms, pregnancy outcomes, lipid abnormalities, and cardiovascular function.

Wartofsky L and Dickey RA. The evidence for a narrower thyrotropin reference range is compelling. J Clin Endocrinol Metab. 2005 Sep; 90(9):5483-8. Debate and controversy currently surround the recommendations of a recent consensus conference that considered issues related to the management of early, mild, or so-called subclinical hypothyroidism and hyperthyroidism. Intimately related to the controversy is the definition of the normal reference range for TSH. It has become clear that previously accepted reference ranges are no longer valid as a result of both the development of more highly sensitive TSH assays and the appreciation that reference populations previously considered normal were contaminated with individuals with various degrees of thyroid dysfunction that served to increase mean TSH levels for the group. Recent laboratory guidelines from the National Academy of Clinical Biochemistry indicate that more than 95% of normal individuals have TSH levels below 2.5 mU/liter. The remainder with higher values are outliers, most of whom are likely to have underlying Hashimoto thyroiditis or other causes of elevated TSH. Importantly, data indicating that African-Americans with very low incidence of Hashimoto thyroiditis have a mean TSH level of 1.18 mU/liter strongly suggest that this value is the true normal mean for a normal population. Recognition and establishment of a more precise and true normal range for TSH have important implications for both screening and treatment of thyroid disease in general and subclinical thyroid disease in particular.

Weinsier RL et al. Do adaptive changes in metabolic rate favor weight regain in weight-reduced individuals? An examination of the set-point theory. Am J Clin Nutr 2000 Nov; 72(5):1088-94 BACKGROUND: Obese persons generally regain lost weight, suggesting that adaptive metabolic changes favor return to a preset weight. OBJECTIVE: Our objective was to determine whether adaptive changes in resting metabolic rate (RMR) and thyroid hormones occur in weight-reduced persons, predisposing them to long-term weight gain. DESIGN: Twenty-four overweight, postmenopausal women were studied at a clinical research center in four 10-d study phases: the overweight state (phase 1, energy balance; phase 2, 3350 kJ/d) and after reduction to a normal-weight state (phase 3, 3350 kJ/d; phase 4, energy balance). Weight-reduced women were matched with 24 never-overweight control subjects. After each study phase, assessments included RMR (by indirect calorimetry), body composition (by hydrostatic weighing), serum triiodothyronine (T (3)), and reverse T (3) (rT (3)). Body weight was measured 4 y later, without intervention. RESULTS: Body composition-adjusted RMR and T (3): rT (3) fell during acute (phase 2) and chronic (phase 3) energy restriction (P: < 0.01), but returned to baseline in the normal-weight, energy-balanced state (phase 4; mean weight loss: 12.9 +/- 2.0 kg). RMR among weight-reduced women (4771 +/- 414 kJ/d) was not significantly different from that in control subjects (4955 +/- 414 kJ/d; P: = 0.14), and lower RMR did not predict greater 4-y weight regain (r = 0.27, NS). CONCLUSIONS: Energy restriction produces a transient hypothyroid-hypometabolic state that normalizes on return to energy-balanced conditions. Failure to establish energy balance after weight loss gives the misleading impression that weight-reduced persons are energy conservative and predisposed to weight regain. Our findings do not provide evidence in support of adaptive metabolic changes as an explanation for the tendency of weight-reduced persons to regain weight.

Yoneda K et al. Direct effects of thyroid hormones on rat coronary artery: nongenomic effects of triiodothyronine and thyroxine. Thyroid 1998 Jul;8(7):609-13 To determine whether thyroid hormones, triiodothyronine (T3) and thyroxine (T4), have any direct, nongenomic effects on vascular smooth muscle cells, we evaluated the effects of these hormones on rat coronary arteries. Bolus injection of T3 or T4 elicited a transient, dose-dependent decrease in coronary perfusion pressure (CPP), as well as an increase in arterial vasodilation. Vasodilation occurred immediately after injection, peaked at 15 seconds, and lasted 80 seconds. Reverse T3 had no effect on CPP or vasodilation. The rapidity of these effects suggests that they are not mediated by the T3-nuclear receptor, but are direct, nongenomic effects of thyroid hormones. Our results also suggest that thyroid hormones may play a role in preventing myocardial ischemia by inducing coronary artery vasodilation.

CHAPTER 4

Testosterone

Physiology:

Testosterone decline can begin as early as 30 years of age. Comparing a 25 year old man to a 75 year old man there is a decrease of 30% in total and 50% decrease in bioavailable testosterone. In addition, Traviston (2006) found that the in the average population, testosterone levels are getting lower every year. There are different methods of measuring and expressing testosterone levels, each with advantages and disadvantages. Total testosterone includes the amount bound to Sex Hormone Binding Globulin, (SHBG), loosely bound to albumin and free in the serum, Advantages of this test are that it is inexpensive, available at all labs and reproducible. Free testosterone excludes the portions bound to SHBG and loosely bound to albumin. Advantages of this measurement are that it may more accurately express physiologic levels as compared to total. The disadvantages are that it does not contain the amount that is loosely bound to albumin and that the results are not as reliable. Bioavailable testosterone is the most useful physiological measurement. It includes free testosterone, loosely bound to albumin and excludes tightly bound to SHBG. It can be calculated if the total testosterone, SHBG and albumin levels are known. There is a free calculator available at www.issam.ch/freetesto.htm. Despite this available technology hormone optimization is a **clinical** specialty and we are not titrating to get to a specific numerical value.

There are multiple feedback loops that are involved in testosterone metabolism (see diagram). Gonadotropin Releasing Hormone (GnRH) stimulates the anterior pituitary to release FSH and LH. FSH stimulates the Sertoli cells to produce sperm. LH stimulates the Leydig cells to produce testosterone. Testosterone can be bio transformed to estradiol (E2) via aromatase and to dihydrotestosterone (DHT) via 5- alpha reductase. There are negative feedback loops to the hypothalamus and anterior pituitary by testosterone, DHT and E2. TRT will require the understanding that when you treat with testosterone, you are in effect treating with the metabolites of E2 and DHT as well.

Testosterone is an essential hormone in men and women. The androgen receptor is widely found in most tissues. Bioidentical testosterone replacement therapy has dramatic benefits on health, mood, well-being and sexuality. Korenman et al. found that half of healthy men between the ages of 50 and 70 years have a bioavailable testosterone level below the lowest level seen in healthy men aged 20 to 40 years old. Normal for age testosterone levels are not optimal and may represent a significant deficiency. Andropause is defined as a stage in life in which inadequate testosterone production for optimal health and well-being. Andropause can be a gradual process and varies from one man to the next, but just like female menopause can have severe health consequences in the long-term. In fact in the Shores study from the *Archives of Internal Medicine* in 2006, men with low testosterone died 88% sooner than men with high testosterone. Khaw et al. study in *Circulation* showed that high endogenous testosterone was correlated with lower mortality for cardiovascular disease, cancer and all cause. In fact, there was a 41 % decrease in mortality in men with testosterone level of 564 as compared to levels of 350 ng/dl. The authors point out that, ironically, fear of prostate cancer has kept men from getting testosterone treatment.

The central controversy in Testosterone replacement therapy is whether TRT increases the risks of developing or exacerbating prostate cancer. Current research by Morgantaler (2006) concludes that "there is not now – nor has there ever been a scientific basis for the belief that T causes PC to grow." There appears to be a paradox because it is known that castration causes metastatic prostate cancer to regress. A saturation model can explain this seemingly counterintuitive situation. According to Morgantaler, it takes a testosterone level of around 90 to saturate the receptors that could accelerate prostate cancer growth, (personal communication). A hypogonadic man with a testosterone of 200 is already saturated and treating this hypogonadism and raising his level to 700 would not further impact the cancer growth if present.

Testosterone deficiency has pleiotropic deleterious effects. There is increased cardiovascular system dysfunction, which can lead to the increased incidence of AMI's and strokes. Cognitive dysfunctions associated with hypogonadism include decreased memory and the increased rate of non-Alzheimer's and Alzheimer's dementia. There is a strong association between decreased testosterone levels and type II diabetes in men. Decreased testosterone in men is also associated with dyslipidemia, osteoporosis, arthritis and depression.

Women, as well, require optimal testosterone. Women have about 10% of the male circulating testosterone levels. Optimal testosterone is needed for sense of well-being, strength (especially upper body strength), nipple and clitoral sensitivity, body composition, and bone density. DHEA supplementation may increase testosterone to optimal levels in women with borderline testosterone deficiency. Women produce 40 to 50% of their circulating testosterone in their adrenals and ovaries. There can be relative androgen deficiency with normal levels in women. A syndrome of RAD has been described in the medical literature. Clinical symptoms, including reduced libido, may be the main diagnostic criteria and these patients will benefit from treatment.

Symptoms:

Testosterone Deficiency symptoms in men may be subtle or overt including:
- Fatigue
- Depression
- Irritability "Grumpy old men" syndrome
- Reduced libido and erectile function
- Decreased sexual desire and decreased sexual fantasies
- Decreased morning erections
- Decreased firmness of erections
- Longer recovery time between orgasms
- Loss of drive and competitive edge
- Stiffness and pain in muscles and joints
- Decreased effectiveness of exercise workouts

Symptoms of female androgen deficiency syndrome (FADS) include:

- Impaired sexual function
- Loss of libido
- Fatigue
- Loss of well being

- Decreased muscle mass and strength and lowered bone density
- Depression
- Anxiety
- Lack of self confidence,
- An "imbalanced" feeling
- Memory loss
- Abdominal fat and weight gain

Literature Review:

Testosterone replacement therapy (TRT) improves libido, erections, cardiovascular status, body composition, cognitive function, mood, depression, glycemic control and inflammation. It is well documented that testosterone replacement improves libido. A study by Jain et al. showed that testosterone replacement given as a transdermal, oral, or intramuscular injection, and significantly improved erectile function. Testosterone levels correlated with cognitive function, and replacement improved cognitive function. Moffat et al. found that serum free testosterone concentration can be used to predict memory performance and cognitive status in elderly men. Gouras et al showed that testosterone replacement therapy prevents the production of beta amyloid precursor protein in men, which suggests that testosterone replacement may play a role in the prevention of Alzheimer's disease. A pilot study by Tan on the effects of testosterone in hypo gonadal aging male patients with Alzheimer's disease revealed that mental status of those given testosterone replacement therapy improved over one year, whereas the mental status of those given a placebo declined. Testosterone replacement has also been shown to significantly improve mood and erections. Low testosterone levels are associated with fatigue, irritability, and depression.

There is a common misconception that testosterone has adverse cardiovascular effects. However, the opposite has been shown with current research. The lower the free testosterone level the more likely coronary artery disease will be present. Testosterone replacement improves ST depression and dilates coronary arteries. TRT also may improve lipids and low testosterone is associated with dyslipidemia. English et al. found that low-dose transdermal testosterone therapy improves angina threshold in men with chronic stable angina. Rosano et al. (1999) found that "Short-term administration of testosterone induces a beneficial effect on exercise-induced myocardial ischemia in men with coronary artery disease." Rosano et al. (1999) also concluded that intracoronary testosterone has direct dilating effects on the coronary arteries. Finally, Hak et al. (2002) found that low levels of endogenous androgens increase the risk of atherosclerosis in elderly men.

Testosterone optimization is anti-inflammatory. Testosterone prevents cytokine production and initiates the acute phase response, which elevates C-reactive protein, serum amyloid A and fibrinogen. Testosterone also prevents the formation of the adhesion molecules vascular cell adhesive molecule (VCAM) and intercellular adhesive molecule, (CD 54/ICAM), which are necessary components of the process of atherosclerosis. Thus, testosterone replacement is a very powerful anti-inflammatory treatment that can help to prevent atherosclerosis. Testosterone has also been shown to be of benefit in the treatment of chronic heart failure. Pugh et al. found that testosterone increases cardiac output, decreases left ventricular load, and has no adverse cardiovascular effects. Malkin et al. show that testosterone replacement moderates inflammatory cytokines and improves heart failure outcomes. Turhan et al. found that men with low free testosterone levels have greater than 3 times the risk for the development of coronary artery disease.

Rhoden et al. point out that benign prostatic hyperplasia (BPH) symptoms are not exacerbated with testosterone supplementation. Cooper et al. studied the effect of exogenous testosterone on prostate volume, serum and semen prostate specific antigen (PSA) levels in healthy young men. Participants were given testosterone intramuscularly at doses of 100, 250, or 500 mg a week. Serum testosterone increased, and there was no change in prostate volume or serum and semen PSA. Morales and Prehn both concluded that there is no evidence to suggest that exogenous androgens promote the development of prostate cancer. Morley states in the January 2000 issue of *Mayo Clinic Proceedings*, "There is no clinical evidence that the risk of either prostate cancer or BPH increases with testosterone replacement therapy." A collaborative analysis published in the *Journal of the National Cancer Institute* in 2008 found that there was no association between the risk of prostate cancer and any hormone measured, including testosterone, DHT, estradiol and others. Gould et al. review of 15 studies of testosterone replacement, up to 15 years in duration, showed no increase of prostate cancer risk. Agarwal (2005) and Sarosdy (2007) found that testosterone treatment studies of patients with prostate cancer after radical prostatectomy and brachytherapy have shown no recurrences or significant increases of PSA. Morgantaler's study in the *Journal of Urology* in 2011 has produced dramatic evidence on the safety profile of TRT. 13 testosterone deficient men with biopsy proven prostate cancer were treated with TRT. After 2.5 years repeat biopsies were done and no cancer was found in 54%, there was also no local progression or metastasis found.

Testosterone is the major predictor of skeletal mass, and it is synergistic with growth hormone (GH) and insulin-like growth factor-1 (IGF-1). Bhasin et al. show that testosterone can improve strength even without exercise, but there is a marked improvement if testosterone is taken in combination with exercise. Declining testosterone levels are associated with accelerated osteoporosis, decreased muscle mass, and anemia - frailty.

Testosterone can be a very powerful tool for the control of insulin resistance. Replacement doses decrease insulin resistance. Low levels of testosterone play a role in the development of type 2 diabetes. Low testosterone is associated with metabolic syndrome, hypertension, type II diabetes, fibromyalgia, and coronary artery disease. Boyanov et al. studied the effect of testosterone supplementation in men with type 2 diabetes, visceral obesity, and partial androgen deficiency. Subjects received testosterone undecanoate, and the results reflect that supplementary testosterone reduced hemoglobin A1C levels by 17.3%, led to a decrease in visceral obesity, and improved symptoms of androgen deficiency including erectile dysfunction.

Kaczmarek et al. showed that decreased testosterone and free testosterone are associated with coronary artery disease in women independent of other risk factors. Dimitrakasis et al. found that women given traditional HRT plus TRT had a lower incidence of breast cancer than those given HRT alone.

Management:

If a male patient presents with clinical symptoms of testosterone deficiency and the Total and /or Free testosterone is suboptimal then replacement therapy is indicated. Baseline laboratory evaluation should include free/total/bioavailable testosterone, estradiol, hemogram and PSA. The Hemogram is evaluated because increased red cell production may occur and monitoring for erythrocytosis is important. This increase in red cell mass may need to be addressed with either blood donation or phlebotomy. A baseline estradiol indicates excess aromatization, which will need to be addressed prior to treatment. If estradiol levels are elevated prior to testosterone supplementation, the effects of aromatization are exacerbated and the addition of supplements to reduce aromatization may be indicated. Currently PSA measurements are controversial in their value to reduce mortality. The review of literature shows that testosterone therapy does not increase the risk of prostate cancer. However, with standard of care in medicine, (which may lead to more harm than good), we still suggest the monitoring of the PSA levels and annual digital rectal exams (DRE). PSA values > 4 are considered elevated. PSA velocity is defined as a > 1.0 increase in a year, so even if normal < 4, if velocity is present, further evaluation is needed. Some patients chronically have levels above 4 that are stable and do not require further evaluation. There are many controversies surrounding PSA testing and it is a non-specific test. If abnormal values are found, repeat testing will often show values that are back to the patient's baseline. Testosterone replacement therapy is generally not given to men with known prostate cancer and is discontinued if there is a diagnosis of prostate cancer as a rule, but exceptions are often made when quality of life issues arise. The current work of Morgantaler explains that testosterone replacement does not cause prostate cancer to grow and even reports a case of a patient with prostate cancer being treated with testosterone. Since this is so controversial we are not recommending this at this time. Although If a patient has had a radical prostatectomy or brachytherapy and their PSA remains <0.1, treatment may be initiated after one year. Ideally, this is best done in consultation with his urologist.

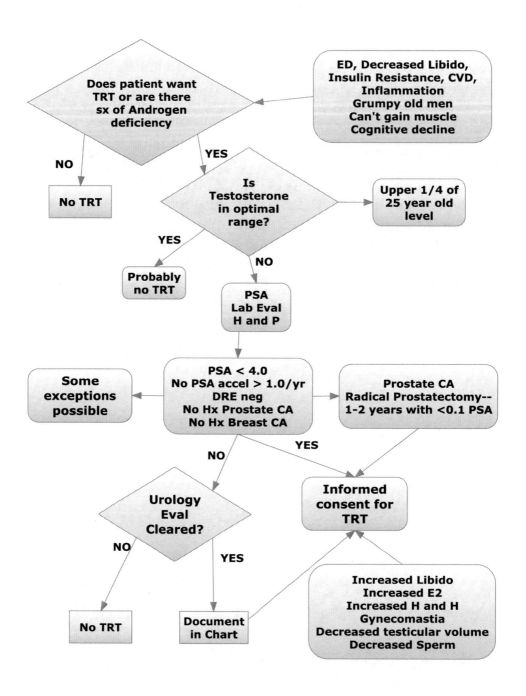

Does patient want TRT or are there sx of Androgen deficiency

ED, Decreased Libido, Insulin Resistance, CVD, Inflammation Grumpy old men Can't gain muscle Cognitive decline

NO

No TRT

YES

Is Testosterone in optimal range?

Upper 1/4 of 25 year old level

YES

Probably no TRT

NO

PSA Lab Eval H and P

Some exceptions possible

PSA < 4.0 No PSA accel > 1.0/yr DRE neg No Hx Prostate CA No Hx Breast CA

Prostate CA Radical Prostatectomy-- 1-2 years with <0.1 PSA

NO

YES

Urology Eval Cleared?

Informed consent for TRT

NO

YES

No TRT

Document in Chart

Increased Libido Increased E2 Increased H and H Gynecomastia Decreased testicular volume Decreased Sperm

Testosterone can be given in the form of weekly injections either intramuscular or subcutaneous, of testosterone esters, which become bioidentical in the blood. Stable serum levels can be obtained for a week, but longer intervals between injections lead to roller coaster effects. Testosterone cypionate is available commercially or compounded at 200 mg/ ml. A starting dosage of 50-100 mg weekly is recommended. Another method of testosterone replacement therapy is by transdermal creams or gels. There are several commercial products but we prefer a skin cream custom-made by a compounding pharmacist. A measured amount of transdermal testosterone cream is applied to the skin daily. There are many different delivery systems for compounded creams. There are tubs, syringes, pumps and click devices. There are standardized in measuring a gram of cream. Any concentration can be created in compounding pharmacies. We recommend starting doses of 50- 100 mg. A written prescription, for a 100 mg dose, would be Testosterone cream 10% = 100 mg/gm, apply 1 gm topically daily in the morning. This 1 gm could be ¼ tsp. for tubs, 1 ml for syringe, 2 pumps or 4 clicks. We recommend you contact your compounding pharmacy to discuss the benefits of each delivery system and to confirm the concentration of hormones in the devices. Caution is needed to avoid accidental transfer to women, children and pets as this can occur with contact to the application area within the first 2 hours. Commercial transdermal products include patches or the skin cream or gel in prepackaged envelopes that is to be used daily. Testosterone pellets can also be inserted subcutaneously with duration of action of three months or longer.

Testosterone Dose Men

- Cream 50-150 mg/day
- Cypionate 50-150 mg/week
- Pellets 75 mg x 5-10 every 3 months
- HCG 1000-5000 IU per week with
  Possible dosing:
    - 250 IU/day
    - 1000 IU twice a week
    - T cypionate 100 mg IM day 1
      HCG 250 IU days 5 and 6

In some men, human chorionic gonadotropin (HCG) may be prescribed instead of testosterone. HCG can be effective as TRT since the alpha subunit of HCG is identical to the alpha subunit of LH and can stimulate the testosterone production in the Leydig cells. Side effects of testosterone replacement therapy can be a decrease in testicular volume and sperm count. If these are issues HCG usage may be an effective alternative. HCG is usually most effective when there is still possible Leydig cell function. FSH and LH levels of 5 or greater are considered elevated. When evaluating whether HCG is an option, evaluate FSH and LH; if elevated HCG treatment most likely will not be effective. The pituitary has already responded but Leydig cell response has been insufficient. If they are not elevated then HCG 250-500 IU subcutaneously daily or comparable dosing of 2000 to 5000 IU weekly can stimulate the Leydig cells to produce more testosterone. An alternate management of TRT reducing these two side effects could be to combine an injection or cream with 500 IU HCG/weekly.

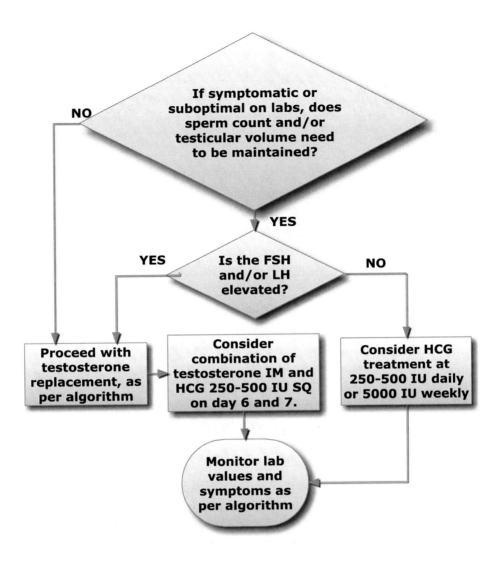

Follow-up lab testing, with serum total/free/bioavailable Testosterone, estradiol and hemogram usually 3 months after the testosterone has been prescribed and every three months thereafter for the first year is recommended. Annual digital rectal exams and PSA are recommended. The dose and concentration of the testosterone can be titrated as needed, according to lab test results and clinical response. Optimal lab values for total testosterone are typically 600-1200. It must be stressed that lab tests are clinical guidelines, and not absolute parameters. For example if total testosterone started at 300 and at 3 months is 580 and clinical evaluation is optimal, we do not need to increase dosing to get to a precise lab value. We wish to stress that this is a clinical specialty and that lab values help to establish our clinical diagnosis. For example, if a patient is being treated with testosterone cream and the serum testing does not show an increase in value, but there is a significant clinical response there are other explanations. Possible explanations could include increases in DHT without significant or even decrease in testosterone, and the patient experiences a clinical response to androgen replacement through DHT. This may be acceptable clinical treatment depending on differing philosophies concerning DHT. Another possibility is the rare situation serum testing does not reflect intracellular testosterone levels and other testing such as salivary or 24 hour urine testing may give you additional information.

Sometimes testosterone replacement therapy causes an erythropoietin- like effect with increased production of red blood cells or erythrocytosis. If a patient's hematocrit increases above 55, he can donate one unit of blood every 6-12 months to keep the hematocrit level 55 or less. If he is unable to donate blood, a therapeutic phlebotomy can be performed.

Biotransformation of Testosterone to Estradiol is catalyzed by aromatase. Optimal testosterone replacement therapy in men requires management of Estradiol as well. The medical literature suggests that that optimal Estradiol level is around 25 mg/dl. Lifestyle, nutritional and pharmacologic treatments can control aromatization and achieve desired Estradiol levels. Minimizing body fat, reducing alcohol consumption, replacing zinc in zinc deficiency can decrease aromatization. For optimal zinc levels, supplementation with 50 mg per day of zinc is recommended. Chrysin, a plant extract flavonoid is claimed to reduce aromatization. Using 500 mg, either oral or transdermal, of Chrysin once or twice daily can reduce aromatization. Anastrozole prescribed in small doses of 0.5 mg 1-2 times a week, will consistently decrease aromatization and Estradiol. Estradiol levels need to be reassessed periodically since adipose reduction may decrease aromatization and anastrozole may no longer be required.

In some patients testosterone replacement therapy can increase DHT via the actions of 5-Alpha-Reductase. DHT may correlate with unwanted scalp hair loss or increased prostatic hyperplasia. Progesterone at 10 mg daily transdermal can have a mild 5-Alpha-Reductase inhibitory action as well as aromatase inhibition. Progesterone treatment when used in doses greater than 25 mg may produce an anti-libido effect. Even low dosage Progesterone of 10 mg can help induce restful sleep. Saw palmetto can act as a mild 5-Alpha-Reductase inhibitor.

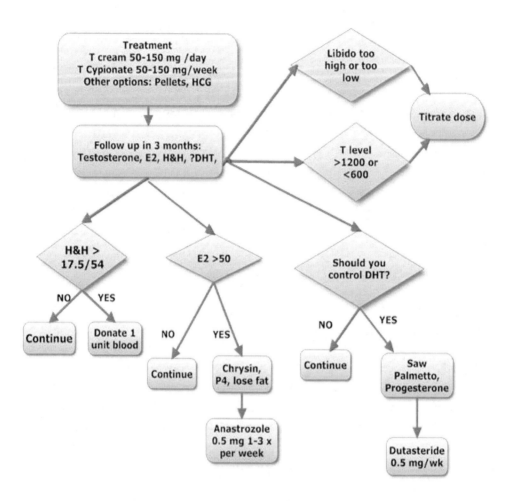

The dose we recommend for saw palmetto is 160 mg two times per day. It is often combined with pygeum (50 mg two times per day) and urtica (120 mg two times per day) two other herbal medicines that have synergistic effects on the prostate. Potent pharmaceutical 5 Alpha- Reductase inhibitors like finasteride or dutasteride can be used to lower the DHT level, but the side effects can include decreases in libido, erectile function and cognitive functions as well as depression. This therapy may be more detrimental than beneficial and natural methods are preferred. There is debate in the medical literature whether finasteride and dutasteride can act as chemoprevention of prostate cancer or can it induce high grade prostate cancer.

At 6-12 months check repeat PSA and DRE are reevaluated. As we stressed above, if there has been a PSA abnormality, a repeat PSA will often return to baseline. If continues abnormal, a urology consult is recommended.

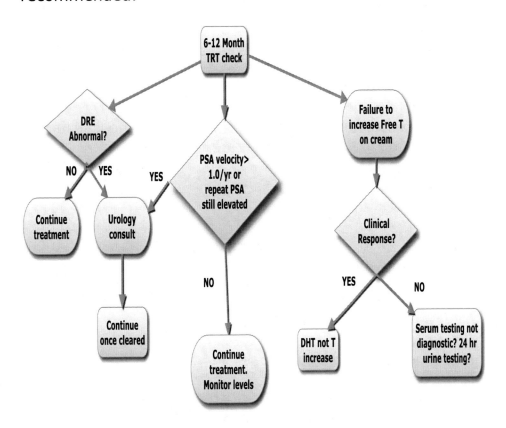

TESTOSTERONE IN Women

Testosterone, in women, is produced in the ovaries and in the adrenals via DHEA. Bioidentical testosterone replacement can dramatically increase libido in women with Relative Androgen Deficiency. Bioidentical testosterone replacement therapy can also decrease inflammation, improve energy levels, increase bone density, decrease blood pressure, decrease cardiovascular disease, lower LDL cholesterol levels, raise HDL cholesterol levels, improve blood glucose levels, improve muscle strength, improve brain function and decrease body fat. Testosterone doses for women are much lower than testosterone doses for men, about 2.5-10% of male doses. Symptoms of testosterone excess in women include oily skin, acne, scalp hair loss, unwanted body hair, "too much" libido, aggressive behavior and salt or sugar cravings. Elevated testosterone levels in women can be caused by PCOS or overtreatment of Testosterone.

Female Testosterone Management:

DHEA may raise testosterone levels in women (not in men) and is useful for treating borderline low testosterone and when minimal clinical symptoms are present. Optimal testosterone values in women are variable. These levels are determined by clinical response of improved libido and without the side effects such as acne and each woman will determine her specific dose in association with her provider. Treatment is clinical however optimal levels for total usually are between 50-80 ng/dl and free is usually 1-6 pg/ml. Bioavailable levels run 10-30 ng/dl.

We recommend an initial starting dose of testosterone transdermal cream .5%, which is 5 mg/gm of cream. When the dispensing system is a click device and each click equals ¼ gm of cream. The dosing we start at is ½ to 1 gm = 2.5 - 5 mg = 2 - 4 clicks daily. It should initially be applied behind the knees and down the calf in the morning. About 10 % of women may get some abnormal coarse hair growth in the area they apply the testosterone. If this occurs, it usually will occur within the first month. If they apply on their legs, this side effect is minimal as most women shave anyway. An occasional female patient will not absorb the cream and require injections of testosterone cypionate usually 5-10 mg IM or subcutaneously weekly or pellets. It is important to educate your patient about side effects.

Lab evaluation should be done in 3 months to assess Free and Total Testosterone, SHBG, DHEA sulfate. If clinical deficiency symptoms persist and lab testing was suboptimal, then we would consider increasing the dosing. Maximum testosterone dosing in women is usually 20 mg in women.

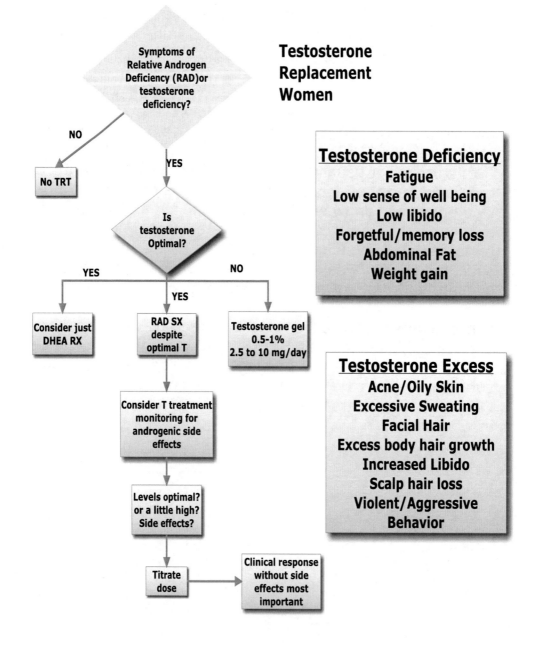

Testosterone Replacement Women

Symptoms of Relative Androgen Deficiency (RAD)or testosterone deficiency?

NO → **No TRT**

YES

Is testosterone Optimal?

YES — **Consider just DHEA RX**

YES — **RAD SX despite optimal T**

NO — **Testosterone gel 0.5-1% 2.5 to 10 mg/day**

Consider T treatment monitoring for androgenic side effects

Levels optimal? or a little high? Side effects?

Titrate dose → **Clinical response without side effects most important**

Testosterone Deficiency
Fatigue
Low sense of well being
Low libido
Forgetful/memory loss
Abdominal Fat
Weight gain

Testosterone Excess
Acne/Oily Skin
Excessive Sweating
Facial Hair
Excess body hair growth
Increased Libido
Scalp hair loss
Violent/Aggressive Behavior

Men and women need testosterone for optimal health and to treat the signs and symptoms of hormone deficiency. Testosterone replacement can result in a healthier brain, a healthier heart, increased muscle mass, greater bone density, improved mood, improved sense of well-being and an improved sexual life. Optimal replacement can lead to a reversal of diabetes and metabolic syndrome. Replacing lowered testosterone levels as we age, when a deficiency is present, is a powerful preventive/regenerative medical treatment.

TESTOSTERONE ABSTRACTS:

Agarwal PK et al. Testosterone replacement therapy after primary treatment for prostate cancer. J Urol. 2005 Feb; 173(2):533-6. PURPOSE: A history of prostate cancer has been an absolute contraindication for testosterone supplementation. We studied a cohort of hypogonadal patients treated with radical retropubic prostatectomy (RRP) for organ confined prostate cancer to determine if testosterone replacement therapy (TRT) could be efficacious and administered safely without causing recurrent prostate tumor. MATERIALS AND METHODS: Ten hypogonadal patients previously treated with RRP for organ confined prostate cancer were identified. They presented with low serum total testosterone (TT) and symptoms of hypogonadism after RRP. Patients had baseline serum determinations of prostate specific antigen (PSA) and TT, and were started on testosterone supplementation. They were assessed periodically for changes in PSA and TT, and for symptomatic improvement using the hormone domain of the Extended Prostate Inventory Composite Health Related Quality of Life questionnaire. RESULTS: At a median followup of 19 months no patient had detectable (greater than 0.1 ng/ml) PSA. TT increased significantly after starting TRT from a mean +/- SD of 197 +/- 67 to 591 +/- 180 ng/dl (p = 0.0002). The Hormone Domain of the Extended Prostate Inventory Composite Health Related Quality of Life questionnaire increased significantly from 38 +/- 5 to 49 +/- 3 (p = 0.00005), primarily due to a decrease in hot flashes and an increase in energy level. CONCLUSIONS: At a median of 19 months of TRT hypogonadal patients with a history of prostate cancer had no PSA recurrence and had statistically significant improvements in TT and hypogonadal symptoms. In highly select patients after RRP TRT can be administered carefully and with benefit to hypogonadal patients with prostate cancer.

Alexander GM, Swerdloff RS, Wang C, et al. Androgen-behavior correlations in hypogonadal men and eugonadal men. II. Cognitive abilities. Hormones and Behavior 1998; 33(2):85-94. Sex-typed cognitive abilities were assessed in 33 hypogonadal men receiving testosterone replacement therapy, 10 eugonadal men receiving testosterone in a male contraceptive clinical trial, and 19 eugonadal men not administered testosterone. Prior to and following hormone administration, men completed four tests measuring visuospatial ability, three tests measuring verbal fluency, two tests measuring perceptual speed, and a measure of verbal memory. Group differences in testosterone levels were unrelated to performance on most cognitive measures, including visuospatial ability. Relative to other men, hypogonadal men were impaired in their verbal fluency and showed improved verbal fluency following treatment with testosterone. These data suggest that testosterone may enhance verbal fluency in hypogonadal men and support the general hypothesis that current levels of testosterone may influence some aspects of cognitive function.

Algarte-Genin M et al. Prevention of Prostate Cancer by Androgens: Experimental paradox or clinical reality? European Urology 46 (Sept 2004) 285-295 Androgen replacement therapy in the aging male with partial androgen deficiency improved quality of life. However, such treatment is prohibited for men with a preexisting prostate cancer. The possibility of an increased risk of prostate cancer for healthy men has also been suggested on theoretical basis but recent experimental data showed that androgens may act in prevention of prostate cancer. In this review, we try to evaluate benefits and risks associated to a hormonal replacement therapy in regard to recent data. Several studies analyzing the role of testosterone for prostatic epithelial cells evidenced that testosterone acts in prostatic cell differentiation but does not have a direct role for induction of cell proliferation. Moreover, clinical studies have shown that low free testosterone levels in serum is associated with aggressive prostate cancer, like that has been observed in men with prostate cancer under prostate cancer chemoprevention by finasteride. These data suggest that an androgen pathway disruption in prostate is responsible of cell deregulations that may be associated not only with apoptosis of differentiated prostatic cells but also with potential cell transformation. The effects of androgens withdrawal for prostate cancer therapy induced in a short time the tumor arrest growth. However with time, cells adapt to low levels of androgens leading to the evolution of an androgen-independent tumor, which is more aggressive and most often fatal. The molecular mechanisms of this evolution begin to merge. A hypothesis is that such mechanisms could be initiated in elderly men with an androgen deficiency. The question is raised of whether hormonal replacement therapy could prevent prostate cancer. An encouraging recent study performed on rats demonstrated a protective effect of DHEA for prostate cancer. However, the putative role of the normalization of DHEA or other androgen levels in prevention of prostate cancer should be evaluated in clinical trials.

Araujo Ab et al Prevalence and incidence of androgen deficiency in middle-aged and older men: estimates from the Massachusetts Male Aging Study. J Clinical Endocrinol Metabolism 2004 Dec; 89(12):5920-6. Little is known about the descriptive epidemiology of androgen deficiency. In this study, we sought to address this issue by providing estimates of the crude and age-specific prevalence and incidence rates of androgen deficiency in a randomly sampled population-based cohort of middle-aged and older men. Data on androgen deficiency (defined using both signs/symptoms plus total and calculated free testosterone) were available for n = 1691 (baseline) and n = 1087 (follow-up) men from the Massachusetts Male Aging Study. Crude and age-specific prevalence and incidence rates were calculated. Based on these estimates, projections for the number of cases of androgen deficiency in the 40- to 69-yr-old U.S. male population were computed. Estimates of the crude prevalence of androgen deficiency at baseline and follow-up were 6.0 and 12.3%, respectively. Prevalence increased significantly with age. From baseline age-specific prevalence data, it is estimated that there are approximately 2.4 million 40- to 69-yr-old U.S. males with androgen deficiency. The crude incidence rate of androgen deficiency was 12.3 per 1,000 person-years, and the rate increased significantly (P < 0.0001) with age. Based on these incidence data, we can expect approximately 481,000 new cases of androgen deficiency per year in U.S. men 40-69 yr old.

Arnlov J et al. Endogenous sex hormones and cardiovascular disease incidence in men. Ann Intern Med. 2006 Aug 1; 145(3):176-84 BACKGROUND: Data suggest that endogenous sex hormones (testosterone, dehydroepiandrosterone sulfate [DHEA-S], and estradiol) influence cardiovascular disease (CVD) risk factors and vascular function. Yet, prospective studies relating sex hormones to CVD incidence in men have yielded inconsistent results. OBJECTIVE: To examine the association of circulating sex hormone levels and CVD risk in men. DESIGN: Prospective cohort study. SETTING: Community-based study in Framingham, Massachusetts. PARTICIPANTS: 2084 middle-aged white men without CVD at baseline. MEASUREMENTS: The authors used multivariable Cox regression to relate baseline levels of testosterone, DHEA-S, and estradiol to the incidence of CVD (coronary, cerebrovascular, or peripheral vascular disease or heart failure) during 10 years of follow-up. RESULTS: During follow-up, 386 men (18.5%) experienced a first CVD event. After adjustment for baseline standard CVD risk factors, higher estradiol level was associated with lower risk for CVD (hazard ratio per SD increment in log estradiol, 0.90 [95% CI, 0.82 to 0.99]; P = 0.035). The authors observed effect modification by age: Higher estradiol levels were associated with lower CVD risk in older (median age >56 years) men (hazard ratio per SD increment, 0.86 [CI, 0.78 to 0.96]; P = 0.005) but not in younger (median age < or =56 years) men (hazard ratio per SD increment, 1.11 [CI, 0.89 to 1.38]; P = 0.36). The association of higher estradiol level with lower CVD incidence remained robust in time-dependent

Cox models (updating standard CVD risk factors during follow-up). Serum testosterone and DHEA-S levels were not statistically significantly associated with incident CVD. LIMITATIONS: Sex hormone levels were measured only at baseline, and the findings may not be generalizable to women and nonwhite people. CONCLUSIONS: In the community-based sample, a higher serum estradiol level was associated with lower risk for CVD events in older men. The findings are consistent with the hypothesis that endogenous estrogen has vasculoprotective influences in men.

Barrett-Connor E et al. Endogenous sex hormones and cognitive function in older men. J Clin Endocrinol Metab 1999 Oct; 84(10):3681-5 the objective of this study was to determine whether endogenous sex hormone levels predict cognitive functions in older men. Our study design was an exploratory analysis in a population-based cohort in Rancho Bernardo, California. The study participants were 547 community-dwelling men 59-89 yr of age at baseline who were not using testosterone or estrogen therapy. Between 1984 and 1987, sera were collected for measurement of endogenous total and bioavailable testosterone and estradiol levels. Between 1988 and 1991, 12 standard neuropsychological instruments were administered, including two items from the Blessed Information-Memory-Concentration (BIMC) Test, three measures of retrieval from the Buschke-Fuld Selective Reminding Test, a category fluency test, immediate and delayed recall from the Visual Reproduction Test, the Mini-Mental State Examination with individual analysis of the Serial Sevens and the "World" Backwards components, and the Trail-Making Test Part B. In age- and education-adjusted analyses, men with higher levels of total and bioavailable estradiol had poorer scores on the BIMC Test and Mini-Mental State Examination. Men with higher levels of bioavailable testosterone had better scores on the BIMC Test and the Selective Reminding Test (long-term storage). Five associations were U-shaped: total testosterone and total and bioavailable estradiol with the BIMC Test; bioavailable testosterone with the "World" test; and total estradiol with the Trail-Making Test. All associations were relatively weak but independent of age, education, body mass index, alcohol use, cigarette smoking and depression. In these older men, low estradiol and high testosterone levels predicted better performance on several tests of cognitive function. Linear and nonlinear associations were also found, suggesting that an optimal level of sex hormones may exist for some cognitive functions.

Basaria et al. November 2001 Anabolic-Androgenic Steroid Therapy in the Treatment of Chronic Diseases. The Journal of Clinical Endocrinology & Metabolism Vol. 86, No. 11 5108-5117 The purpose of this study was to review the preclinical and clinical literature relevant to the efficacy and safety of anabolic androgen steroid therapy for palliative treatment of severe weight loss associated with chronic diseases. Data sources were published literature identified from the Medline database from January 1966 to December 2000, bibliographic references, and textbooks. Reports from preclinical and clinical trials were selected. Study designs and results were extracted from trial reports. Statistical evaluation or meta-analysis of combined results was not attempted. Androgenic anabolic steroids (AAS) are widely prescribed for the treatment of male hypogonadism; however, they may play a significant role in the treatment of other conditions as well, such as cachexia associated with human immunodeficiency virus, cancer, burns, renal and hepatic failure, and anemia associated with leukemia or kidney failure. A review of the anabolic effects of androgens and their efficacy in the treatment of these conditions is provided. In addition, the numerous and sometimes serious side effects that have been known to occur with androgen use are reviewed. Although the threat of various side effects is present, AAS therapy appears to have a favorable anabolic effect on patients with chronic diseases and muscle catabolism. We recommend that AAS can be used for the treatment of patients with acquired immunodeficiency syndrome wasting and in severely catabolic patients with severe burns. Preliminary data in renal failure-associated wasting are also positive. Advantages and disadvantages should be weighed carefully when comparing AAS therapy to other weight-gaining measures. Although a conservative approach to the use of AAS in patients with chronic diseases is still recommended, the utility of AAS therapy in the attenuation of severe weight loss associated with disease states such as cancer, postoperative recovery, and wasting due to pulmonary and hepatic disease should be more thoroughly investigated.

Bhasin S. et al. Testosterone replacement increases fat-free mass and muscle size in hypogonadal men. J Clin Endocrinol Metab. 1997 Feb; 82(2):407-13. Testosterone-induced nitrogen retention in castrated male animals and sex-related differences in the size of the muscles in male and female animals have been cited as evidence that testosterone has anabolic effects. However, the effects of testosterone on body composition and muscle size have not been rigorously studied. The objective of this study was to determine the effects of replacement doses of testosterone on fat-free mass and muscle size in healthy hypogonadal men in the setting of controlled nutritional intake and exercise level. Seven hypogonadal men, 19-47 yr of age, after at least a 12-week washout from previous androgen therapy, were treated for 10 weeks with testosterone enanthate (100 mg/week) by im injections. Body weight, fat-free mass measured by underwater weighing and deuterated water dilution, and muscle size measured by magnetic resonance imaging were assessed before and after treatment. Energy and protein intake were standardized at 35 Cal/kg.day and 1.5 g/kg.day, respectively. Body weight increased significantly from 79.2 +/- 5.6 to 83.7 +/- 5.7 kg after 10 weeks of testosterone replacement therapy (weight gain, 4.5 +/- 0.6 kg; P = 0.0064). Fat-free mass, measured by underwater weighing, increased from 56.0 +/- 2.5 to 60.9 +/- 2.2 kg (change, +5.0 +/- 0.7 kg; P = 0.0004), but percent fat did not significantly change. Similar increases in fat-free mass were observed with the deuterated water method. The cross-sectional area of the triceps arm muscle increased from 2421 +/- 317 to 2721 +/- 239 mm2 (P = 0.045), and that of the quadriceps leg muscle increased from 7173 +/- 464 to 7720 +/- 454 mm2 (P = 0.0427), measured by magnetic resonance imaging. Muscle strength, assessed by one repetition maximum of weight-lifting exercises increased significantly after testosterone treatment. L-[1-13C] Leucine turnover, leucine oxidation, and nonoxidative disappearance of leucine did not significantly change after 10 weeks of treatment. There was no significant change in hemoglobin, hematocrit, creatinine, and transaminase levels. Replacement doses of testosterone increase fat-free mass and muscle size and strength in hypogonadal men. Whether androgen replacement in wasting states characterized by low testosterone levels will have similar anabolic effects remains to be studied.

Bhasin S. The dose-dependent effects of testosterone on sexual function and on muscle mass and function. Mayo Clin Proc. 2000 Jan; 75 Suppl: S70-5 Testosterone dose-response relationships are central to the issue of testosterone replacement therapy, within the context of both hypogonadal men and older men with declining testosterone levels. Dosages are also important when considering anabolic applications of testosterone for treating sarcopenia associated with chronic illness. The critical issue is whether increases in muscle mass and function can be achieved with dosages that will not adversely affect lipid profile, cardiovascular risk, and the prostate. The dose-response relationship and mechanisms of androgen action on the muscle for controlling it are being investigated.

Bhasin S et al. Testosterone therapy in adult men with androgen deficiency syndromes: an endocrine society clinical practice guideline. J Clin Endocrinol Metab. 2006 Jun; 91(6):1995-2010. OBJECTIVE: The objective was to provide guidelines for the evaluation and treatment of androgen deficiency syndromes in adult men. PARTICIPANTS: The Task Force was composed of a chair, selected by the Clinical Guidelines Subcommittee of The Endocrine Society, five additional experts, a methodologist, and a professional writer. The Task Force received no corporate funding or remuneration. EVIDENCE: The Task Force used systematic reviews of available evidence to inform its key recommendations. The Task Force used consistent language and graphical descriptions of both the strength of recommendation and the quality of evidence, using the recommendations of the Grading of Recommendations, Assessment, Development, and Evaluation group. CONSENSUS PROCESS: Consensus was guided by systematic reviews of evidence and discussions during three group meetings, several conference calls, and e-mail communications. The drafts prepared by the panelists with the help of a professional writer were reviewed successively by The Endocrine Society's Clinical Guidelines Subcommittee, Clinical Affairs Committee, and Council. The version approved by the Council was placed on The Endocrine Society's web site for comments by members. At each stage of review, the Task Force received written comments and incorporated needed changes. CONCLUSIONS: We recommend making a diagnosis of androgen deficiency only in men with consistent symptoms and signs and unequivocally low serum testosterone levels. We suggest the measurement of morning total testosterone level by a reliable assay as the initial diagnostic test. We recommend confirmation of the diagnosis by repeating the measurement of morning total testosterone and in some patients by measurement of free or bioavailable testosterone level, using accurate assays. We recommend testosterone therapy for symptomatic men with androgen deficiency, which have low testosterone levels, to induce and maintain secondary sex characteristics and to improve their sexual function, sense of well-being, muscle mass and strength, and bone mineral density. We recommend against starting testosterone therapy in patients with breast or prostate cancer, a palpable prostate nodule or induration or prostate-specific antigen greater than 3 ng/ml without further urological evaluation, erythrocytosis (hematocrit > 50%), hyperviscosity, untreated obstructive sleep apnea, severe lower urinary tract symptoms with International Prostate Symptom Score (IPSS) greater than 19, or class III or IV heart failure. When testosterone therapy is instituted, we suggest aiming at achieving testosterone levels during treatment in the mid-normal range with any of the approved formulations, chosen on the basis of the patient's preference, consideration of pharmacokinetics, treatment burden, and cost. Men receiving testosterone therapy should be monitored using a standardized plan.

Boyanov MA et al. Testosterone supplementation in men with type 2 diabetes, visceral obesity and partial androgen deficiency. Aging Male. 2003 Mar;6(1):1-7. The objective of this study was to assess the effects of oral testosterone supplementation therapy on glucose homeostasis, obesity and sexual function in middle-aged men with type 2 diabetes and mild androgen deficiency. Forty-eight middle-aged men, with type 2 diabetes, (visceral) obesity and symptoms of androgen deficiency, were included in this open-label study. Twenty-four subjects received testosterone undecanoate (TU; 120 mg daily, for 3 months); 24 subjects received no treatment. Body composition was analyzed by bio-impedance. Parameters of metabolic control were determined. Symptoms of androgen deficiency and erectile dysfunction were scored by self-administered questionnaires. TU had a positive effect on (visceral) obesity: statistically significant reduction in body weight (2.66%), waist-hip ratio (-3.96%) and body fat (-5.65%); negligible changes were found in the control group. TU significantly improved metabolic control: decrease in blood glucose values and mean glycated hemoglobin (HbA1c) (from 10.4 to 8.6%). TU treatment significantly improved symptoms of androgen deficiency (including erectile dysfunction), with virtually no change in the control group. There were no adverse effects on blood pressure or hematological, biochemical and lipid parameters, and no adverse events. Oral TU treatment of type 2 diabetic men with androgen deficiency improves glucose homeostasis and body composition (decrease in visceral obesity), and improves symptoms of androgen deficiency (including erectile dysfunction). In these men, the benefit of testosterone supplementation therapy exceeds the correction of symptoms of androgen deficiency and also includes glucose homeostasis and metabolic control.

Burris A et al. A long-term, prospective study of the physiologic and behavioral effects of hormone replacement in untreated hypogonadal men. J Androl 1992 Jul-Aug;13(4):297-304 This study describes sexual activity, nocturnal penile erections, and mood states as a function of serum levels of androgens in previously untreated hypogonadal men before and during hormone replacement, selected infertile men (elevated serum follicle-stimulating hormone levels), and normal men. Nocturnal penile tumescence and rigidity were measured with a portable monitor, and sexual activity and mood were assessed by prospective, self-reported written forms. Nocturnal erections were absent or of very low amplitude and duration in the untreated hypogonadal men compared to the infertile and normal men. Nocturnal erections increased steadily during hormone replacement and were in the normal range within 6 to 12 months of treatment. In contrast, serum testosterone concentration rapidly reached the upper range of normal. During treatment, the hypogonadal men reported increases in several aspects of sexual activity, including sexual interest and the number of spontaneous erections. On mood inventories, the untreated hypogonadal men scored significantly higher in ratings of depression, anger, fatigue, and confusion than did infertile and normal men. During hormonal replacement therapy these scores decreased, although the hypogonadal men continued to score higher in "depression" than did infertile and normal men. In most instances, the men with infertility and the normal men were statistically indistinguishable in nocturnal penile tumescence and rigidity parameters, self-reported sexual activity, and mood state. These data support the hypothesis that androgen treatment increases nocturnal and spontaneous erections, and sexual interest, and has some capacity to improve mood.

Caminiti G et al. Effect of long-acting testosterone treatment on functional exercise capacity, skeletal muscle performance, insulin resistance, and baroreflex sensitivity in elderly patients with chronic heart failure a double-blind, placebo-controlled, randomized study. J Am Coll Cardiol. 2009 Sep 1;54(10):919-27 OBJECTIVES: This study investigated the effect of a 12-week long-acting testosterone administration on maximal exercise capacity, ventilatory efficiency, muscle strength, insulin resistance, and baroreflex sensitivity (BRS) in elderly patients with chronic heart failure (CHF).BACKGROUND: CHF is characterized by a metabolic shift favoring catabolism and impairment in skeletal muscle bulk and function that could be involved in the pathophysiology of heart failure.METHODS: Seventy elderly patients with stable CHF-median age 70 years, ejection fraction 31.8 +/- 7%-were randomly assigned to receive testosterone (n = 35, intramuscular injection every 6 weeks) or placebo (n = 35), both on top of optimal medical therapy. At baseline and at the end of the study, all patients underwent echocardiogram, cardiopulmonary exercise test, 6-min walk test (6MWT), quadriceps maximal voluntary contraction (MVC), and isokinetic strength (peak torque) and BRS assessment (sequences technique).RESULTS: Baseline peak oxygen consumption (VO(2)) and quadriceps isometric strength showed a direct relation with serum testosterone concentration. Peak VO (2) significantly improved in testosterone but was unchanged in placebo. Insulin sensitivity was significantly improved in testosterone. The MVC and peak torque significantly increased in testosterone but not in placebo. The BRS significantly improved in testosterone but not in placebo. Increase in testosterone levels was significantly related to improvement in peak VO (2) and MVC. There were no significant changes in left ventricular function either in testosterone or placebo.CONCLUSIONS: These results suggest that long-acting testosterone therapy improves exercise capacity, muscle strength, glucose metabolism, and BRS in men with moderately severe CHF. Testosterone benefits seem to be mediated by metabolic and peripheral effects.

Caretta N et al. Erectile dysfunction in aging men: testosterone role in therapeutic protocols. J Endocrinol Invest. 2005; 28 (11 Suppl Proceedings):108-11 Aging in men is accompanied by a decrease in libido and sexual activity. Recently, it has been demonstrated that a significant proportion of men >60 yr of age has biochemical hypogonadism. Hypoandrogenism, which is associated with other conditions that negatively influence erectile activity, may be an important cofactor in the induction of erectile dysfunction and in the response to phosphodiesterase type 5 (PDE5) inhibitors in aging. In these patients, administration of 50 mg sildenafil or 3 mg apomorphine has no influence on erectile function. Recently we showed that, in hypogonadal subjects, testosterone treatment might stimulate endothelial and neuronal production of vasoactive substances like nitric oxide (NO). Furthermore it can improve endothelial repair mechanisms by increasing bone marrow-derived endothelial progenitor cell (EPC) number in the peripheral circulation. Finally, the normal response to pharmacological stimulation with apomorphine or sildenafil, observed in hypogonadal men treated with testosterone, indicates a positive role of this hormone in the central and peripheral control of erection, confirming the possible positive influence on endothelial function and PDE5 expression. Therefore, we suggest measuring plasma testosterone levels in aged men with erectile dysfunction and recommend treating those barring clinical contraindications. Testosterone plus PDE5 inhibitors may be beneficial in improving erectile function in hypogonadal men with erectile dysfunction who were unresponsive to PDE5 inhibitors alone.

Cassidenti D et al. Effects of sex steroids on skin 5 alpha-reductase activity in vitro Obstetrics & Gynecology 1991; 78:103-107 Skin 5 alpha-reductase activity is the major factor influencing the manifestation of androgen excess. Although oral contraceptives have been useful for the treatment of androgen excess, little is known of the independent effects of the various progestins and estrogens on inhibition of skin 5 alpha-reductase activity. We incubated minces of normal genital and pubic skin with physiologic concentrations of 3H-testosterone to assess 5 alpha-reductase activity by its conversion to 3H-dihydrotestosterone. In separate experiments, 5 alpha-reductase activity was assessed before and after the addition of progesterone, medroxyprogesterone acetate, levonorgestrel, norethindrone, 17 beta-estradiol, and ethinyl estradiol. Progesterone, levonorgestrel, and norethindrone demonstrated 97 +/- 5.3%, 47.9 +/- 6.3%, and 59 +/- 4.6% inhibition, respectively, of genital skin 5 alpha-reductase activity at 10(-4) mol/L (P less than .01). Medroxyprogesterone acetate, however, failed to affect 5 alpha-reductase activity at similar doses. Estradiol exhibited 40.8 +/- 14.2% inhibition at 10(-4) mol/L (P less than .01), whereas ethinyl estradiol at concentrations from 10(-8) to 10(-4) mol/L failed to inhibit 5 alpha-reductase activity. We conclude that progesterone and the 19-nor-derivatives inhibit 5 alpha-reductase activity at high doses, whereas medroxyprogesterone acetate does not. Therefore, the 19-nor-progestin component may expand the usefulness of oral contraceptives in the treatment of hirsutism by an inhibitory action on skin 5 alpha-reductase activity.

Channer KS, Jones TH Cardiovascular effects of testosterone: implications of the "male menopause"? Heart. 2003 Feb; 89(2):121-2. A relatively low blood concentration of testosterone in the older man may have adverse effects on atherosclerosis, and explain the higher incidence of coronary heart disease in the male.

Chen C et al. Cancer Epidemiol Biomarkers Prev. Endogenous sex hormones and prostate cancer risk: a case-control study nested within the Carotene and Retinol Efficacy Trial. 2003 Dec; 12(12):1410-6. To examine whether endogenous androgens influence the occurrence of prostate cancer, we conducted a nested case-control study among participants enrolled in the Carotene and Retinol Efficacy Trial. We analyzed serum samples of 300 cases diagnosed between 1987 and 1998, and 300 matched controls. Higher concentrations of testosterone (T) were not associated with increased prostate cancer risk. Relative to men with levels in the lowest fourth of the distribution, men in the upper fourth of total T had a risk of 0.82 [95% confidence interval (CI), 0.52-1.29]. The corresponding relative risks for free T (0.72; 95% CI, 0.45-1.14), percentage of free T (0.74; 95% CI, 0.46-1.19), and total T: sex hormone binding globulin ratio (0.52; 95% CI, 0.32-0.83) similarly were not elevated. Higher concentrations of androstenedione, dehydroepiandrosterone sulfate, and 3 alpha-androstanediol glucuronide were weakly associated with risk. Relative risks associated with being in the highest fourth for androstenedione, dehydroepiandrosterone sulfate, and 3 alpha-androstanediol glucuronide were 1.20 (95% CI, 0.76-1.89), 1.38 (95% CI, 0.86-2.21), and 1.27 (95% CI, 0.80-2.00), respectively. Men in the upper fourth of total estradiol (E2), free E2 and percentage of free E2 had relative risks of 0.71 (95% CI, 0.42-1.13), 0.52 (95% CI, 0.33-0.82), and 0.65 (95% CI, 0.40-1.05), respectively. The inverse association between E2 and prostate cancer risk was largely restricted to men with blood collection within 3 years of diagnosis. Our results add to the evidence that serum testosterone is unrelated to prostate cancer incidence. The suggestions that intraprostatic androgen activity may increase risk and that serum estrogens may decrease risk, warrant additional study.

Cooper CS et al. Effect of exogenous testosterone on prostate volume, serum and semen prostate specific antigen levels in healthy young men J Urol 1998 Feb; 159(2):441-3 PURPOSE: We investigate and define the effects of exogenous testosterone on the normal prostate. MATERIALS AND METHODS: A total of 31 healthy volunteers 21 to 39 years old were randomized to receive either 100, 250 or 500 mg. testosterone via intramuscular injection once a week for 15 weeks. Baseline measurements of serum testosterone, free testosterone and prostate specific antigen (PSA) were taken at week 1. Semen samples were also collected for PSA content and prostate volumes were determined by transrectal ultrasound before testosterone injection. Blood was then drawn every other week before each testosterone injection for the 15 weeks, every other week thereafter until week 28 and again at week 40. After the first 15 weeks semen samples were again collected and prostate volumes were determined by repeat transrectal ultrasound. RESULTS: Free and total serum testosterone levels increased significantly in the 250 and 500 mg. dose groups. No significant change occurred in the prostate volume or serum PSA levels at any dose of exogenous testosterone. Total semen PSA levels decreased following administration of testosterone but did not reach statistical significance. CONCLUSIONS: Despite significant elevations in serum total and free testosterone, healthy young men do not demonstrate increased serum or semen PSA levels, or increased prostate volume in response to exogenous testosterone injections.

Daniell HW et al. Hypogonadism in men consuming sustained-action oral opioids. J Pain. 2002 Oct; 3(5):377-84. Naturally occurring opiates (endorphins) diminish testosterone levels by inhibiting both hypothalamic gonadotrophin releasing hormone production and testicular testosterone synthesis. Heroin addicts treated with a single daily dose of methadone and nonaddicts receiving continuous intrathecal opioids quickly develop low luteinizing hormone and total testosterone levels. A similar pattern was sought in men consuming commonly prescribed oral opioids. Free testosterone (FT), total testosterone (TT), estradiol (E(2)), dihydrotestosterone (DHT), luteinizing hormone (LH), and follicle-stimulating hormone (FSH) were measured in 54 community-dwelling outpatient men consuming oral sustained-action dosage forms of opioids several times daily for control of nonmalignant pain. Hormone levels were related to the opioid consumed, dosage and dosage form, nonopioid medication use, and several personal characteristics and were compared with the hormone analyses of 27 similar men consuming no opioids. Hormone levels averaged much lower in opioid users than in control subjects in a dose-related pattern (P < .0001 for all comparisons). FT, TT, and E (2) levels were subnormal in 56%, 74%, and 74%, respectively, of opioid consumers. Forty-eight men (89%) exhibited subnormal levels of either FT or E (2). Either TT or E (2) level was subnormal in all 28 men consuming the equivalent of 100 mg of methadone daily and in 19 of 26 (73%) consuming smaller opioid doses. Eighty-seven percent (39 of 45) of opioid-ingesting men who reported normal erectile function before opioid use reported severe erectile dysfunction or diminished libido after beginning their opioid therapy. Commonly prescribed opioids in sustained-action dosage forms usually produce subnormal sex hormone levels, which may contribute to a diminished quality of life for many patients with painful chronic illness.

Dimitrakakis C et al. Breast cancer incidence in women using testosterone in addition to usual hormone therapy. Menopause 11 (5) 2004 OBJECTIVE: There is now convincing evidence that usual hormone therapy for ovarian failure increases the risk for breast cancer. We have previously shown that ovarian androgens normally protect mammary epithelial cells from excessive estrogenic stimulation, and therefore we hypothesized that the addition of testosterone to usual hormone therapy might protect women from breast cancer. DESIGN: This was a retrospective, observational study that followed 508 postmenopausal women receiving testosterone in addition to usual hormone therapy in South Australia. Breast cancer status was ascertained by mammography at the initiation of testosterone treatment and biannually thereafter. The average age at the start of follow-up was 56.4 years, and the mean duration of follow-up was 5.8 years. Breast cancer incidence in this group was compared with that of untreated women and women using usual hormone therapy reported in the medical literature and to age-specific local population rates. RESULTS: There were seven cases of invasive breast cancer in this population of testosterone users, for an incidence of 238 per 100,000 woman-years. The rate for estrogen/progestin and testosterone users was 293 per 100,000 woman-years--substantially less than women receiving estrogen/pro-gestin in the Women's Health Initiative study (380 per 100,000 woman-years) or in the "Million Women" Study (521 per 100,000 woman-years). The breast cancer rate in our testosterone users was closest to that reported for hormone therapy never-users in the latter study (283 per 100,000 woman-years), and their age-standardized rate was the same as for the general population in South Australia. CONCLUSIONS: These observations suggest that the addition of testosterone to conventional hormone therapy for postmenopausal women does not increase and may indeed reduce the hormone therapy-associated breast cancer risk-thereby returning the incidence to the normal rates observed in the general, untreated population.

Edinger KL et al. Testosterone's anti-anxiety and analgesic effects may be due in part to actions of its 5alpha-reduced metabolites in the hippocampus. Psychoneuroendocrinology. 2005 Jun; 30(5):418-30 Although testosterone (T) may have effects to enhance analgesia and reduce anxiety, its effects and mechanisms are not well understood. We hypothesized that if T's anti-anxiety and analgesic effects are due in part to actions of its 5alpha-reduced metabolite (dihydrotestosterone-DHT) and/or its 3alpha-hydroxysteroid dehydrogenase reduced metabolite (3alpha-androstanediol-3alpha-diol), in the hippocampus, then androgen regimens that increase levels of these metabolites in the hippocampus should produce anti-anxiety behavior, and analgesic effects, in gonadectomized (GDX) male rats. In Experiment 1, GDX rats were administered T, DHT, 3alpha-diol (1 mg/kg, SC), or vehicle. In Experiment 2, GDX rats had T, DHT, 3alpha-diol-containing inserts, or empty control inserts applied to the dorsal hippocampus immediately prior to behavioral testing. Androgen-administered rats (SC or intrahippocampal) showed significantly more exploratory behavior in the open field and elevated plus maze, less freezing in response to shock, and longer tailflick and pawlick latencies. These findings suggest that T's anti-anxiety effects may be due in part to actions of its 5alpha-reduced metabolites in the dorsal hippocampus.

El-Sakka AI et al. Prostatic specific antigen in patients with hypogonadism: effect of testosterone replacement. J Sex Med. 2005 Mar; 2(2):235-40, INTRODUCTION: The effect of parenteral testosterone replacement therapy on prostatic specific antigen (PSA) level or the development or growth of prostate cancer is unclear. AIM: To assess the effect of testosterone replacement on PSA level in patients with hypogonadism associated with erectile dysfunction (ED). METHODS: A total of 187 male patients above the age of 45 with hypogonadism associated with ED were enrolled in this study. Patients were screened for ED by the erectile function domain of the International Index of Erectile Function (IIEF). Patients underwent routine laboratory investigations, plus total testosterone, and PSA assessment. Replacement treatment with parenteral testosterone every 2-4 weeks for 1 year was instituted. Total testosterone and PSA serum levels were assessed every 3 months during the treatment course. RESULTS: Mean age +/- SD was 62.8 +/- 11.4. Of the patients 87.7% were sexually active. Of the patients 10.2% had mild, 40.6% had moderate and 49.2% had severe ED. Of the study population, 62.5% had ED complaints for less than 5 years and 84.5% had gradual onset of their complaint. The majority of the patients (91.4%) had either progressive or stationary course while the minority reported regressive course and improvement of the condition. There was a significant increase of the post-treatment testosterone level in comparison to pretreatment level (P < 0.05). No significant increase in the post-treatment PSA level in comparison to pretreatment (P > 0.05). No significant difference between pre- and post-treatment categories of PSA level (normal, borderline, high) in relation to the severity of ED (P > 0.05). There was no significant association between PSA level and the duration of testosterone replacement therapy in the study population (P > 0.05). CONCLUSION: The current study demonstrated that the level of PSA was not significantly changed after 1 year of testosterone replacement therapy in patients with hypogonadism associated with ED.

Endogenous Sex Hormones and Prostate Cancer: A Collaborative Analysis of 18 Prospective Studies Endogenous Hormones and Prostate Cancer Collaborative Group. J Natl Cancer Inst 2008 100: 170-183 BACKGROUND: Sex hormones in serum have been hypothesized to influence the risk of prostate cancer. We performed a collaborative analysis of the existing worldwide epidemiologic data to examine these associations in a uniform manner and to provide more precise estimates of risks.METHODS: Data on serum concentrations of sex hormones from 18 prospective studies that included 3886 men with incident prostate cancer and 6438 control subjects were pooled by the Endogenous Hormones and Prostate Cancer Collaborative Group. Relative risks (RRs) of prostate cancer by fifths of serum hormone concentration were estimated by use of conditional logistic regression with stratification by study, age at recruitment, and year of recruitment. All statistical tests were two-sided.RESULTS: No associations were found between the risk of prostate cancer and serum concentrations of testosterone, calculated free testosterone, dihydrotestosterone, dehydroepiandrosterone sulfate, androstenedione, androstanediol glucuronide, estradiol, or calculated free estradiol. The serum concentration of sex hormone-binding globulin was modestly inversely associated with prostate cancer risk (RR in the highest vs lowest fifth = 0.86, 95% confidence interval = 0.75 to 0.98; P (trend) = .01). There was no statistical evidence of heterogeneity among studies, and adjustment for potential confounders made little difference to the risk estimates.CONCLUSIONS: In this collaborative analysis of the worldwide data on endogenous hormones and prostate cancer risk, serum concentrations of sex hormones were not associated with the risk of prostate cancer.

English KM et al. Low-dose transdermal testosterone therapy improves angina threshold in men with chronic stable angina: A randomized, double-blind, placebo-controlled study. Circulation 2000 Oct 17; 102(16):1906-11 BACKGROUND: Experimental studies suggest that androgens induce coronary vasodilatation. We performed this pilot project to examine the clinical effects of long-term low-dose androgens in men with angina. METHODS AND RESULTS: Forty-six men with stable angina completed a 2-week, single-blind placebo run-in, followed by double-blind randomization to 5 mg testosterone daily by transdermal patch or matching placebo for 12 weeks, in addition to their current medication. Time to 1-mm ST-segment depression on treadmill exercise testing and hormone levels were measured and quality of life was assessed by SF-36 at baseline and after 4 and 12 weeks of treatment. Active treatment resulted in a 2-fold increase in androgen levels and an increase in time to 1-mm ST-segment depression from (mean+/-SEM) 309+/-27 seconds at baseline to 343+/-26 seconds after 4 weeks and to 361+/-22 seconds after 12 weeks. This change was statistically significant compared with that seen in the placebo group (from 266+/-25 seconds at baseline to 284+/-23 seconds after 4 weeks and to 292+/-24 seconds after 12 weeks; P:=0.02 between the 2 groups by ANCOVA). The magnitude of the response was greater in those with lower baseline levels of bioavailable testosterone (r=-0. 455, P :< 0.05). There were no significant changes in prostate specific antigen, hemoglobin, lipids, or coagulation profiles during the study. There were significant improvements in pain perception (P: =0.026) and role limitation resulting from physical problems (P: =0.024) in the testosterone-treated group. CONCLUSIONS: Low-dose supplemental testosterone treatment in men with chronic stable angina reduces exercise-induced myocardial ischemia.

Fink B et al. The 2nd-4th digit ratio (2D:4D) and neck circumference: implications for risk factors in coronary heart disease. Int J Obes (Lond). 2006 Apr; 30(4):711-4. BACKGROUND: The ratio of the lengths of the 2nd and 4th digit (2D:4D) is negatively related to prenatal and adult concentrations of testosterone (T). Testosterone appears to be a protective against myocardial infarction (MI) in men as men with low 2D:4D are older at first MI than men with high 2D:4D and men with coronary artery disease have lower T levels than men with normal angiograms. Neck circumference (NC), a simple and time-saving screening measure to identify obesity is reported to be positively correlated with the factors of the metabolic syndrome, a complex breakdown of normal physiology characterized by obesity, insulin resistance, hyperlipidemia, and hypertension, and is therefore likely to increase the risk of coronary heart disease (CHD). OBJECTIVE: To investigate possible associations between 2D:4D ratios and NC in men and women. RESEARCH METHODS AND PROCEDURES: 2D:4D ratios, NC, along with measures of waist and hip circumferences, body mass index (BMI), and waist-to-hip ratio was recorded from 127 men and 117 women. RESULTS: A significant positive correlation between 2D:4D and NC and was found for men but not for women after controlling for body mass index (BMI); the higher the ratio the higher the NC. DISCUSSION: This finding supports the suggestion of NC to serve as a predictor for increased risk for CHD as previously suggested. In addition, the present association suggests a predisposition for men towards CHD via 2D:4D as proxy to early sex-steroid exposure.

Foresta C et al. Reduced Number of Circulating Endothelial Progenitor Cells in Hypogonadal Men. Journal of Clinical Endocrinology & Metabolism 91(11):4599–4602 CONTEXT: Endothelial dysfunction seems to be the first step of the atherosclerotic process. In the past few years, it has been demonstrated that injured endothelial monolayer is restored by a premature pool of circulating progenitor cells (PCs) and a more mature one of circulating endothelial PCs (EPCs). Even though there is increasing evidence that estrogens play a beneficial role on EPCs and, even if debated, on the cardiovascular system, less is known about androgens.OBJECTIVE: Our objective was to evaluate the levels of circulating PCs and EPCs in men with hypogonadotropic hypogonadism (HH) and the effect of prolonged testosterone (T) replacement therapy on these cells.DESIGN AND SETTING: We conducted a prospective study on males with HH at a university andrological center.PATIENTS: The study included 10 young HH patients (28.6 +/- 3.1 yr) and 25 age-matched controls.INTERVENTIONS: Idiopathic HH patients were treated with T gel therapy, 50 mg/d for 6 months.MAIN OUTCOME MEASURES: We assessed circulating PC and EPC concentrations and immunocytochemistry for androgen receptor expression on cultured EPCs.RESULTS: At baseline, HH patients showed a significant reduction of both PCs and EPCs with respect to controls. T replacement therapy induced a significant increase of these cells with respect to baseline. Immunocytochemistry on cultured EPCs showed strong expression of the androgen receptor.CONCLUSIONS: Hypotestosteronemia is associated with a low number of circulating PCs and EPCs in young HH subjects. T treatment is able to induce an increase in these cells through a possible direct effect on the bone marrow.

Fukui, M et al. Diabetes Care 26:1869–1873, June, 2003
Association between serum testosterone concentration and carotid atherosclerosis in men with type 2 diabetes. OBJECTIVE: There is evidence to suggest that low concentrations of testosterone are associated with an increased risk of cardiovascular disease in men. The aim of this study was to evaluate the relationship between serum testosterone concentration and carotid atherosclerosis as well as major cardiovascular risk factors in men with type 2 diabetes. RESEARCH DESIGN AND METHODS: Serum free and total testosterone concentrations were measured in 253 consecutive men with type 2 diabetes. The relationships between serum testosterone concentration and carotid atherosclerosis, determined by ultrasonographically evaluated intima-media thickness (IMT) and plaque score (PS) in a subgroup of 154 diabetic patients, as well as major cardiovascular risk factors, including age, blood pressure, and lipid concentrations, were evaluated. RESULTS: Inverse correlations were found between free testosterone (F-tes) concentration and IMT (r = -0.206, P = 0.0103) and between F-tes concentration and PS (r = -0.334, P < 0.001). The IMT and PS were significantly greater in patients with lower concentrations of F-tes (<10 pg/ml) than in patients with higher concentrations of F-tes (1.01 +/- 0.29 vs. 0.91 +/- 0.26 mm, P = 0.038; 4.5 +/- 3.8 vs. 2.4 +/- 3.2, P = 0.0003; respectively). An inverse correlation was found between serum F-tes concentration and age (r = -0.420, P < 0.0001). A positive correlation was found between serum F-tes and total cholesterol concentrations (r = 0.145, P = 0.0238). CONCLUSIONS: Serum F-tes concentration is inversely associated with carotid atherosclerosis determined by ultrasonographically evaluated IMT and PS in men with type 2 diabetes. nd carotid atherosclerosis in men with type 2 diabetes.

Gould DC, Kirby RS Testosterone replacement therapy for late onset hypogonadism: what is the risk of inducing prostate cancer?Prostate Cancer Prostatic Dis. 2006;9(1):14-8 Prescription sales of testosterone have risen considerably over the last decade and are likely to continue to grow as further preparations become available. Testosterone promotes existing prostate cancer; however, concern does exist as to whether or not testosterone therapy induces prostate cancer. The aim of this article is to review the evidence for such a link.

Gouras GK et al. Proc Natl Acad Sci U S A 2000 Feb 1; 97(3):1202-5

Testosterone reduces neuronal secretion of Alzheimer's beta-amyloid peptides Alzheimer's disease (AD) is characterized by the age-related deposition of beta-amyloid (Abeta) 40/42 peptide aggregates in vulnerable brain regions. Multiple levels of evidence implicate a central role for Abeta in the pathophysiology of AD. Abeta peptides are generated by the regulated cleavage of an approximately 700-aa Abeta precursor protein (betaAPP). Full-length betaAPP can undergo proteolytic cleavage either within the Abeta domain to generate secreted sbetaAPPalpha or at the N- and C-terminal domain(s) of Abeta to generate amyloidogenic Abeta peptides. Several epidemiological studies have reported that estrogen replacement therapy protects against the development of AD in postmenopausal women. We previously reported that treating cultured neurons with 17beta-estradiol reduced the secretion of Abeta40/42 peptides, suggesting that estrogen replacement therapy may protect women against the development of AD by regulating betaAPP metabolism. Increasing evidence indicates that testosterone, especially bioavailable testosterone, decreases with age in older men and in postmenopausal women. We report here that treatment with testosterone increases the secretion of the nonamyloidogenic APP fragment, sbetaAPPalpha, and decreases the secretion of Abeta peptides from N2a cells and rat primary cerebrocortical neurons. These results raise the possibility that testosterone supplementation in elderly men may be protective in the treatment of AD.

Gunawardena, K et al. Testosterone is a potential augmentor of antioxidant induced apoptosis in human prostate cancer cells. Cancer Detect Prev. 2002; 26(2):105-13

We have investigated the effect of antioxidant-induced apoptosis in human prostate cancer cell lines that is augmented by testosterone (T). In this study, DU-145 (androgen unresponsive), ALVA-101 (partially androgen responsive), and LNCaP (androgen responsive) were grown in tissue culture with RPMI 1640 medium, 5–10% fetal bovine serum (FBS), antibiotics and 5% CO_2. Treatment with 2.5–20 μg/ml of PDTC significantly (P<0.05, n=6) lowered cell growth in all three cells 2–60% following treatment for 1–7 days. T (10−12 M) alone enhances cell growth in androgen responsive cells. In contrast, the combination of PDTC and T significantly (P<0.05, n=6) augmented the PDTC induction of apoptosis in the androgen responsive cells, (ALVA-101 and LNCaP), but not in the androgen unresponsive cells (DU-145). PDTC reduced the nuclear NF-κB, as determined with an electrophoretic mobility shift assay (EMSA), to 50% of the control in LNCaP cells, 65% in ALVA-101 cells and 45% in DU-145 cells, but the combination of PDTC and T was not more potent than

PDTC alone in any of the cell lines. PDTC suppressed both the AR mRNA and protein expression and reversed the stimulatory effect of T on androgen receptor (AR) protein synthesis in LNCaP and AVLA-101 cells. In conclusion, PDTC is a potent growth inhibitor and an inducer of apoptosis in human prostate cancer cells by reducing nuclear NF-κB and AR protein expression. PDTCs suppression of AR synthesis and nuclear NF-κB in response to T may contribute to its enhancement of apoptosis observed with T and PDTC compared to PDTC alone.

Habib FK, et al. Serenoa repens (Permixon) inhibits the 5alpha-reductase activity of human prostate cancer cell lines without interfering with PSA expression. Int J Cancer. 2005 Mar 20; 114(2):190-4. The phytotherapeutic agent Serenoa repens is an effective dual inhibitor of 5alpha-reductase isoenzyme activity in the prostate. Unlike other 5alpha-reductase inhibitors, Serenoa repens induces its effects without interfering with the cellular capacity to secrete PSA. Here, we focussed on the possible pathways that might differentiate the action of Permixon from that of synthetic 5alpha-reductase inhibitors. We demonstrate that Serenoa repens, unlike other 5alpha-reductase inhibitors, does not inhibit binding between activated AR and the steroid receptor-binding consensus in the promoter region of the PSA gene. This was shown by a combination of techniques: assessment of the effect of Permixon on androgen action in the LNCaP prostate cancer cell line revealed no suppression of AR and maintenance of PSA protein expression at control levels. This was consistent with reporter gene experiments showing that Permixon failed to interfere with AR-mediated transcriptional activation of PSA and that both testosterone and DHT were equally effective at maintaining this activity. Our results demonstrate that despite Serenoa repens effective inhibition of 5alpha-reductase activity in the prostate; it did not suppress PSA secretion. Therefore, we confirm the therapeutic advantage of Serenoa repens over other 5alpha-reductase inhibitors as treatment with the phytotherapeutic agent will permit the continuous use of PSA measurements as a useful biomarker for prostate cancer screening and for evaluating tumour progression.

Hak, Elisabeth et al. Low Levels of Endogenous Androgens Increase the Risk of Atherosclerosis in Elderly Men: The Rotterdam Study. The Journal of Clinical Endocrinology & Metabolism Vol. 87, 2002, No. 8 3632-3639 In both men and women, circulating androgen levels decline with advancing age. Until now, results of several small studies on the relationship between endogenous androgen levels and atherosclerosis have been inconsistent. In the population-based Rotterdam Study, we investigated the association of levels of dehydroepiandrosterone sulfate (DHEAS) and total and bioavailable testosterone with aortic atherosclerosis among 1,032 nonsmoking men and women aged 55 yr and over. Aortic atherosclerosis was assessed by radiographic detection of calcified deposits in the abdominal aorta, which have been shown to reflect intimal atherosclerosis. Relative to men with levels of total and bioavailable testosterone in the lowest tertile, men with levels of these hormones in the highest tertile had age-adjusted relative risks of 0.4 [95% confidence interval (CI), 0.2–0.9] and 0.2 (CI, 0.1–0.7), respectively, for the presence of severe aortic atherosclerosis. The corresponding relative risks for women were 3.7 (CI, 1.2–11.6) and 2.3 (CI, 0.7–7.8). Additional adjustment for cardiovascular disease risk factors did not materially affect the results in men, whereas in women the associations diluted. Men with levels of total and bioavailable testosterone in subsequent tertiles were also protected against progression of aortic atherosclerosis measured after 6.5 yr (SD ± 0.5 yr) of follow-up (P for trend = 0.02). No clear association between levels of DHEAS and presence of severe aortic atherosclerosis was found, either in men or in women. In men, a protective effect of higher levels of DHEAS against progression of aortic atherosclerosis was suggested, but the corresponding test for trend did not reach statistical significance. In conclusion, we found an independent inverse association between levels of testosterone and aortic atherosclerosis in men. In women, positive associations between levels of testosterone and aortic atherosclerosis were largely due to adverse cardiovascular disease risk factors.

Hatzoglou A. et al. Membrane androgen receptor activation induces apoptotic regression of human prostate cancer cells in vitro and in vivo. (Journal of Clinical Endocrinology & Metabolism 2004, 10.1210/jc.2004-0801) Nongenomic androgen actions imply mechanisms different from the classical intracellular androgen receptor (iAR) activation. We have recently reported the identification of a membrane androgen receptor (mAR) on LNCaP human prostate cancer cells, mediating testosterone signal transduction within minutes. In the present study we provide evidence that activation of mAR by nonpermeable, BSA-coupled testosterone results in 1) inhibition of LNCaP cell growth (with a 50% inhibitory concentration of 5.08 nM, similar to the affinity of testosterone for membrane sites); 2) induction in LNCaP cells of both apoptosis and the proapoptotic Fas protein; and 3) a significant decrease in migration, adhesion, and invasion of iAR-negative DU145 human prostate cancer cells. These actions persisted in the presence of antiandrogen flutamide or after decreasing the content of iAR in LNCaP cells by iAR antisense oligonucleotides. Testosterone-BSA was also effective in inducing apoptosis of DU145 human prostate cancer cells, negative for iAR, but expressing mAR sites. In LNCaP cell-inoculated nude mice, treatment with testosterone-BSA (4.8 mg/kg body weight) for 1 month resulted in a 60% reduction of tumor size compared with that in control animals receiving only BSA, an effect that was not affected by the antiandrogen flutamide. Our findings suggest that activators of mAR may represent a new class of antitumoral agents of prostate cancer.

Hau M et al. Testosterone reduces responsiveness to nociceptive stimuli in a wild bird. Horm Behav. 2004 Aug;

46(2):165-70. The hormone testosterone (T) is involved in the control of aggressive behavior in male vertebrates. T enhances the frequency and intensity of aggressive behaviors during competitive interactions among males. By promoting high-intensity aggression, T also increases the risk of injury and presumably the perception of painful stimuli. However, perception of painful stimuli during fights could counteract the expression of further aggressive behavior. We therefore hypothesize that one function of T during aggressive interactions is to reduce nociception (pain sensitivity). Here, we experimentally document that T indeed reduces behavioral responsiveness to a thermal painful stimulus in captive male house sparrows (Passer domesticus). Skin nociception was quantified by foot immersion into a hot water bath, a benign thermal stimulus. Males treated with exogenous testosterone left their foot longer in hot water than control birds. Conversely, males in which the physiological actions of testosterone were pharmacologically blocked withdrew their foot faster than control birds. Testosterone might exert its effects on pain sensitivity through conversion into estradiol in the dorsal horn of the spinal cord. Decreased nociception during aggressive encounters may promote the immediate and future willingness of males to engage in high-intensity fights.

Hoffman MA. Is low serum free testosterone a marker for high grade prostate cancer? J Urol 2000 Mar; 163(3):824-7 PURPOSE: The association of free and total testosterone with prostate cancer is incompletely understood. We investigated the relationship of serum free and total testosterone to the clinical and pathological characteristics of prostate cancer. MATERIALS AND METHODS: We retrospectively reviewed the clinical records of 117 consecutive patients treated by 1 physician and diagnosed with prostate cancer at our medical center between 1994 and 1997. Low free and total testosterone levels were defined as 1.5 or less and 300 ng. /dl. respectively. RESULTS: After evaluating all 117 patients we noted no correlation of free and total testosterone with prostate specific antigen, patient age, prostatic volume, percent of positive biopsies, biopsy Gleason score or clinical stage. However, in patients with low versus normal free testosterone there were an increased mean percent of biopsies that showed cancer (43% versus 22%, p = 0.013) and an increased incidence of a biopsy Gleason score of 8 or greater (7 of 64 versus 0 of 48, p = 0.025). Of the 117 patients 57 underwent radical retropubic prostatectomy. In those with low versus normal free testosterone an increased mean percent of biopsies demonstrated cancer (47% versus 28%, p = 0.018). Pathological evaluation revealed stage pT2ab, pT2c, pT3 and pT4 disease, respectively, in 31%, 64%, 8% and 0% of patients with low and in 40%, 40.6%, 12.5% and 6.2% in those with normal free testosterone (p>0.05). CONCLUSIONS: In our study patients with prostate cancer and low free testosterone had more extensive disease. In addition, all men with a biopsy Gleason score of 8 or greater had low serum free testosterone. This finding suggests that low serum free testosterone may be a marker for more aggressive disease.

Hogervorst E et al. Low free testosterone is an independent risk factor for Alzheimer's disease. Exp Gerontol. 2004 Nov-Dec; 39(11-12):1633-9. The purpose of this study was to assess pituitary gonadotropins and free testosterone levels in a larger cohort of men with Alzheimer's disease (AD, n=112) and age-matched controls (n=98) from the Oxford Project to Investigate Memory and Ageing (OPTIMA). We measured gonadotropins (follicle stimulating hormone, FSH, and luteinizing hormone, LH), sex hormone binding globulin (SHBG, which determines the amount of free testosterone) and total testosterone (TT) using enzyme immunoassays. AD cases had significantly higher LH and FSH and lower free testosterone levels. LH, FSH and SHBG all increased with age, while free testosterone decreased. Low free testosterone was an independent predictor for AD. Its variance was overall explained by high SHBG, low TT, high LH, an older age and low body mass index (BMI). In controls, low thyroid stimulating hormone levels were also associated with low free testosterone. Elderly AD cases had raised levels of gonadotropins. This response may be an attempt to normalize low free testosterone levels. In non-demented participants, subclinical hyperthyroid disease (a risk factor for AD) which can result in higher SHBG levels was associated with low free testosterone. Lowering SHBG and/or screening for subclinical thyroid disease may prevent cognitive decline and/or wasting in men at risk for AD.

Iczkowski, K. et al. The Dual 5 alpha reductase inhibitor dutasteride induces atrophic changes and decreases cancer volume in the human prostate. Urology 65:76-82, 2005 OBJECTIVES: To perform the first evaluation of the effects of the 5-alpha-reductase inhibitor class of drugs on cancer histopathologic features at radical prostatectomy in a placebo-controlled multicenter trial. METHODS: We analyzed prostatectomy slides in a blinded manner from 17 men treated with dutasteride, an inhibitor of types 1 and 2 isoenzymes of 5-alpha-reductase, and 18 men treated with placebo for 5 to 11 weeks before radical prostatectomy. The histopathologic features of benign epithelium, high-grade prostatic intraepithelial neoplasia, and cancer were recorded, and the treatment effect was scored. Digital imaging analysis was used to measure the stroma/epithelium ratio and epithelial height, as well as the nuclear area in cancer. RESULTS: In benign epithelium, treatment caused distinctive cytoarchitectural changes of atrophy and a decrease in the epithelial height (P = 0.053). The peripheral zone showed the most marked response to treatment. In cancer tissue, the tumor volume was significantly lower in the dutasteride-treated men than in the placebo-treated men (mean 15% versus 24%, respectively, P = 0.025), the percentage of atrophic epithelium was increased (P = 0.041), and the stroma/gland ratio was doubled (P = 0.046). The treatment alteration effect score was doubled (P = 0.055) and did not correlate with any Gleason score changes. CONCLUSIONS: After short-term dutasteride treatment, benign epithelium showed involution and epithelial shrinkage, and prostate cancer tissue demonstrated a decrease in epithelium relative to stroma. These findings indicate that dutasteride induces significant phenotypic alterations in both the benign and the neoplastic prostate, supportive of a chemopreventive or chemoactive role.

Jankowska EA. Circulating estradiol and mortality in men with systolic chronic heart failure. JAMA. 2009 May 13; 301(18):1892-901. CONTEXT: Androgen deficiency is common in men with chronic heart failure (HF) and is associated with increased morbidity and mortality. Estrogens are formed by the aromatization of androgens; therefore, abnormal estrogen metabolism would be anticipated in HF. OBJECTIVE: To examine the relationship between serum concentration of estradiol and mortality in men with chronic HF and reduced left ventricular ejection fraction (LVEF). DESIGN, SETTING, AND PARTICIPANTS: A prospective observational study at 2 tertiary cardiology centers (Wroclaw and Zabrze, Poland) of 501 men (mean [SD] age, 58 [12] years) with chronic HF, LVEF of 28% (SD, 8%), and New York Heart Association [NYHA] classes 1, 2, 3, and 4 of 52, 231, 181, and 37, respectively, who were recruited between January 1, 2002, and May 31, 2006. Cohort was divided into quintiles of serum estradiol (quintile 1, < 12.90 pg/mL; quintile 2, 12.90-21.79 pg/mL; quintile 3, 21.80-30.11 pg/mL; quintile 4, 30.12-37.39 pg/mL; and quintile 5, > or = 37.40 pg/mL). Quintile 3 was considered prospectively as the reference group. MAIN OUTCOME MEASURES: Serum concentrations of estradiol and androgens (total testosterone and dehydroepiandrosterone sulfate [DHEA-S]) were measured using immunoassays.
RESULTS: Among 501 men with chronic HF, 171 deaths (34%) occurred during the 3-year follow-up. Compared with quintile 3, men in the lowest and highest estradiol quintiles had increased mortality (adjusted hazard ratio [HR], 4.17; 95% confidence interval [CI], 2.33-7.45 and HR, 2.33; 95% CI, 1.30-4.18; respectively; $P < .001$). These 2 quintiles had different clinical characteristics (quintile 1: increased serum total testosterone, decreased serum DHEA-S, advanced NYHA class, impaired renal function, and decreased total fat tissue mass; and quintile 5: increased serum bilirubin and liver enzymes, and decreased serum sodium; all $P < .05$ vs quintile 3). For increasing estradiol quintiles, 3-year survival rates adjusted for clinical variables and androgens were 44.6% (95% CI, 24.4%-63.0%), 65.8% (95% CI, 47.3%-79.2%), 82.4% (95% CI, 69.4%-90.2%), 79.0% (95% CI, 65.5%-87.6%), and 63.6% (95% CI, 46.6%-76.5%); respectively ($P < .001$).CONCLUSION: Among men with chronic HF and reduced LVEF, high and low concentrations of estradiol compared with the middle quintile of estradiol are related to an increased mortality.

Jeong, HJ et al. Inhibition of aromatase activity by flavinoids. ArchPharm Res. 1999 Jun; 22(3):309-12 In searching for potent cancer chemopreventive agents from synthetic or natural products, 28 randomly selected flavonoids were screened for inhibitory effects against partially purified aromatase prepared from human placenta. Over 50% of the flavonoids significantly inhibited aromatase activity, with greatest activity being demonstrated with apigenin (IC50: 0.9 microg/mL), chrysin (IC50: 1.1 microg/mL), and hesperetin (IC50: 1.0 microg/mL).

Kaczmarek A et al. The association of lower testosterone level with coronary artery disease in postmenopausal women.Int J Cardiol 2003 Jan; 87(1):53-7 OBJECTIVE: Testosterone (T) is assumed to be a risk factor for coronary artery disease (CAD). However, recent studies have demonstrated a beneficial effect of T on myocardial ischaemia in men with CAD. To assess the potential role of T in CAD in postmenopausal women we investigated the association between T level and CAD and relationship between T and other CAD metabolic risk factors. RESULTS: Within the 12-month study period, 108 consecutive, postmenopausal women (age 62+/-7 years) referred for diagnostic coronary angiography were prospectively included in the study. In all patients serum level of T, sex hormone-binding globulin (SHBG), total cholesterol (T-chol), LDL-chol, HDL-chol, triglycerides (TG), apolipoproteins A(1) and B (apo A(1), apo B), lipoprotein a [Lp(a)], and C reactive protein were measured. Testosterone free index (TFI) was calculated as Tx100/SHBG. CAD was documented in 51 (47%) patients (CAD+). Women with CAD had decreased T level and lower TFI (T: 0.99+/-0.4 vs. 1.41+/-0.7 nmol/l, P=0.005; TFI: 3.2+/-1.4 vs. 4.2+/-2.2, P=0.04, CAD+ vs. CAD-, respectively). No difference in SHBG was found between the two groups. In 16 women (six CAD+, 10 CAD-) who were on hormonal replacement therapy (HRT+) we observed significantly elevated T level and TFI (T: 1.62+/-0.5 vs. 1.15+/-0.7 nmol/l; TFI: 5.0+/-2.2 vs. 3.5+/-1.8, HRT+ vs. HRT-, respectively, P<0.05). When these women were excluded from the analysis, T level remained decreased in CAD+ group (0.96+/-0.4 vs. 1.22+/-0.5 nmol/l, CAD+ vs. CAD- respectively, P<0.02). CAD+ group had an unfavourable profile of metabolic CAD risk factors as evidenced by elevated T-chol, LDL-chol, Lp(a), apoB, and decreased apoA(1) (P<0.05 vs. CAD- in all comparisons). Neither T nor TFI correlated with CAD metabolic risk factors (r<0.2, P>0.1 for all correlations), apart from an inverse correlation between T and Lp (a) (r=-0.24, P=0.04). CONCLUSION: In postmenopausal women decreased T level is associated with CAD independently of the other CAD metabolic risk factors. Hormonal replacement therapy tends to increase T level which may further support the beneficial role of HRT in postmenopausal women.

Keogh E Can a sexually dimorphic index of prenatal hormonal exposure be used to examine cold pressor pain perception in men and women? : Eur J Pain. 2006 Apr 4

There is considerable evidence to suggest that important differences exist between men and women in their experience of pain. Research has now turned to determine what the mechanisms of such differences actually are. One potential explanation is the effect of sex hormones, especially those typically found in greater concentration within women, e.g., estrogen, progesterone. However, it is also possible that other hormones, such as testosterone may be important. The current study employed a non-invasive sexually dimorphic index (digit ratio) that is believed to reflect prenatal exposure to testosterone, and related this to the cold pressor pain experiences of 23 men and 27 healthy women. As expected, females had greater symmetry between the second and fourth digits, and also reported lower pain tolerance levels. Although some significant relationships were found between digit ratio/digit length and cold pressor pain reports they were relatively inconsistent. Furthermore, the main finding, that pain thresholds were positively related to digit ratio in women but not men, is somewhat inconsistent with predictions. The results are discussed in light of methods for investigating the effect of prenatal hormonal exposure on pain sensitivity in men and women.

Khaw KT, Barrett-Connor EJ. Blood pressure and endogenous testosterone in men: an inverse relationship. Hypertens. 1988 Apr; 6(4):329-32. Exogenous sex hormone use, including oral contraceptives, post-menopausal hormonal therapy and anabolic steroids, has been associated with blood pressure changes in both sexes, but little is known about the relationship between blood pressure and endogenous sex hormones. We examined this relationship in men in the Rancho Bernardo population study. Out of 1132 men aged 30-79 years, those with hypertension, categorically defined as systolic blood pressure (SBP) greater than 160 mmHg and/or diastolic blood pressure (DBP) greater than 95 mmHg had significantly lower testosterone levels than non-hypertensives. Systolic and diastolic blood pressure inversely correlated with testosterone levels ($r = 0.17$, P less than 0.001 for systolic; $r = -0.15$, P less than 0.001 for diastolic) in the whole cohort. This association was present over the whole range of blood pressures and sex hormone levels with a stepwise decrease in mean SBP and DBP per increasing quartile of testosterone. Obesity accounted for some, but not all, of this relationship, which was reduced, but still apparent after adjusting for age and body mass index. No other hormone (androstendione, estrone, and estradiol) or sex hormone-binding globulin showed a consistent relationship with blood pressure. The clinical and physiological significance of this relationship merits further investigation.

Khaw KT. et al. Endogenous testosterone and mortality due to all causes, cardiovascular disease, and cancer in men. Circulation. 2007; 116:2694-2701 BACKGROUND: The relation between endogenous testosterone concentrations and health in men is controversial.METHODS AND RESULTS: We examined the prospective relationship between endogenous testosterone concentrations and mortality due to all causes, cardiovascular disease, and cancer in a nested case-control study based on 11 606 men aged 40 to 79 years surveyed in 1993 to 1997 and followed up to 2003. Among those without prevalent cancer or cardiovascular disease, 825 men who subsequently died were compared with a control group of 1489 men still alive, matched for age and date of baseline visit. Endogenous testosterone concentrations at baseline were inversely related to mortality due to all causes (825 deaths), cardiovascular disease (369 deaths), and cancer (304 deaths). Odds ratios (95% confidence intervals) for mortality for increasing quartiles of endogenous testosterone compared with the lowest quartile were 0.75 (0.55 to 1.00), 0.62 (0.45 to 0.84), and 0.59 (0.42 to 0.85), respectively (P<0.001 for trend after adjustment for age, date of visit, body mass index, systolic blood pressure, blood cholesterol, cigarette smoking, diabetes mellitus, alcohol intake, physical activity, social class, education, dehydroepiandrosterone sulfate, androstanediol glucuronide, and sex hormone binding globulin). An increase of 6 nmol/L serum testosterone (approximately 1 SD) was associated with a 0.81 (95% confidence interval 0.71 to 0.92, P<0.01) multivariable-adjusted odds ratio for mortality. Inverse relationships were also observed for deaths due to cardiovascular causes and cancer and after the exclusion of deaths that occurred in the first 2 years.

CONCLUSIONS: In men, endogenous testosterone concentrations are inversely related to mortality due to cardiovascular disease and all causes. Low testosterone may be a predictive marker for those at high risk of cardiovascular disease.

Korbonits M, Slawik M A comparison of a novel testosterone bioadhesive buccal system, striant, with a testosterone adhesive patch in hypogonadal males J Clin Endocrinol Metab. 2004 May; 89(5):2039-43. A novel delivery system has been developed for testosterone replacement. This formulation, COL-1621 (Striant), a testosterone-containing buccal mucoadhesive system, has been shown in preliminary studies to replace testosterone at physiological levels when used twice daily. Therefore, the current study compared the steady-state pharmacokinetics and tolerability of the buccal system with a testosterone-containing skin patch (Andropatch or Androderm) in an international multicenter study of a group of hypogonadal men. Sixty-six patients were randomized into two groups; one applied the buccal system twice daily, whereas the other applied the transdermal patch daily, in each case for 7 d. Serum total testosterone and dihydrotestosterone concentrations were measured at d 1, 3 or 4, and 6, and serially over the last 24 h of the study. Pharmacokinetic parameters for each formulation were calculated, and the two groups were compared. The tolerability of both formulations was also evaluated. Thirty-three patients were treated with the buccal preparation, and 34 were treated with the transdermal patch. The average serum testosterone concentration over 24 h showed a mean of 18.74 nmol/liter (SD =; 5.90) in the buccal system group and 12.15 nmol/liter (SD =; 5.55) in the transdermal patch group (P < 0.01). Of the patients treated with the buccal system, 97% had average steady-state testosterone concentrations within the physiological range (10.41-36.44 nmol/liter); whereas only 56% of the transdermal patch patients achieved physiological total testosterone concentrations (P < 0.001 between groups). Testosterone concentrations were within the physiological range in the buccal system group for a significantly greater portion of the 24-h treatment period than in the transdermal patch group (mean, 84.9% vs. 54.9%; P < 0.001). Testosterone/dihydrotestosterone ratios were physiological and similar in both groups. Few patients experienced major adverse effects from either treatment. No significant local tolerability problems were noted with the buccal system, other than a single patient withdrawal. We conclude that this buccal system is superior to the transdermal patch in achieving testosterone concentrations within the normal range. It may, therefore, be a valuable addition to the range of choices for testosterone replacement therapy.

Korenman SG, Morley JE, Mooradian AD, et al. 1990 Secondary hypogonadism in older men: its relationship to impotence. J Clin Endocrinol Metab. 71:963–969. The relation of the reproductive endocrine system to impotence in older men was examined by measuring the concentrations of testosterone (T), bioavailable testosterone (BT), LH, and PRL and body mass index (BMI) in 57 young controls (YC), 50 healthy potent older controls attending a health fair (HF), and 267 impotent patients (SD). The SD and HF had markedly reduced mean T and BT values compared to YC. When adjusted for age and BMI there was no difference in BT between potent and impotent older men. The percent BT was much higher in YC than in the older groups. While the percent BT rose significantly with increased T in YC, it was inversely related to T in the older subjects, suggesting that increased sex hormone-binding globulin binding was a primary event leading to a low BT. Forty-eight percent of HF and 39% of SD were hypogonadal, as defined by a mean BT of 2.5 SD or more below the mean of YC (less than or equal to 2.3 nmol/L). Ninety percent of these had LH values in the normal range, suggesting hypothalamic-pituitary dysfunction. Thirty-four SD and six each of YC and older control volunteers (OC) underwent GnRH testing. Older subjects showed impaired responsiveness to GnRH compared to YC. A low basal LH level correlated very highly with hyporesponsiveness to GnRH. Thus, secondary hypogonadism and impotence are two common, independently distributed conditions of older men.

Kupelian V et al. Low sex hormone-binding globulin, total testosterone, and symptomatic androgen deficiency are associated with development of the metabolic syndrome in nonobese men. J Clin Endocrinol Metab. 2006 Mar; 91(3):843-50. BACKGROUND: The metabolic syndrome (MetS), characterized by central obesity, lipid and insulin dysregulation, and hypertension, is a precursor state for cardiovascular disease. The purpose of this analysis was to determine whether low serum sex hormone levels or clinical androgen deficiency (AD) predict the development of MetS. METHODS: Data were obtained from the Massachusetts Male Aging Study, a population-based prospective cohort of 1709 men observed at three time points (T1, 1987-1989; T2, 1995-1997; T3, 2002-2004). MetS was defined using a modification of the ATP III guidelines. Clinical AD was defined using a combination of testosterone levels and clinical signs and symptoms. The association between MetS and sex hormone levels or clinical AD was assessed using relative risks (RR), and 95% confidence intervals (95% CI) were estimated using Poisson regression models. RESULTS: Analysis was conducted in 950 men without MetS at T1. Lower levels of total testosterone and SHBG were predictive of MetS, particularly among men with a body mass index (BMI) below 25 kg/m2 with adjusted RRs for a decrease in 1 sd of 1.41 (95% CI, 1.06-1.87) and 1.65 (95% CI, 1.12-2.42). Results were similar for the AD and MetS association, with RRs of 2.51 (95% CI, 1.12-5.65) among men with a BMI less than 25 compared with an RR of 1.22 (95% CI, 0.66-2.24) in men with a BMI of 25 or greater. CONCLUSIONS: Low serum SHBG, low total testosterone, and clinical AD are associated with increased risk of developing MetS over time, particularly in nonoverweight, middle-aged men (BMI, <25). Together, these results suggest that low SHBG and/or AD may provide early warning signs for cardiovascular risk and an opportunity for early intervention in nonobese men.

Laaksonen DE et al. Sex hormones, inflammation and the metabolic syndrome: a population-albased study.Eur J Endocrinol. 2003 Dec; 149(6):601-8. OBJECTIVE: Mild hypoandrogenism in men is associated with features of the metabolic syndrome, but the association with the metabolic syndrome itself using an accepted definition has not been described. DESIGN: Men with the metabolic syndrome were identified and testosterone and sex hormone-binding globulin (SHBG) levels were determined in a population-based cohort of 1896 non-diabetic middle-aged Finnish men. RESULTS: Calculated free testosterone and SHBG were 11% and 18% lower (P<0.001) in men with the metabolic syndrome (n=345, World Health Organisation definition). After categorisation by tertiles and adjusting for age and body mass index, total and free testosterone and SHBG were inversely associated with concentrations of insulin, glucose, triglycerides, C-reactive protein (CRP) and CRP-adjusted ferritin and positively associated with high-density lipoprotein cholesterol. Men with free testosterone levels in the lowest third were 2.7 (95% confidence interval (CI) 2.0-3.7) times more likely to have the metabolic syndrome in age-adjusted analyses, and 1.7 (95% CI 1.2-2.4) times more likely even after further adjusting for body mass index. Exclusion of men with cardiovascular disease did not alter the association. The inverse association of SHBG with the metabolic syndrome was somewhat stronger. CONCLUSIONS: Low testosterone and SHBG levels were strongly associated not only with components of the metabolic syndrome, but also with the metabolic syndrome itself, independently of body mass index. Furthermore, sex hormones were associated with inflammation and body iron stores. Even in the absence of late-stage consequences such as diabetes and cardiovascular disease, subtle derangements in sex hormones are present in the metabolic syndrome, and may contribute to its pathogenesis.

Laaksonen DE et al. Testosterone and Sex Hormone-Binding Globulin Predict the Metabolic Syndrome and Diabetes in Middle-Aged Men.Diabetes Care. 2004 May;27(5):1036-1041 OBJECTIVE: In men, hypoandrogenism is associated with features of the metabolic syndrome, but the role of sex hormones in the pathogenesis of the metabolic syndrome and diabetes is not well understood. We assessed the association of low levels of testosterone and sex hormone-binding globulin (SHBG) with the development of the metabolic syndrome and diabetes in men. RESEARCH DESIGN AND METHODS: Concentrations of SHBG and total and calculated free testosterone and factors related to insulin resistance were determined at baseline in 702 middle-aged Finnish men participating in a population-based cohort study. These men had neither diabetes nor the metabolic syndrome. RESULTS: After 11 years of follow-up, 147 men had developed the metabolic syndrome (National Cholesterol Education Program criteria) and 57 men diabetes. Men with total testosterone, calculated free testosterone, and SHBG levels in the lower fourth had a severalfold increased risk of developing the metabolic syndrome (odds ratio [OR] 2.3, 95% CI 1.5-3.4; 1.7, 1.2-2.5; and 2.8, 1.9-4.1, respectively) and diabetes (2.3, 1.3-4.1; 1.7, 0.9-3.0; and 4.3, 2.4-7.7, respectively) after adjustment for age. Adjustment for potential confounders such as cardiovascular disease, smoking, alcohol intake, and socioeconomic status did not alter the associations. Factors related to insulin resistance attenuated the associations, but they remained significant, except for free testosterone. CONCLUSIONS: Low total testosterone and SHBG levels independently predict development of the metabolic syndrome and diabetes in middle-aged men. Thus, hypoandrogenism is an early marker for disturbances in insulin and glucose metabolism that may progress to the metabolic syndrome or frank diabetes and may contribute to their pathogenesis.

Leder BZ et al. Effects of aromatase inhibition in elderly men with low or borderline-low serum testosterone levels.J Clin Endocrinol Metab. 2004 Mar; 89(3):1174-80. As men age, serum testosterone levels decrease, a factor that may contribute to some aspects of age-related physiological deterioration. Although androgen replacement has been shown to have beneficial effects in frankly hypogonadal men, its use in elderly men with borderline hypogonadism is controversial. Furthermore, current testosterone replacement methods have important limitations. We investigated the ability of the orally administered aromatase inhibitor, anastrozole, to increase endogenous testosterone production in 37 elderly men (aged 62-74 yr) with screening serum testosterone levels less than 350 ng/dl. Subjects were randomized in a double-blind fashion to the following 12-wk oral regimens: group 1: anastrozole 1 mg daily (n = 12); group 2: anastrozole 1 mg twice weekly (n = 11); and group 3: placebo daily (n = 14). Hormone levels, quality of life (MOS Short-Form Health Survey), sexual function (International Index of Erectile Function), benign prostate hyperplasia severity (American Urological Association Symptom Index Score), prostate-specific antigen, and measures of safety were compared among groups. Mean +/- SD bioavailable testosterone increased from 99 +/- 31 to 207 +/- 65 ng/dl in group 1 and from 115 +/- 37 to 178 +/- 55 ng/dl in group 2 (P < 0.001 vs. placebo for both groups and P = 0.054 group 1 vs. group 2). Total testosterone levels increased from 343 +/- 61 to 572 +/- 139 ng/dl in group 1 and from 397 +/- 106 to 520 +/- 91 ng/dl in group 2 (P < 0.001 vs. placebo for both groups and P = 0.012 group 1 vs. group 2). Serum estradiol levels decreased from 26 +/- 8 to 17 +/- 6 pg/ml in group 1 and from 27 +/- 8 to 17 +/- 5 pg/ml in group 2 (P < 0.001 vs. placebo for both groups and P = NS group 1 vs. group 2). Serum LH levels increased from 5.1 +/- 4.8 to 7.9 +/- 6.5 U/liter and from 4.1 +/- 1.6 to 7.2 +/- 2.8 U/liter in groups 1 and 2, respectively (P = 0.007 group 1 vs. placebo, P = 0.003 group 2 vs. placebo, and P = NS group 1 vs. group 2). Scores for hematocrit, MOS Short-Form Health Survey, International Index of Erectile Function, and American Urological Association Symptom Index Score did not change. Serum prostate-specific antigen levels increased in group 2 only (1.7 +/- 1.0 to 2.2 +/- 1.5 ng/ml, P = 0.031, compared with placebo). These data demonstrate that aromatase inhibition increases serum bioavailable and total testosterone levels to the youthful normal range in older men with mild hypogonadism. Serum estradiol levels decrease modestly but remain within the normal male range. The physiological consequences of these changes remain to be determined.

Lunenfeld B Endocrinology of the aging male. Minerva Ginecol. 2006 Apr; 58(2):153-70 Despite enormous medical progress during the past few decades, the last years of life are still accompanied by increasing ill health and disability. The ability to maintain active and independent living for as long as possible is a crucial factor for ageing healthily and with dignity. The most important and drastic gender differences in aging are related to the reproductive organs. In distinction to the course of reproductive ageing in women, with the rapid decline in sex hormones expressed by the cessation of menses, men experience a slow and continuous decline. This decline in endocrine function involves: a decrease of testosterone, dehydro epiandrosterone (DHEA), oestrogens, thyroid stimulating hormone (TSH), growth hormone (GH), IGF1, and melatonin. The decrease of sex hormones is concomitant with a temporary increase of luteinizing hormone (LH) and follicle-stimulating hormone (FSH). In addition sex hormone binding globulins (SHBG) increase with age resulting in further lowering the concentrations of free biologically active androgens. These hormonal changes are directly or indirectly associated with changes in body constitution, fat distribution (visceral obesity), muscle weakness, osteopenia, osteoporosis, urinary incontinence, loss of cognitive functioning, reduction in well being, depression, as well as sexual dysfunction. The laboratory and clinical findings of partial endocrine deficiencies in the aging male will be described and discussed in detail. With the prolongation of life expectancy both women and men today live 1/3 of their life with endocrine deficiencies. Interventions such as hormone replacement therapy may alleviate the debilitating conditions of secondary partial endocrine deficiencies by preventing the preventable and delaying the inevitable.

Maggio M et al. Correlation between testosterone and the inflammatory marker soluble interleukin-6 receptor (sIL-6r) in older men.J Clin Endocrinol Metab. 2005 Nov 1 CONTEXT: An age-associated decline in testosterone (T) levels and an increase in proinflammatory cytokines contribute to chronic diseases in older men.

Whether and how these changes are related is unclear. OBJECTIVE: We hypothesized that T and inflammatory markers are negatively correlated in older men. DESIGN: This was a cross-sectional study. SETTING: A population-based sample of older men was studied. PARTICIPANTS AND MEASURES: After excluding participants taking glucocorticoids or antibiotics or those with recent hospitalization, 467 men, aged 65 yr or older, had complete determinations of total T, bioavailable T, SHBG, albumin, IL-6, soluble IL-6 receptor (sIL-6r), TNF-alpha, IL-1beta, and C-reactive protein. RESULTS: After adjusting for potential confounders, sIL-6r was significantly and inversely correlated with total T ($r = -0.20$; $P < 0.001$) and bioavailable T ($r = -0.12$; $P < 0.05$). T was not correlated with any other inflammatory marker. CONCLUSIONS: These preliminary findings suggest an inverse relationship between T and sIL-6r. Longitudinal studies are needed to establish the causality of this association.

Makinen J et al. Increased carotid atherosclerosis in andropausal middle-aged men. J Am Coll Cardiol. 2005 May 17; 45(10) OBJECTIVES: This study examined the association between carotid artery intima-media thickness (IMT), serum sex hormone levels, and andropausal symptoms in middle-aged men. BACKGROUND: Male sex hormones may play a dual role in the pathogenesis of atherosclerosis in men by carrying both proatherogenic and atheroprotective effects. METHODS: We studied 239 40- to 70-year-old men (mean +/- SD: 57 +/- 8 years) who participated in the Turku Aging Male Study and underwent serum lipid and sex hormone measurements. Ninety-nine men (age 58 +/- 7 years) were considered andropausal (i.e., serum testosterone <9.8 nmol/l or luteinizing hormone [LH] >6.0 U/l and testosterone in the normal range), and in both situations, they had subjective symptoms of andropause (a high symptom score in questionnaire). Three were excluded because of diabetes. The rest of the men (age 57 +/- 8 years) served as controls. Carotid IMT was determined using high-resolution B-mode ultrasound, and serum testosterone, estradiol (E2), LH, and sex hormone-binding globulin were measured using standard immunoassays. RESULTS: Andropausal men had a higher maximal IMT compared with controls in the common carotid (1.08 +/- 0.34 vs. 1.00 +/- 0.23, $p < 0.05$) and in the carotid bulb (1.44 +/- 0.48 vs. 1.27 +/- 0.35, $p = 0.003$). Common carotid IMT correlated inversely with serum testosterone ($p = 0.003$) and directly with LH ($p = 0.006$) in multivariate models adjusted for age, total cholesterol, body mass index, blood pressure, and smoking. CONCLUSIONS: Middle-aged men with symptoms of andropause, together with absolute or compensated (as reflected by high normal to elevated LH) testosterone deficiency, show increased carotid IMT. These data suggest that normal testosterone levels may offer protection against the development of atherosclerosis in middle-aged men.

Malkin CJ et al. Testosterone as a protective factor against atherosclerosis--immunomodulation and influence upon plaque development and stability. J Endocrinol. 2003 Sep; 178(3):373-

80 Inflammation plays a central pathogenic role in the initiation and progression of coronary atheroma and its clinical consequences. Cytokines are the mediators of cellular inflammation and promote local inflammation in the arterial wall, which may lead to vascular smooth muscle apoptosis, degradation of the fibrin cap and plaque rupture. Platelet adhesion and thrombus formation then occur, resulting clinically in unstable angina or myocardial infarction. Recent studies have suggested that cytokines are pathogenic, contributing directly to the disease process. 'Anti-cytokine' therapy may, therefore, be of benefit in preventing or slowing the progression of cardiovascular disease. Both oestrogens and testosterone have been shown to have immune-modulating effects; testosterone in particular appears to suppress activation of pro-inflammatory cytokines. Men with low testosterone levels are at increased risk of coronary artery disease. An anti-inflammatory effect of normal physiological levels of sex hormones may, therefore, be important in atheroprotection. In this Article, we discuss some of the mechanisms involved in atherosclerotic coronary artery disease and the putative link between testosterone deficiency and atheroma formation. We present the hypothesis that the immune-modulating properties of testosterone may be important in inhibiting atheroma formation and progression to acute coronary syndrome.

Malkin CJ et al. The effect of testosterone replacement on endogenous inflammatory cytokines and lipid profiles in hypogonadal men J Clin Endocrinol Metab. 2004 Jul; 89(7):3313-8. Testosterone has immune-modulating properties, and current in vitro evidence suggests that testosterone may suppress the expression of the proinflammatory cytokines TNFalpha, IL-1beta, and IL-6 and potentiate the expression of the antiinflammatory cytokine IL-10. We report a randomized, single-blind, placebo-controlled, crossover study of testosterone replacement (Sustanon 100) vs. placebo in 27 men (age, 62 +/- 9 yr) with symptomatic androgen deficiency (total testosterone, 4.4 +/- 1.2 nmol/liter; bioavailable testosterone, 2.4 +/- 1.1 nmol/liter). Compared with placebo, testosterone induced reductions in TNFalpha (-3.1 +/- 8.3 vs. 1.3 +/- 5.2 pg/ml; P = 0.01) and IL-1beta (-0.14 +/- 0.32 vs. 0.18 +/- 0.55 pg/ml; P = 0.08) and an increase in IL-10 (0.33 +/- 1.8 vs. -1.1 +/- 3.0 pg/ml; P = 0.01); the reductions of TNFalpha and IL-1beta were positively correlated (r(S) = 0.588; P = 0.003). In addition, a significant reduction in total cholesterol was recorded with testosterone therapy (-0.25 +/- 0.4 vs. -0.004 +/- 0.4 mmol/liter; P = 0.04). In conclusion, testosterone replacement shifts the cytokine balance to a state of reduced inflammation and lowers total cholesterol. Twenty of these men had established coronary disease, and because total cholesterol is a cardiovascular risk factor, and proinflammatory cytokines mediate the development and complications associated with atheromatous plaque, these properties may have particular relevance in men with overt vascular disease.

Malkin CJ et al. Testosterone replacement in hypogonadal men with angina improves ischaemic threshold and quality of life. Heart. 2004 Aug; 90(8):871-6. BACKGROUND: Low serum testosterone is associated with several cardiovascular risk factors including dyslipidaemia, adverse clotting profiles, obesity, and insulin resistance. Testosterone has been reported to improve symptoms of angina and delay time to ischaemic threshold in unselected men with coronary disease. OBJECTIVE: This randomised single blind placebo controlled crossover study compared testosterone replacement therapy (Sustanon 100) with placebo in 10 men with ischaemic heart disease and hypogonadism. RESULTS: Baseline total testosterone and bioavailable testosterone were respectively 4.2 (0.5) nmol/l and 1.7 (0.4) nmol/l. After a month of testosterone, delta value analysis between testosterone and placebo phase showed that mean (SD) trough testosterone concentrations increased significantly by 4.8 (6.6) nmol/l (total testosterone) ($p = 0.05$) and 3.8 (4.5) nmol/l (bioavailable testosterone) ($p = 0.025$), time to 1 mm ST segment depression assessed by Bruce protocol exercise treadmill testing increased by 74 (54) seconds ($p = 0.002$), and mood scores assessed with validated questionnaires all improved. Compared with placebo, testosterone therapy was also associated with a significant reduction of total cholesterol and serum tumour necrosis factor alpha with delta values of -0.41 (0.54) mmol/l ($p = 0.04$) and -1.8 (2.4) pg/ml ($p = 0.05$) respectively. CONCLUSION: Testosterone replacement therapy in hypogonadal men delays time to ischaemia, improves mood, and is associated with potentially beneficial reductions of total cholesterol and serum tumour necrosis factor alpha.

Malkin CJ et al. Testosterone therapy in men with moderate severity heart failure: a double-blind randomized placebo controlled trial. Eur Heart J. 2005 Aug 10 AIMS: Chronic heart failure is associated with maladaptive and prolonged neurohormonal and pro-inflammatory cytokine activation causing a metabolic shift favouring catabolism, vasodilator incapacity, and loss of skeletal muscle bulk and function. In men, androgens are important determinants of anabolic function and physical strength and also possess anti-inflammatory and vasodilatory properties. METHODS AND RESULTS: We conducted a randomized, double-blind, placebo-controlled parallel trial of testosterone replacement therapy (5 mg Androderm) at physiological doses in 76 men (mean+/-SD, age 64+/-9.9) with heart failure (ejection fraction 32.5+/-11%) over a maximum follow-up period of 12 months. The primary endpoint was functional capacity as assessed by the incremental shuttle walk test (ISWT). At baseline, 18 (24%) had serum testosterone below the normal range and bioavailable testosterone correlated with distance walked on the initial ISWT (r=0.3, P=0.01). Exercise capacity significantly improved with testosterone therapy compared with placebo over the full study period (mean change +25+/-15 m) corresponding to a 15+/-11% improvement from baseline (P=0.006 ANOVA). Symptoms improved by at least one functional class on testosterone in 13 (35%) vs. 3 (8%) on placebo (P=0.01). No significant changes were found in handgrip strength, skeletal muscle bulk by cross-sectional computed tomography, or in tumour necrosis factor levels. Testosterone therapy was safe with no excess of adverse events although the patch preparation was not well tolerated by the study patients. CONCLUSION: Testosterone replacement therapy improves functional capacity and symptoms in men with moderately severe heart failure.

Marks LS et al. Effect of testosterone replacement therapy on prostate tissue in men with late-onset hypogonadism: a randomized controlled trial JAMA. 2006 Nov 15; 296(19):2369-71.

CONTEXT: Prostate safety is a primary concern when aging men receive testosterone replacement therapy (TRT), but little information is available regarding the effects of TRT on prostate tissue in men.
OBJECTIVE: To determine the effects of TRT on prostate tissue of aging men with low serum testosterone levels.DESIGN, SETTING, AND PARTICIPANTS: Randomized, double-blind, placebo-controlled trial of 44 men, aged 44 to 78 years, with screening serum testosterone levels lower than 300 ng/dL (<10.4 nmol/L) and related symptoms, conducted at a US community-based research center between February 2003 and November 2004.INTERVENTION: Participants were randomly assigned to receive 150 mg of testosterone enanthate or matching placebo intramuscularly every 2 weeks for 6 months.MAIN OUTCOME MEASURES: The primary outcome measure was the 6-month change in prostate tissue androgen levels (testosterone and dihydrotestosterone). Secondary outcome measures included 6-month changes in prostate-related clinical features, histology, biomarkers, and epithelial cell gene expression.RESULTS: Of the 44 men randomized, 40 had prostate biopsies performed both at baseline and at 6 months and qualified for per-protocol analysis (TRT, n = 21; placebo, n = 19). Testosterone replacement therapy increased serum testosterone levels to the mid-normal range (median at baseline, 282 ng/dL [9.8 nmol/L]; median at 6 months, 640 ng/dL [22.2 nmol/L]) with no significant change in serum testosterone levels in matched, placebo-treated men. However, median prostate tissue levels of testosterone (0.91 ng/g) and dihydrotestosterone (6.79 ng/g) did not change significantly in the TRT group. No treatment-related change was observed in prostate histology, tissue biomarkers (androgen receptor, Ki-67, CD34), gene expression (including AR, PSA, PAP2A, VEGF, NXK3, CLU [Clusterin]), or cancer incidence or severity. Treatment-related changes in prostate volume, serum prostate-specific antigen, voiding symptoms, and urinary flow were minor.
CONCLUSIONS: These preliminary data suggest that in aging men with late-onset hypogonadism, 6 months of TRT normalizes serum androgen levels but appears to have little effect on prostate tissue androgen levels and cellular functions. Establishment of prostate safety for large populations of older men undergoing longer duration of TRT requires further study.

Moffat SD, Resnick SM. Long-term measures of free testosterone predict regional cerebral blood flow patterns in elderly men.Neurobiol Aging. 2006 May 11 We previously reported that high circulating free testosterone (T) was associated with better performance on tests of memory, executive function, and spatial ability, and with a reduced risk for Alzheimer's disease. In this study, we report that free T levels, measured on multiple occasions over 14 years, predict regional cerebral blood flow (rCBF) measured by PET in 40 older men. Voxel-based regression, indicated that higher Free T was associated with increased rCBF in the hippocampus bilaterally (extending to the parahippocampal gyrus on the right), anterior cingulate gyrus, and right inferior frontal cortex. Total T concentrations were positively correlated with rCBF in the left putamen, bilateral thalamus, and left inferior frontal cortex and negatively correlated with amygdala rCBF bilaterally. These findings suggest that endogenous T influences brain physiology in regions critical for memory and attention and provide one mechanism through which T may affect cognitive function.

Morales A.Androgen replacement therapy and prostate safety.Eur Urol 2002 Feb; 41(2):113-20 Progress in the understanding of the action of exogenous testosterone has diminished many of the concerns that existed regarding its safety. The major interest is now focused on the effects of androgen supplementation on the prostate gland. Many such concerns have been addressed but others remain to be fully elucidated. It is well established that hypogonadal men receiving adequate androgen therapy develop a prostate with a volume similar to what would be expected from their eugonadal counterparts. Androgen therapy results in modest elevations in the PSA and minor changes in flow parameters. Prostate cancer, on the other hand, remains the most prominent of the safety concerns. Although there is no evidence that normal levels of testosterone promote the development of cancer of the prostate, it is clear that the administration of testosterone enhances a pre-existing prostatic malignancy. Androgen supplementation studies have been, in most cases, of short duration and lacked a control cohort. The current evidence does not support the view that appropriate treatment of hypogonadal elderly men with androgens has a causal relationship with prostate cancer. Larger experience, however, is needed. The same criteria applies to the use of other hormones such as dehydrotestosterone, dehydroepiandrosterone follicle stimulating and growth hormone. A set of recommendations regarding androgen replacement therapy and prostate safety is proposed.

Morales A. Monitoring androgen replacement therapy: testosterone and prostate safety.J Endocrinol Invest. 2005; 28(3 Suppl):122-7 The aging of the world population has brought to the forefront of medical practice the diagnosis and treatment of hypogonadism in adult men. There is an increasing interest on the use of testosterone (T) and other androgens to manage men with clinical and biochemical evidence of hypogonadism. Although treatment with T has been used for 70 yr and it is, generally, safe and effective, there are a number of safety issues--ranging from cardiovascular and lipid alterations to hematological changes--that the physician needs to be aware of. Unquestionably, prostate safety constitutes the most important one. No evidence exists that appropriate androgen administration with knowledgeable monitoring carries significant or potentially serious adverse effects on the prostate gland. Men with symptomatic lower urinary obstruction need to be assessed carefully prior to androgen administration. The suspicion of prostate cancer is an absolute contraindication for T use. Recommendations are available for the judicious and safe use of T in aging men.

Morgentaler A Testosterone and Prostate Cancer: An Historical Perspective on a Modern Myth. Eur Urol. 2006 Jul 26; OBJECTIVES: To review the historical origins and current evidence for the belief that testosterone (T) causes prostate cancer (pCA) growth. METHODS: Review of the historical literature regarding T administration and pCA, as well as more recent studies investigating the relationship of T and pCA. RESULTS: In 1941 Huggins and Hodges reported that marked reductions in T by castration or estrogen treatment caused metastatic pCA to regress, and administration of exogenous T caused pCA to grow. Remarkably, this latter conclusion was based on results from only one patient. Multiple subsequent reports revealed no pCA progression with T administration, and some men even experienced subjective improvement, such as resolution of bone pain. More recent data have shown no apparent increase in pCA rates in clinical trials of T supplementation in normal men or men at increased risk for pCA, no relationship of pCA risk with serum T levels in multiple longitudinal studies, and no reduced risk of pCA in men with low T. The apparent paradox in which castration causes pCA to regress yet higher T fails to cause pCA to grow is resolved by a saturation model, in which maximal stimulation of pCA is reached at relatively low levels of T. CONCLUSIONS: This historical perspective reveals that there is not now-nor has there ever been-a scientific basis for the belief that T causes pCA to grow. Discarding this modern myth will allow exploration of alternative hypotheses regarding the relationship of T and pCA that may be clinically and scientifically rewarding.

Morgentaler A Testosterone replacement therapy and prostate risks: where's the beef? Can J Urol. 2006 Feb; 13 Suppl 1:40-3. It has been part of the conventional medical wisdom for six decades that higher testosterone in some way increases the risk of prostate cancer. This belief is derived largely from the well-documented regression of prostate cancer in the face of surgical or pharmacological castration. However, there is an absence of scientific data supporting the concept that higher testosterone levels are associated with an increased risk of prostate cancer. Specifically, no increased risk of prostate cancer was noted in 1) clinical trials of testosterone supplementation, 2) longitudinal population-based studies, or 3) in a high-risk population of hypogonadal men receiving testosterone treatment. Moreover, hypogonadal men have a substantial rate of biopsy-detectable prostate cancer, suggesting that low testosterone has no protective effect against development of prostate cancer. These results argue against an increased risk of prostate cancer with testosterone replacement therapy.

Morgentaler, M. Guideline for Male Testosterone therapy. A clinician's perspective. J. Clin Endo Metab. 92 (2) 416-417, 2007 no abstract available

Morgentaler A. et al Two years of testosterone therapy associated with decline in prostate-specific antigen in a man with untreated prostate cancer. J Sex Med. 2009 Feb; 6(2):574-7. INTRODUCTION: Testosterone (T) therapy has long been considered contraindicated in men with prostate cancer (PCa). However, the traditional view regarding the relationship of T to PCa has come under new scrutiny, with recent reports suggesting that PCa growth may not be greatly affected by variations in serum T within the near-physiologic range.AIM: This report details the clinical and prostate-specific antigen (PSA) response of a man with untreated PCa treated with T therapy for 2 years.METHODS: Measurements of serum PSA, total and free T concentrations were obtained at regular intervals at baseline and following initiation of T therapy.MAIN OUTCOME MEASURE: Serum PSA during T therapy.
RESULTS: An 84-year-old man was seen for symptoms of hypogonadism, with serum total T within the normal range at 400 ng/dL, but with a reduced free T of 7.4 pg/mL (radioimmunoassay [RIA], reference range 10.0-55.0). PSA was 8.5 ng/mL, and 8.1 ng/mL when repeated. Prostate biopsy revealed Gleason 6 cancer in both lobes. He refused treatment for PCa, but requested T therapy, which was initiated with T gel after informed consent regarding possible cancer progression. Serum T increased to a mean value of 699 ng/dL and free T to 17.1 pg/mL. PSA declined to a nadir of 5.2 ng/mL at 10 months, increased slightly to 6.2 ng/mL at 21 months, and then declined to 3.8 ng/mL at 24 months after addition of dutasteride for voiding symptoms. No clinical PCa progression was noted.CONCLUSION: A decline in PSA was noted in a man with untreated PCa who received T therapy for 2 years. This case provides support for the notion that PCa growth may not be adversely affected by changes in serum T beyond the castrate or near-castrate range.

Morgentler A et al. Testosterone therapy in men with untreated prostate cancer. J Urol. 2011 Apr;185(4):1256-60. PURPOSE: A history of prostate cancer has been a longstanding contraindication to the use of testosterone therapy due to the belief that higher serum testosterone causes more rapid prostate cancer growth. Recent evidence has called this paradigm into question. In this study we investigate the effect of testosterone therapy in men with untreated prostate cancer.

MATERIALS AND METHODS:

We report the results of prostate biopsies, serum prostate specific antigen and prostate volume in symptomatic testosterone deficient cases receiving testosterone therapy while undergoing active surveillance for prostate cancer. RESULTS:A total of 13 symptomatic testosterone deficient men with untreated prostate cancer received testosterone therapy for a median of 2.5 years (range 1.0 to 8.1). Mean age was 58.8 years. Gleason score at initial biopsy was 6 in 12 men and 7 in 1. Mean serum concentration of total testosterone increased from 238 to 664 ng/dl (p <0.001). Mean prostate specific antigen did not change with testosterone therapy (5.5 ± 6.4 vs 3.6 ± 2.6 ng/ml, p = 0.29). Prostate volume was unchanged. Mean number of followup biopsies was 2. No cancer was found in 54% of followup biopsies. Biopsies in 2 men suggested upgrading, and subsequent biopsies in 1 and radical prostatectomy in another indicated no progression. No local prostate cancer progression or distant disease was observed.CONCLUSIONS:Testosterone therapy in men with untreated prostate cancer was not associated with prostate cancer progression in the short to medium term. These results are consistent with the saturation model, ie maximal prostate cancer growth is achieved at low androgen concentrations. The longstanding prohibition against testosterone therapy in men with untreated or low risk prostate cancer or treated prostate cancer without evidence of metastatic or recurrent disease merits reevaluation.

Morley J. Testosterone and frailty. Clin Geriatr Med 1997 Nov;13(4):685-95 Although estrogen replacement therapy has become well established in the management of postmenopausal women, most physicians pay much less attention to the testosterone status of their older male patients. There is now increasing evidence that testosterone deficiency-Low Testosterone Syndrome-occurs in older men and is associated with decreased muscle strength and bone density, as well as memory problems. This article reviews the evidence for the existence of Low Testosterone Syndrome, often characterized as the male menopause or viropause, and the emerging evidence that testosterone therapy may ameliorate some of the symptoms and signs of frailty in men beyond 50 years of age.

Morley JE. Testosterone replacement and the physiologic aspects of aging in men.Mayo Clin Proc. 2000 Jan; 75 Suppl: S83-7 Clinical and epidemiologic studies, along with basic scientific research, have shown a trend toward androgen deficiency in aging males. The focus of the clinical investigations described here is to determine whether testosterone deficiency is a physiologic cause of the aging process and whether testosterone replacement might prevent or ameliorate a decline in quality of life associated with age-related decline in physical and psychological functioning.

Mudali S, Dobs AS Effects of testosterone on body composition of the aging male. Mech Ageing Dev. 2004 Apr; 125(4):297-304

The aging process is accompanied by significant changes in body composition characterized by decreased fat free mass and increased and redistributed fat mass. Muscle loss results from the atrophy of muscle fibers and decreased synthesis of muscle proteins. Increased number of adipocytes and fat accumulation in non-adipose tissue leads to adiposity. These changes can impose functional limitations and increase morbidity. In men, declining testosterone levels that occur with aging can be a contributing factor to these changes. Studies in hypogonadal men have shown that testosterone replacement is effective in increasing muscle mass and strength and decreasing fat mass. The molecular mechanisms of testosterone's influence on muscle and adipose are not fully elucidated. However, testosterone appears to stimulate IGF-1 expression directly and indirectly leading to increased muscle protein synthesis and growth. It may also counter the inhibitory effects of myostatin, cytokines, and glucocorticoids. The predominant effects of testosterone on fat mass are increased lipolysis and decreased adipogenesis. Current evidence suggests that testosterone replacement may be effective in reversing age-dependent body composition changes and associated morbidity. However, hypogonadism must be diagnosed carefully, and therapy should be monitored regularly in order to avoid the adverse effects associated with testosterone supplementation.

Muller M et al. Endogenous sex hormones and progression of carotid atherosclerosis in elderly men. Circulation. 2004 May 4; 109(17):2074-9.

BACKGROUND: The burden of atherosclerosis especially afflicts the increasing older segment of the population. Recent evidence has emphasized a protective role of endogenous sex hormones in the development of atherosclerosis in aging men. METHODS AND RESULTS: We studied the association between endogenous sex hormones and progression of atherosclerosis in 195 independently living elderly men. Participants underwent measurements of carotid intima-media thickness (IMT) at baseline in 1996 and again in 2000. At baseline, serum concentrations of testosterone (total and free) and estradiol (total and free E2) were measured. Serum free testosterone concentrations were inversely related to the mean progression of IMT of the common carotid artery after adjustment for age (beta=-3.57; 95% CI, -6.34 to -0.80). Higher serum total and free E2 levels were related to progression of IMT of the common carotid artery after adjustment for age (beta=0.38; 95% CI, -0.11 to 0.86; and beta=0.018; 95% CI, -0.002 to 0.038, respectively). These associations were independent of body mass index, waist-to-hip ratio, presence of hypertension and diabetes, smoking, and serum cholesterol levels CONCLUSIONS: Low free testosterone levels were related to IMT of the common carotid artery in elderly men independently of cardiovascular risk factors.

Muniyappa R et al. Long-Term Testosterone Supplementation Augments Overnight Growth Hormone Secretion in Healthy Older Men. Am J Physiol Endocrinol Metab. 2007 Circulating testosterone (T) and GH/IGF-I are diminished in healthy aging men. Short-term administration of high doses of T augments GH secretion in older men. However, effects of long-term, low-dose T supplementation on GH secretion are unknown. Our objective was to evaluate effects of long-term, low-dose T administration on nocturnal GH secretory dynamics and AM concentrations of IGF-I and IGFBP-3 in healthy older men (65-88 yr, n = 34) with low-normal T and IGF-I. In a double-masked, placebo-controlled, randomized study we assessed effects of low-dose T supplementation (100 mg im every 2 wk) for 26 wk on nocturnal GH secretory dynamics [8 PM to 8 AM, Q(20) min sampling, analyzed by multiparameter deconvolution and approximate entropy (ApEn) algorithms]. The results were that T administration increased serum total T by 33% (P = 0.004) and E (2) by 31% (P = 0.009) and decreased SHBG by 17% (P = 0.002) vs. placebo. T supplementation increased nocturnal integrated GH concentrations by 60% (P = 0.02) and pulsatile GH secretion by 79% (P = 0.05), primarily due to a twofold increase in GH secretory burst mass (P = 0.02) and a 1.9-fold increase in basal GH secretion rate (P = 0.05) vs. placebo. There were no significant changes in GH burst frequency or orderliness of GH release (ApEn). IGF-I levels increased by 22% (P = 0.02), with no significant change in IGFBP-3 levels after T vs. placebo. We conclude that low-dose T supplementation for 26 wk increases spontaneous nocturnal GH secretion and morning serum IGF-I concentrations in healthy older men.

Nathan L et al. Testosterone inhibits early atherogenesis by conversion to estradiol: critical role of aromatase. Proc Natl Acad Sci U S A. 2001 Mar 13;98(6):3589-93 The effects of testosterone on early atherogenesis and the role of aromatase, an enzyme that converts testosterone to estrogens, were assessed in low density lipoprotein receptor-deficient male mice fed a Western diet. Castration of male mice increased the extent of fatty streak lesion formation in the aortic origin compared with testes-intact animals. Administration of anastrazole, a selective aromatase inhibitor, to testes-intact males increased lesion formation to the same extent as that observed with orchidectomized animals. Testosterone supplementation of orchidectomized animals reduced lesion formation when compared with orchidectomized animals receiving the placebo. This attenuating effect of testosterone was not observed when the animals were treated simultaneously with the aromatase inhibitor. The beneficial effects of testosterone on early atherogenesis were not explained by changes in lipid levels. Estradiol administration to orchidectomized males attenuated lesion formation to the same extent as testosterone administration. Aromatase was expressed in the aorta of these animals as assessed by reverse transcription-PCR and immunohistochemistry. These results indicate that testosterone attenuates early atherogenesis most likely by being converted to estrogens by the enzyme aromatase expressed in the vessel wall.

Oettel M et al. Progesterone: the forgotten hormone in men? Aging Male. 2004 Sep; 7(3):236-57 'Classical' genomic progesterone receptors appear relatively late in phylogenesis, i.e. it is only in birds and mammals that they are detectable. In the different species, they mediate manifold effects regarding the differentiation of target organ functions, mainly in the reproductive system. Surprisingly, we know little about the physiology, endocrinology, and pharmacology of progesterone and progestins in male gender or men respectively, despite the fact that, as to progesterone secretion and serum progesterone levels, there are no great quantitative differences between men and women (at least outside the luteal phase). In a prospective cohort study of 1026 men with and without cardiovascular disease, we were not able to demonstrate any age-dependent change in serum progesterone concentrations. Progesterone influences spermiogenesis, sperm capacitation/acrosome reaction and testosterone biosynthesis in the Leydig cells. Other progesterone effects in men include those on the central nervous system (CNS) (mainly mediated by 5alpha-reduced progesterone metabolites as so-called neurosteroids), including blocking of gonadotropin secretion, sleep improvement, and effects on tumors in the CNS (meningioma, fibroma), as well as effects on the immune system, cardiovascular system, kidney function, adipose tissue, behavior, and respiratory system. A progestin may stimulate weight gain and appetite in men as well as in women. The detection of progesterone receptor isoforms would have a highly diagnostic value in prostate pathology (benign prostatic hypertrophy and prostate cancer). The modulation of progesterone effects on typical male targets is connected with a great pharmacodynamic variability. The reason for this is that, in men, some important effects of progesterone are mediated non-genomically through different molecular biological modes of action. Therefore, the precise therapeutic manipulation of progesterone actions in the male requires completely new endocrine-pharmacological approaches.

Padero MC et al. Androgen supplementation in older women: too much hype, not enough data. J Am Geriatr Soc 2002 Jun; 50(6):1131-40 Androgen supplementation in women has received enormous attention in the scientific and lay communities. That it enhances some aspects of cognitive function, sexual function, muscle mass, strength, and sense of well-being is not in question. What is not known is whether physiological testosterone replacement can improve health-related outcome in older women without its virilizing side effects. Although it is assumed that the testosterone dose-response relationship is different in women than in men and that clinically relevant outcomes on the above-mentioned effects can be achieved at lower testosterone doses, these assumptions have not been tested rigorously. Androgen deficiency has no clear-cut definition. Clinical features may include impaired sexual function, low energy, depression, and a total testosterone level of less than 15 ng/dL, the lower end of the normal range. Measurement of free testosterone is ideal, because it provides a better estimate of the biologically relevant fraction. It is not widely used in clinical practice, because some methods of measuring free testosterone assay are hampered by methodological difficulties. In marked contrast to the abrupt decline in estrogen and progesterone production at menopause, serum testosterone is lower in older women than in menstruating women, with the decline becoming apparent a decade before menopause. This article reviews testosterone's effects on sexual function, cognitive function, muscle mass, body composition, and immune function in postmenopausal women.

Pantuck AJ et al. Phase II Study of Pomegranate Juice for Men with Rising Prostate-Specific Antigen following Surgery or Radiation for Prostate Cancer.Clin Cancer Res. 2006 Jul 1;12(13):4018-4026 PURPOSE: Phytochemicals in plants may have cancer preventive benefits through antioxidation and via gene-nutrient interactions. We sought to determine the effects of pomegranate juice (a major source of antioxidants) consumption on prostate-specific antigen (PSA) progression in men with a rising PSA following primary therapy.
EXPERIMENTAL DESIGN: A phase II, Simon two-stage clinical trial for men with rising PSA after surgery or radiotherapy was conducted. Eligible patients had a detectable PSA > 0.2 and < 5 ng/mL and Gleason score < or = 7. Patients were treated with 8 ounces of pomegranate juice daily (Wonderful variety, 570 mg total polyphenol gallic acid equivalents) until disease progression. Clinical end points included safety and effect on serum PSA, serum-induced proliferation and apoptosis of LNCaP cells, serum lipid peroxidation, and serum nitric oxide levels.RESULTS: The study was fully accrued after efficacy criteria were met. There were no serious adverse events reported and the treatment was well tolerated. Mean PSA doubling time significantly increased with treatment from a mean of 15 months at baseline to 54 months posttreatment (P < 0.001). In vitro assays comparing pretreatment and posttreatment patient serum on the growth of LNCaP showed a 12% decrease in cell proliferation and a 17% increase in apoptosis (P = 0.0048 and 0.0004, respectively), a 23% increase in serum nitric oxide (P = 0.0085), and significant (P < 0.02) reductions in oxidative state and sensitivity to oxidation of serum lipids after versus before pomegranate juice consumption.CONCLUSIONS: We report the first clinical trial of pomegranate juice in patients with prostate cancer. The statistically significant prolongation of PSA doubling time, coupled with corresponding laboratory effects on prostate cancer in vitro cell proliferation and apoptosis as well as oxidative stress, warrant further testing in a placebo-controlled study.

Phillips GB Relationship between serum sex hormones and coronary artery disease in postmenopausal women. Arterioscler Thromb Vasc Biol. 1997 Apr; 17(4):695-701

Although sex hormones appear to be importantly involved in the development of coronary heart disease, apparently no study has yet reported an alteration in an endogenous sex hormone level in relation to coronary heart disease in women. In an attempt to determine whether any sex hormone abnormality might be a factor in the development of myocardial infarction in women, estradiol and testosterone, as well as sex hormone-binding globulin, insulin, dehydroepiandrosterone sulfate, and risk factors for myocardial infarction, were measured in relation to the degree of coronary artery disease (CAD) in 60 postmenopausal women undergoing coronary angiography. In a multiple-regression analysis with the degree of CAD as the dependent variable and free testosterone (FT), estradiol, age, body mass index, systolic blood pressure, cholesterol, smoking, and insulin as independent variables in the model, only FT ($P < .008$) and cholesterol ($P = .01$) were significantly related to the degree of CAD, both positively. To exclude a possible confounding effect due to prior myocardial infarction, the multiple-regression analysis was repeated for the subgroup of 49 patients remaining after excluding the 11 patients who had ever had a myocardial infarction; again only FT ($P < .04$) and cholesterol ($P = .05$) were significantly related to the degree of CAD. Neither total testosterone in place of FT nor HDL cholesterol in place of total cholesterol in the model was significantly related to CAD. Sex hormone-binding globulin and dehydroepiandrosterone sulfate, added individually to the model, showed no significant relationship to CAD. These results raise the possibility that in women an elevated FT level may be a risk factor for coronary atherosclerosis.

Phillips GB. Is atherosclerotic cardiovascular disease an endocrinological disorder? The estrogen-androgen paradox. J Clin Endocrinol Metab. 2005 May;90(5):2708-11 The strikingly lower incidence of myocardial infarction (MI) in premenopausal women than in men of the same age suggests an important role for sex hormones in the etiology of MI. Supporting such a role are studies, carried out mostly in men, that report abnormalities of sex hormone levels in patients with MI, correlations of sex hormone levels with degree of atherosclerosis and with levels of risk factors for MI, and changes in the levels of risk factors with administration of sex hormones. Studies have also reported a prospective relationship in men of testosterone level with progression of atherosclerosis, accumulation of visceral adipose tissue, and other risk factors for MI. Puzzling, however, is that neither the level of testosterone nor of estrogen was found to be predictive of coronary events in any of the eight prospective studies that have been carried out. Also puzzling is that whereas the gender difference in incidence of MI would suggest that testosterone promotes and/or estrogen prevents MI, the cross- sectional, hormone administration, and prospective studies have suggested that in men testosterone may prevent and estrogen promote MI. These studies have thus revealed an estrogen-androgen paradox: that endogenous sex hormones may relate both to atherosclerotic cardiovascular disease and its risk factors oppositely in women and men. Recently recognized experiments of nature and their knockout mouse models may present another manifestation of this estrogen-androgen paradox and could help resolve these apparent contradictions.

Prehn RT. On the prevention and therapy of prostate cancer by androgen administration. Cancer Res 1999 Sep 1; 59(17):4161-4 It has been widely suggested that elevated androgen levels may be critically involved in the genesis of prostate cancer. Despite the dependency of the normal prostate and of most prostatic cancers upon androgens and the fact that tumors can be produced in some rodent models by androgen administration, I will argue that, contrary to prevalent opinion, declining rather than high levels of androgens probably contribute more to human prostate carcinogenesis and that androgen supplementation would probably lower the incidence of the disease. I will also consider the possibility that the growth of androgen-independent prostate cancers might be reduced by the administration of androgens.

Rao et al. Effect of testosterone on threshold of pain.Indian J Physiol Pharmacol. 1981 Oct-Dec; 25(4):387-8. Pain threshold for thermal stimulus was studied in male albino rats before and after three days of treatment with testosterone. It was also determined 15 days after castration and three days after testosterone treatment of castrated rats. There was a significant reduction in pain threshold after testosterone treatment and a marked increase in pain threshold after castration. This increase disappeared after administration of testosterone to the castrated rats.

Rosano GM et al. Acute anti-ischemic effect of testosterone in men with coronary artery disease. Circulation 1999 Apr 6; 99(13):1666-70 BACKGROUND: The role of testosterone on the development of coronary artery disease in men is controversial. The evidence that men have a greater incidence of coronary artery disease than women of a similar age suggests a possible causal role of testosterone. Conversely, recent studies have shown that the hormone improves endothelium-dependent relaxation of coronary arteries in men. Accordingly, the aim of the present study was to evaluate the effect of acute administration of testosterone on exercise-induced myocardial ischemia in men. METHODS AND RESULTS: After withdrawal of antianginal therapy, 14 men (mean age, 58+/-4 years) with coronary artery disease underwent 3 exercise tests according to the modified Bruce protocol on 3 different days (baseline and either testosterone or placebo given in a random order). The exercise tests were performed 30 minutes after administration of testosterone (2.5 mg IV in 5 minutes) or placebo. All patients showed at least 1-mm ST-segment depression during the baseline exercise test and after placebo, whereas only 10 patients had a positive exercise test after testosterone. Chest pain during exercise was reported by 12 patients during baseline and placebo exercise tests and by 8 patients after testosterone. Compared with placebo, testosterone increased time to 1-mm ST-segment depression (579+/-204 versus 471+/-210 seconds; P<0. 01) and total exercise time (631+/-180 versus 541+/-204 seconds; P<0. 01). Testosterone significantly increased heart rate at the onset of 1-mm ST-segment depression (135+/-12 versus 123+/-14 bpm; P<0.01) and at peak exercise (140+/-12 versus 132+/-12 bpm; P<0.01) and the rate-pressure product at the onset of 1-mm ST-segment depression (24 213+/-3750 versus 21 619+/-3542 mm Hgxbpm; P<0.05) and at peak exercise (26 746+/-3109 versus 22 527+/-5443 mm Hgxbpm; P<0.05). CONCLUSIONS: Short-term administration of testosterone induces a beneficial effect on exercise-induced myocardial ischemia in men with coronary artery disease. This effect may be related to a direct coronary-relaxing effect.

Sarosdy MF. Testosterone replacement for hypogonadism after treatment of early prostate cancer with brachytherapy. Cancer. 2007 Feb 1;109(3):536-41 BACKGROUND: Controversy and a notable paucity of published clinical data best characterize the current knowledge of testosterone-replacement therapy (TRT) for hypogonadism after treatment for early, localized prostate cancer. The objective of this study was to assess the risk of biochemical failure with TRT after treatment of early prostate cancer with permanent transperineal brachytherapy with or without external beam therapy in patients with low serum levels of testosterone and clinical symptoms of hypogonadism.METHODS: Patients who underwent prostate brachytherapy from 1996 to 2004 and received subsequent TRT for symptomatic hypogonadism were reviewed to detail cancer characteristics and treatment as well as pre- and post-TRT serum testosterone and prostate-specific antigen (PSA) values.
RESULTS: Thirty-one men received TRT after prostate brachytherapy for 0.5 to 8.5 years (median, 4.5 years), with a follow-up that ranged from 1.5 years to 9.0 years (median, 5.0 years) postbrachytherapy. TRT was started from 0.5 years to 4.5 years (median, 2.0 years) after brachytherapy. Serum total testosterone levels ranged from 30 ng/dL to 255 ng/dL (median, 188 ng/dL) before TRT and rose to 365 ng/dL to 1373 ng/dL (median, 498 ng/dL) on TRT. Transient rises in PSA were observed in 1 patient. The most recent PSA level was <0.1 ng/mL in 23 patients (74.2%), <0.5 ng/mL in 30 patients (96.7%), and <1 ng/mL in 31 patients (100%). No patients stopped TRT because of cancer recurrence or documented cancer progression.
CONCLUSIONS: For patients with low serum testosterone levels and symptoms of hypogonadism, TRT may be used with caution and close follow-up after prostate brachytherapy.

Schmidt M, Renner C, Loffler G. Progesterone inhibits glucocorticoid-dependent aromatase induction in human adipose fibroblasts. J Endocrinol. 1998 Sep;158(3):401-7 In fibroblasts derived from human adipose tissue, aromatase induction is observed after exposure to 1 microM cortisol in the presence of serum or platelet-derived growth factor (PDGF). Progesterone suppresses this induction in a dose-dependent manner, 10 microM resulting in complete inhibition. A reduced cortisol concentration (0.1 microM) concomitantly reduces the progesterone concentration required for effective inhibition (10-100 nM). This effect of progesterone is specific, as neither the release of cellular enzymes nor aromatase induction by dibutyryl-cAMP, which acts independently from cortisol, are affected. However, the inhibitory effect of progesterone requires its presence throughout the induction period. Kinetic studies in intact cells reveal a reduced number of aromatase active sites upon progesterone treatment, whereas progesterone at near-physiological concentration (100 nM) does not inhibit aromatase activity in isolated microsomes. Semi-quantitative reverse transcriptase PCR analysis shows reduced amounts of aromatase mRNA in progesterone-treated cells, indicating specific inhibition of the glucocorticoid-dependent pathway of aromatase induction. The inhibitory effect of progesterone is not blocked by the anti-progestin ZK114043, excluding action via progesterone receptors and indicating competition for the glucocorticoid receptor. Progesterone must be considered a potential physiological inhibitor of glucocorticoid-dependent aromatase induction in adipose tissue. It is proposed that it is a suppressor of aromatase induction in adipose tissue in premenopausal women.

Schmidt M et al. Androgen conversion in osteoarthritis and rheumatoid arthritis synoviocytes--androstenedione and testosterone inhibit estrogen formation and favor production of more potent 5alpha-reduced androgens. Arthritis Res Ther. 2005; 7(5):R938-48. In synovial cells of patients with osteoarthritis (OA) and rheumatoid arthritis (RA), conversion products of major anti-inflammatory androgens are as yet unknown but may be proinflammatory. Therefore, therapy with androgens in RA could be a problem. This study was carried out in order to compare conversion products of androgens in RA and OA synoviocytes. In 26 OA and 24 RA patients, androgen conversion in synovial cells was investigated using radiolabeled substrates and analysis by thin-layer chromatography and HPLC. Aromatase expression was studied by immunohistochemistry. Dehydroepiandrosterone (DHEA) was converted into androstenediol, androstenedione (ASD), 16alphaOH-DHEA, 7alphaOH-DHEA, testosterone, estrone (E1), estradiol (E2), estriol (E3), and 16alphaOH-testosterone (similar in OA and RA). Surprisingly, levels of E2, E3, and 16alpha-hydroxylated steroids were as high as levels of testosterone. In RA and OA, 5alpha-dihydrotestosterone increased conversion of DHEA into testosterone but not into estrogens. The second androgen, ASD, was converted into 5alpha-dihydro-ASD, testosterone, and negligible amounts of E1, E2, E3, or 16alphaOH-testosterone. 5alpha-dihydro-ASD levels were higher in RA than OA. The third androgen, testosterone, was converted into ASD, 5alpha-dihydro-ASD, 5alpha-dihydrotestosterone, and negligible quantities of E1 and E2. 5alpha-dihydrotestosterone was higher in RA than OA. ASD and testosterone nearly completely blocked aromatization of androgens. In addition, density of aromatase-positive cells and concentration of released E2, E3, and free testosterone from superfused synovial tissue was similar in RA and OA but estrogens were markedly higher than free testosterone. In conclusion, ASD and testosterone might be favorable anti-inflammatory compounds because they decrease aromatization and increase anti-inflammatory 5alpha-reduced androgens. In contrast, DHEA did not block aromatization but yielded high levels of estrogens and proproliferative 16alpha-hydroxylated steroids. Androgens were differentially converted to pro- and anti-inflammatory steroid hormones via diverse pathways.

Schubert M et al. Intramuscular testosterone undecanoate: pharmacokinetic aspects of a novel testosterone formulation during long-term treatment of men with hypogonadism. J Clin Endocrinol Metab. 2004 Nov; 89(11):5429-34. In an open-label, randomized, prospective trial, we investigated pharmacokinetics and several efficacy and safety parameters of a novel, long-acting testosterone (T) undecanoate (TU) formulation in 40 hypogonadal men (serum testosterone concentrations < 5 nmol/liter). For the first 30 wk (comparative study), the patients were randomly assigned to receive either 10 x 250 mg T enanthate (TE) im every 3 wk (n = 20) or 3 x 1000 mg TU im every 6 wk (loading dose) followed by 1 x 1000 mg after an additional 9 wk (n = 20). In a follow-up study, observation continued in those patients who completed the comparative part and opted for TU treatment (8 x 1000 mg TU every 12 wk in former TU patients and 2 x 1000 mg TU every 8 wk plus 6 x 1000 mg every 12 wk in former TE patients) for an additional 20-21 months. Here we report only the pharmacokinetic aspects of the new TU formulation for the first approximately 2.5 yr of treatment. At baseline, serum T concentrations did not significantly differ between the two study groups. In the TE group, mean trough levels of serum T were always less than 10 nmol/liter before the next injection, whereas in the TU group, mean trough levels of serum T were 14.1 +/- 4.5 nmol/liter after the first two doses (6-wk intervals) and 16.3 +/- 5.7 nmol/liter after the 9-wk interval at wk 30. The mean serum levels of dihydrotestosterone and estradiol also increased in parallel to the serum T pattern and remained within the normal range. In the follow-up study, the former TU patients (n = 20) received eight TU injections at 12-wk intervals, and the TE patients (n = 16) switched to TU and initially received two TU injections at 8-wk intervals (loading) and continued with six TU injections at 12-wk intervals (maintenance). This regimen resulted in stable mean serum trough levels of T (ranging from 14.9 +/- 5.2 to 16.5 +/- 8.0 nmol/liter) and estradiol (ranging from 98.5 +/- 45.2 to 80.4 +/- 14.4 pmol/liter). The present study has shown that 1000 mg TU injected into male patients with hypogonadism at 12-wk intervals is well tolerated and leads to T levels within normal ranges, using four instead of 17 or more TE injections per year. An initial loading dose of either 3 x 1000 mg TU every 6 wk at the beginning of hormone substitution or 2 x 1000 mg TU every 8 wk after switching from the short-acting TE to TU were found to be a adequate dosing regimens for starting of treatment with the long-acting TU preparation.

Shores MM et al. Low serum testosterone and mortality in male veterans. Arch Intern Med. 2006 Aug 14; 166(15):1660-5

BACKGROUND: Low serum testosterone is a common condition in aging associated with decreased muscle mass and insulin resistance. This study evaluated whether low testosterone levels are a risk factor for mortality in male veterans. METHODS: We used a clinical database to identify men older than 40 years with repeated testosterone levels obtained from October 1, 1994, to December 31, 1999, and without diagnosed prostate cancer. A low testosterone level was a total testosterone level of less than 250 ng/dL (<8.7 nmol/L) or a free testosterone level of less than 0.75 ng/dL (<0.03 nmol/L). Men were classified as having a low testosterone level (166 [19.3%]), an equivocal testosterone level (equal number of low and normal levels) (240 [28.0%]), or a normal testosterone level (452 [52.7%]). The risk for all-cause mortality was estimated using Cox proportional hazards regression models, adjusting for demographic and clinical covariates over a follow-up of up to 8 years. RESULTS: Mortality in men with normal testosterone levels was 20.1% (95% confidence interval [CI], 16.2%-24.1%) vs 24.6% (95% CI, 19.2%-30.0%) in men with equivocal testosterone levels and 34.9% (95% CI, 28.5%-41.4%) in men with low testosterone levels. After adjusting for age, medical morbidity, and other clinical covariates, low testosterone levels continued to be associated with increased mortality (hazard ratio, 1.88; 95% CI, 1.34-2.63; P<.001) while equivocal testosterone levels were not significantly different from normal testosterone levels (hazard ratio, 1.38; 95% CI, 0.99%-1.92%; P=.06). In a sensitivity analysis, men who died within the first year (50 [5.8%]) were excluded to minimize the effect of acute illness, and low testosterone levels continued to be associated with elevated mortality. CONCLUSIONS: Low testosterone levels were associated with increased mortality in male veterans. Further prospective studies are needed to examine the association between low testosterone levels and mortality.

Sinha-Hikim I et al. Effects of testosterone supplementation on skeletal muscle fiber hypertrophy and satellite cells in community-dwelling older men. J Clin Endocrinol Metab. 2006 Aug; 91(8):3024-33.

OBJECTIVE: In this study, we determined the effects of graded doses of testosterone on muscle fiber cross-sectional area (CSA) and satellite cell number and replication in older men. PARTICIPANTS: Healthy men, 60-75 yr old, received a long-acting GnRH agonist to suppress endogenous testosterone production and 25, 50, 125, 300, or 600 mg testosterone enanthate im weekly for 20 wk. METHODS: Immunohistochemistry, light and confocal microscopy, and electron microscopy were used to perform fiber typing and quantitate myonuclear and satellite cell number in vastus lateralis biopsies, obtained before and after 20 wk of treatment. RESULTS: Testosterone administration in older men was associated with dose-dependent increases in CSA of both types I and II fibers.

Satellite cell number increased dose dependently at the three highest doses (3% at baseline vs. 6.2, 9.2, and 13.0% at 125, 300, and 600 mg doses, P < 0.05). Testosterone administration was associated with an increase in the number of proliferating cell nuclear antigen+ satellite cells (1.8% at baseline vs. 3.9, 7.5, and 13% at 125, 300, and 600 mg doses, P < 0.005). The expression of activated Notch, examined only in the 300-mg group (baseline, 2.3 vs. 9.0% after treatment, P < 0.005), increased in satellite cells after testosterone treatment. The expression of myogenin (baseline, 6.2 vs. 20.7% after treatment, P < 0.005), examined only in the 300-mg group, increased significantly in muscle fiber nuclei after testosterone treatment, but Numb expression did not change. CONCLUSIONS: Older men respond to graded doses of testosterone with a dose-dependent increase in muscle fiber CSA and satellite cell number. Testosterone-induced skeletal muscle hypertrophy in older men is associated with increased satellite cell replication and activation.

Stattin P et al. High levels of circulating testosterone are not associated with increased prostate cancer risk: a pooled prospective study. Int J Cancer. 2004 Jan 20; 108(3):418-24

Androgens stimulate prostate cancer in vitro and in vivo. However, evidence from epidemiologic studies of an association between circulating levels of androgens and prostate cancer risk has been inconsistent. We investigated the association of serum levels of testosterone, the principal androgen in circulation, and sex hormone-binding globulin (SHBG) with risk in a case-control study nested in cohorts in Finland, Norway and Sweden of 708 men who were diagnosed with prostate cancer after blood collection and among 2,242 men who were not. In conditional logistic regression analyses, modest but significant decreases in risk were seen for increasing levels of total testosterone down to odds ratio for top vs. bottom quintile of 0.80 (95% CI = 0.59-1.06; p(trend) = 0.05); for SHBG, the corresponding odds ratio was 0.76 (95% CI = 0.57-1.01; p(trend) = 0.07). For free testosterone, calculated from total testosterone and SHBG, a bell-shaped risk pattern was seen with a decrease in odds ratio for top vs. bottom quintile of 0.82 (95% CI = 0.60-1.14; p (trend) = 0.44). No support was found for the hypothesis that high levels of circulating androgens within a physiologic range stimulate development and growth of prostate cancer.

Svartberg J. Epidemiology: testosterone and the metabolic syndrome.

Int J Impot Res. 2006 Jul 20 Low levels of testosterone, hypogonadism, have several common features with the metabolic syndrome. In the Tromso Study, a population-based health survey, testosterone levels were inversely associated with anthropometrical measurements, and the lowest levels of total and free testosterone were found in men with the most pronounced central obesity. Total testosterone was inversely associated with systolic blood pressure, and men with hypertension had lower levels of both total and free testosterone. Furthermore, men with diabetes had lower testosterone levels compared to men without a history of diabetes, and an inverse association

120

between testosterone levels and glycosylated hemoglobin was found. Thus, there are strong associations between low levels of testosterone and the different components of the metabolic syndrome. In addition, an independent association between low testosterone levels and the metabolic syndrome itself has recently been presented in both cross-sectional and prospective population-based studies. Thus, testosterone may have a protective role in the development of metabolic syndrome and subsequent diabetes mellitus and cardiovascular disease in aging men. However, clinical trials are needed to confirm this assumption.

Tan RS A pilot study on the effects of testosterone in hypogonadal aging male patients with Alzheimer's disease. Aging Male. 2003 Mar; 6(1):13-7. The male aging process brings about declines in hormonal function including a gradual decline in bioavailable testosterone levels. Animal studies suggest that testosterone modulates cognitive function through enhancing acetylcholine release and up-modulation of nicotinic receptors. Tau protein deposition is also affected by androgen supplementation in animals. We hypothesize that testosterone replacement in elderly hypogonadal males may improve cognition, in particular the visual-spatial domain. Thirty-six male patients with a new diagnosis of Alzheimer's disease had their total and bioavailable testosterone levels measured. None of the patients had been on acetylcholinesterase inhibitors. Ten of the 36 patients (28%) were deemed biochemically hypogonadal (total testosterone < 240 ng/dl or 7 nmol/l). Five of the hypogonadal patients were randomized to testosterone and five to placebo. Initial Alzheimer's Disease Assessment Scale cognitive subscale (ADAScog) and Mini Mental Status Examination (MMSE) ranged from 31 to 19 and from 17 to 22, respectively. The clock drawing test (CDT) and the pentagon-tracing portion of the MMSE were used as measures of visual-spatial abilities. Normal prostate-specific antigen (PSA) levels were essential before treatment with intramuscular testosterone, 200 mg every 2 weeks. Measurement of testosterone, complete blood count, lipids, PSA and neuropsychological cognitive tests were repeated at 3, 6, 9 and 12 months of treatment. In the testosterone-treated group, levels of total testosterone increased from a mean of 126.4 ng/dl to 341 ng/dl or 3.6 nmol/l to 9.7 nmol/l (p = 0.11). Bioavailable testosterone also increased from a mean of 48.7 ng/dl to 142 ng/dl or 1.39 nmol/l to 4.05 nmol/l (p = 0.10). PSA levels were also elevated from a mean of 0.98 to 1.37 ng/ml (p = 0.07). ADAScog improved from a mean of 25 to 16.3 (p = 0.02); MMSE improved from a mean of 19.4 to 23.2 (p = 0.02), CDT also improved from 2.2 to 3.2 (p = 0.07). One patient stopped treatment because of hypersexual behavior. The placebo-treated group deteriorated gradually. This small pilot study performed in aging male patients suggests that testosterone could indeed improve cognition, including visual-spatial skills in mild to moderate Alzheimer's disease.

Tilakaratne A, Soory M. Effects of the anti-androgen finasteride on 5 alpha-reduction of androgens in the presence of progesterone in human gingival fibroblasts. J Periodontal Res.

2000 Aug; 35(4):179-85. Oestrogens and androgens stimulate collagen matrix synthesis, while progesterone is a competitive inhibitor for the 5 alpha-reduction of testosterone to 5 alpha-dihydrotestosterone (DHT). The anti-androgen finasteride is a specific inhibitor of the 5 alpha-reductase type 2 isoenzyme, associated with anabolic functions. The aim of this investigation is to study the effects of progesterone and finasteride on 5 alpha-reduction of androgen substrates by human gingival fibroblasts. Monolayer cultures of human gingival fibroblasts (HGF) of the 4th 9th passage were established in Eagle's minimum essential medium (MEM). Duplicate incubations were performed with 14C-testosterone/14C-4-androstenedione as substrates and progesterone (P) or finasteride (F), at concentrations of 0.5, 1, 3 and 5 microg/ml, alone and in combination, for 24 h. Similarly, the effects of the alkaline phosphatase inhibitor levamisole (L, 30 microg/ml) and P were studied. Steroid metabolites were analysed and quantified, using a radioisotope scanner. Progesterone inhibited DHT synthesis in HGF from 14C-testosterone by 24-62% (n = 8; p < 0.01). Finasteride caused 59 82% inhibition (n=8; p<0.01). The combination of P+F showed a similar degree of inhibition (68-78%) of DHT synthesis to that of F alone (n = 8; p<0.01). There was 35-56% stimulation of 17beta-HSD (hydroxysteroid dehydrogenase) activity by P, F and P + F (n = 8; p < 0.01). When 14C-4-androstenedione was used as substrate there was 47% inhibition of 5 alpha-reductase activity at higher concentrations of P and 63 and 44% stimulation at 0.5 and 1 microg/ml (n = 8; p < 0.01). F and P + F caused 40-67% inhibition of this activity. P, F and P + F caused 2-2.7-fold stimulation of 17beta-HSD activity in response to all concentrations studied. L inhibited DHT synthesis from both substrates by 36-38%, with further inhibition of 55-70% (n = 4; p < 0.01), with P; this is suggestive of ligand-independent alkaline phosphatase activity mediated by 5 alpha-reductase. Inhibition of 5 alpha-reductase activity by finasteride in gingival fibroblasts is suggestive of target tissue anabolic functions in gingivae and competitive inhibition by progesterone, is suggestive of regulation of hormone mediated tissue responses during repair.

Travison TG et al. A population-level decline in serum testosterone levels in American men. J Clin Endocrinol Metab. 2006 Oct 24 CONTEXT: Age-specific estimates of mean testosterone (T) concentrations appear to vary by year of observation and by birth cohort, and estimates of longitudinal declines in T typically outstrip cross-sectional decreases. These observations motivate a hypothesis of a population-level decrease in T over calendar time, independent of chronological aging. OBJECTIVE: The goal of this study was to establish the magnitude of population-level changes in serum T concentrations and the degree to which they are explained by secular changes in relative weight and other factors. DESIGN: We describe a prospective cohort study of health and endocrine functioning in randomly selected men of age 45-79 yr. We provide three data collection waves: baseline (T1: 1987-1999) and two follow-ups (T2: 1995-1997, T3: 2002-2004). SETTING: This was an observational study of randomly selected men residing in greater Boston, Massachusetts. PARTICIPANTS: Data obtained from 1374, 906, and 489 men at T1, T2, and T3, respectively, totaling 2769 observations taken on 1532 men. MAIN OUTCOME MEASURES: The main outcome measures were serum total T and calculated bioavailable T. RESULTS: We observe a substantial age-independent decline in T that does not appear to be attributable to observed changes in explanatory factors, including health and lifestyle characteristics such as smoking and obesity. The estimated population-level declines are greater in magnitude than the cross-sectional declines in T typically associated with age. CONCLUSIONS: These results indicate that recent years have seen a substantial, and as yet unrecognized, age-independent population-level decrease in T in American men, potentially attributable to birth cohort differences or to health or environmental effects not captured in observed data.

Tsujimura A et al. Treatment with human chorionic gonadotropin for PADAM: a preliminary report. Aging Male. 2005 Sep-Dec; 8(3-4):175-9 The purpose of this study was to evaluate the efficacy and safety of human chorionic gonadotropin (hCG) for patients with partial androgen deficiency of the aging male (PADAM). Twenty-one patients over 50 years of age with PADAM symptoms were included in this study. Laboratory and endocrinologic profiles were reviewed as appropriate, and PADAM symptoms were judged by means of several questionnaires such as the Aging Males' Symptoms (AMS) scale, short version of the International Index of Erectile Function (IIEF-5), and the Self-rating Depression Scale (SDS). Laboratory and endocrinologic values and symptom scores were evaluated and compared before and after treatment by hCG injection. The treatment period was 8.0 +/- 5.0 months (3.0-24.0 months). Serum concentrations of testosterone, including total testosterone, calculated free testosterone, and calculated bioavailable testosterone, increased significantly. AMS total scores and subscores decreased significantly after treatment. However, IIEF-5 and SDS scores did not improve. With respect to adverse effects, laboratory tests showed that only red blood cell count, hematocrit and hemoglobin level increased significantly after treatment; however, these values remained within the normal range. No adverse effect was identified after treatment. We conclude that hCG injection may be considered as a treatment for PADAM.

Turhan S et al. The association between androgen levels and premature coronary artery disease in men. Coron Artery Dis. 2007 May; 18(3):159-62. OBJECTIVE: The relationship between androgens and the risk of development of coronary artery disease has not been clarified well. This study was planned to determine the relationship between serum androgen levels and premature development of coronary artery disease in men.METHODS: Sixty-nine men below 45 years of age with documented coronary artery disease (mean age 41.0+/-4.7) constituted the study group. Control group consisted of 56 men with similar age and normal coronary angiograms (mean age 41.3+/-3.8). Total and free testosterone, estradiol, and fasting plasma total, low-density lipoprotein, and high-density lipoprotein cholesterol, and triglyceride levels were measured, and compared between the two groups.RESULTS: Mean age, body mass index, and the frequency of hypertension were similar between the two groups; however, diabetes mellitus, smoking, hyperlipidemia, and family history of coronary artery disease were more frequent in the coronary artery disease group. Total and free testosterone levels of the patients with coronary artery disease were significantly lower than those of controls, whereas estradiol levels did not differ. Multivariate logistic regression analysis revealed that free testosterone levels (P=0.014; odds ratio=0.90; 95% confidence interval=0.87-0.99), hyperlipidemia (P<0.001; odds ratio=8.2; 95% confidence interval=3.17-21.0), and smoking (P=0.026; odds ratio=3.12; 95% confidence interval=1.15-8.48) were independent predictors of premature coronary artery disease. Moreover, using receiver operating characteristic analysis, patients with free testosterone levels below the cut-off value of 17.3 pg/ml had an adjusted 3.3-fold risk of developing premature coronary artery disease compared to those with free testosterone levels above the cut-off level (odds ratio=3.3; 95% confidence interval=1.57-6.87).CONCLUSION: A low level of free testosterone may be related to the development of premature coronary artery disease.

Turna B et al. Women with low libido: correlation of decreased androgen levels with female sexual function index. Int J Impot Res. 2004 Dec 09 The aim of the present study was to investigate a possible correlation between decreased androgen levels and female sexual function index (FSFI) in women with low libido and compare these findings with normal age-matched subjects. In total, 20 premenopausal women with low libido (mean age 36.7; range 24-51 y) and 20 postmenopausal women with low libido (mean age 54; 45-70 y), and 20 premenopausal healthy women (mean age 32.2; range 21-51 y) and 20 postmenopausal healthy women (mean age 53.5; range 48-60 y) as controls were enrolled in the current study. Women with low libido had symptoms for at least 6 months and were in stable relationships. All premenopausal patients had regular menstrual cycles and all postmenopausal patients and controls were on estrogen replacement therapy. None of the patients were taking birth control pills, corticosteroids or had a history of chronic medical illnesses. All completed the FSFI and Beck's Depression Inventory (BDI) questionnaires. Hormones measured included: cortisol; T3, T4 and TSH; estradiol; total and free testosterone; dehydroepiandrosterone sulfate (DHEA-S); sex hormone binding globulin (SHBG). We performed statistical analysis by parametric and nonparametric comparisons and correlations, as appropriate. We found significant differences between the women with low libido and the controls in total testosterone, free testosterone and DHEA-S levels and full-scale FSFI score for both pre- and postmenopausal women (P<0.05). In addition, decreased total testosterone, free testosterone and DHEA-S levels positively correlated with full-scale FSFI score and FSFI-desire, FSFI-arousal, FSFI-lubrication and FSFI-orgasm scores (P<0.05). Our data suggest that women with low libido have lower androgen levels compared to age-matched normal control groups and their decreased androgen levels correlate positively with female sexual function index domains.

van den Beld et al. Measures of bioavailable serum testosterone and estradiol and their relationships with muscle strength, bone density, and body composition in elderly men J Clin Endocrinol Metab 2000 Sep;85(9):3276-82 In the present cross-sectional study of 403 independently living elderly men, we tested the hypothesis that the decreases in bone mass, body composition, and muscle strength with age are related to the fall in circulating endogenous testosterone (T) and estrogen concentrations. We compared various measures of the level of bioactive androgen and estrogen to which tissues are exposed. After exclusion of subjects with severe mobility problems and signs of dementia, 403 healthy men (age, 73-94 yr) were randomly selected from a population-based sample. Total T (TT), free T (FT), estrone (E1), estradiol (E2), and sex hormone-binding globulin (SHBG) were determined by RIA. Levels of non-SHBG-bound T (non-SHBG-T), FT (calc-FT), the TT/SHBG ratio, non-SHBG-bound E2, and free E2 were calculated. Physical characteristics of aging included muscle strength measured using dynamometry, total body bone mineral density (BMD), hip BMD, and body composition, including lean mass and fat mass, measured by dual-energy x-ray absorptiometry. In this population of healthy elderly men, calc-FT, non-SHBG-T, E1, and E2 (total, free, and non-SHBG bound) decreased significantly with age. T (total and non-SHBG-T) was positively related with muscle strength and total body BMD (for non-SHBG-T, respectively, beta = 1.93 +/- 0.52, P < 0.001 and beta = 0.011 +/- 0.002, P < 0.001). An inverse association existed between T and fat mass (beta = -0.53 +/- 0.15, P < 0.001). Non-SHBG-T and calc-FT were more strongly related to muscle strength, BMD, and fat mass than TT and were also significantly related to hip BMD. E1 and E2 were both positively, independently associated with BMD (for E2, beta = 0.21 +/- 0.08, P < 0.01). Non-SHBG-bound E2 was slightly strongly related to BMD than total E2. The positive relation between T and BMD was independent of E2. E1 and E2 were not related with muscle strength or body composition. In summary, bioavailable T, E1, total E2, and bioavailable E2 all decrease with age in healthy old men. In this cross-sectional study in healthy elderly men, non-SHBG-bound T seems to be the best parameter for serum levels of bioactive T, which seems to play a direct role in the various physiological changes that occur during aging. A positive relation with muscle strength and BMD and a negative relation with fat mass was found. In addition, both serum E1 and E2 seem to play a role in the age-related bone loss in elderly men, although the cross-sectional nature of the study precludes a definitive conclusion. Non-SHBG-bound E2 seems to be the best parameter of serum bioactive E2 in describing its positive relation with BMD.

Vermeulen A. Androgens in the aging male. J Clin Endocrinol Metab. 1991. 73:221–224. IN CONTRAST to the situation in women, where the menopause marks the end of the fertile period, in men fertility persists into old age. Nevertheless old age in men is accompanied by clinical signs, such as a decrease in muscle and bone mass, decrease in sexual hair growth, and decreased libido and sexual activity, suggesting decreased virility. These clinical signs are supported by histological evidence for a decreased Leydig mass and function.Evidence for decreased plasma testosterone in elderly men. As to biochemical evidence for decreased androgenicity in elderly men, 25 yr ago the blood production rate of testosterone was reported to be decreased, which at least partially is caused by a decrease of the metabolic clearance. Whether or not aging is also associated with a decrease in plasma testosterone concentrations has long been highly controversial. Indeed, a large series of publications in the 1960s and early 1970s reporting decreased plasma testosterone concentrations in elderly

Vigna GB et al. Testosterone replacement, cardiovascular system and risk factors in the aging male. J Endocrinol Invest. 2005; 28(11 Suppl Proceedings):69-74 Investigations concerning the role of testosterone replacement on cardiovascular risk show conflicting results. Treatments with supraphysiological doses seem detrimental in animal models and men. On the other hand, cross-sectional, prospective and angiographic studies frequently find an inverse, favorable relationship between plasma testosterone and cardiovascular events. Testosterone replacement therapy in the hypogonadic elderly has a positive or at least neutral effect on several coronary disease risk factors. Testosterone appears to decrease LDL-cholesterol without adversely affecting HDL cholesterol, and improve insulin sensibility and the thrombotic/fibrinolytic balance; testosterone does not negatively influence the inflammatory response and arterial wall vasoreactivity. These findings provide a measure of reassurance concerning potential adverse heart effects of testosterone substitutional therapy in older men, even if more specific trials than reported are needed to overcome residual suspicions.

Webb CM et al. Effects of testosterone on coronary vasomotor regulation in men with coronary heart disease. Circulation. 1999 Oct 19; 100(16):1690-6. BACKGROUND: The increased incidence of coronary artery disease in men compared with premenopausal women suggests a detrimental role of male hormones on the cardiovascular system. However, testosterone has direct relaxing effects on coronary arteries in animals, as shown both in vitro and in vivo. The effect of testosterone on the human coronary circulation remains unknown. METHODS AND RESULTS: We studied 13 men (aged 61+/-11 years) with coronary artery disease. They underwent measurement of coronary artery diameter and blood flow after a 3-minute intracoronary infusion of vehicle control (ethanol) followed by 2-minute intracoronary infusions of acetylcholine (10(-7) to 10(-5) mol/L) until peak velocity response. A dose-response curve to 3-minute infusions of testosterone (10(-10) to 10(-7) mol/L) was then determined, and the acetylcholine infusions were repeated. Finally, an intracoronary bolus of isosorbide dinitrate (1000 microgram) was given. Coronary blood flow was calculated from measurements of blood flow velocity using intracoronary Doppler and coronary artery diameter using quantitative coronary angiography. Testosterone significantly increased coronary artery diameter compared with baseline (2.78+/-0. 74 mm versus 2.86+/-0.72 mm [P=0.05], 2.87+/-0.71 mm [P=0.038], and 2.90+/-0.75 mm [P=0.005] for baseline versus testosterone 10(-9) to 10(-7) mol/L, respectively). A significant increase in coronary blood flow occurred at all concentrations of testosterone compared with baseline (geometric mean [95% CI]: 32 [25, 42] versus 36.3 [27, 48] (P=0.006), 35.3 [26, 47] (P=0.029), 36.8 [28, 49] (P=0.002), and 37 [28, 48] (P=0.002), mL/min for baseline versus testosterone 10(-10) to 10(-7) mol/L, respectively). No differences existed in coronary diameter or blood flow responses to acetylcholine before versus after testosterone. CONCLUSIONS: Short-term intracoronary administration of testosterone, at physiological concentrations, induces coronary artery dilatation and increases coronary blood flow in men with established coronary artery disease.

Yeap BB et al. Lower serum testosterone is independently associated with insulin resistance in non-diabetic older men. The Health In Men Study. Eur JEndocrinol. 2009 Aug 18. 2:
OBJECTIVE: Insulin resistance is associated with metabolic syndrome and type 2 diabetes, representing a risk factor for cardiovascular disease. This relationship may be modulated to some extent by age-related changes in sex hormone status. We examined whether lower testosterone or sex hormone-binding globulin (SHBG) levels in older men are associated with insulin resistance independently of measures of central obesity.DESIGN: Cross-sectional analysis of 2470 community-dwelling non-diabetic men aged > or = 70 years.
METHODS: Age, body mass index (BMI) and waist circumference were measured. Early morning sera were assayed for total testosterone, SHBG, LH and insulin levels. Free testosterone was calculated using mass action equations, and insulin resistance was assessed using a homeostatic model (HOMA2-IR).RESULTS: Total testosterone, free testosterone and SHBG declined progressively across increasing quintiles of HOMA2-IR (all P<0.001) and correlated inversely with log HOMA2-IR (r=-0.27, -0.14 and -0.24 respectively, all P<0.001). After adjusting for age, BMI, waist circumference, high-density lipoprotein and triglyceride levels, total testosterone was independently associated with log HOMA2-IR (beta=0.05, P<0.001), while SHBG was not. Serum total testosterone <8 nmol/l was associated with HOMA2-IR in the highest quintile (odds ratio (OR) 1.67, 95% confidence interval (CI) 1.02-2.73) as was total testosterone > or = 8 and <15 nmol/l (OR 1.29, 95% CI 1.03-1.63).CONCLUSIONS: In older men, lower total testosterone is associated with insulin resistance independently of measures of central obesity. This association is seen with testosterone levels in the low to

normal range. Further studies are needed to evaluate interventions that raise testosterone levels in men with reduced insulin sensitivity.

Yeap BB et al.   Lower testosterone levels predict incident stroke and transient ischemic attack in older men. J Clin Endocrinol Metab. 2009 Jul; 94(7):2353-9. CONTEXT: Lower circulating testosterone concentrations are associated with metabolic syndrome, type 2 diabetes, carotid intima-media thickness, and aortic and lower limb arterial disease in men. However, it is unclear whether lower testosterone levels predict major cardiovascular events.OBJECTIVE: We examined whether lower serum testosterone was an independently significant risk factor for symptomatic cerebrovascular events in older men.DESIGN: This was a prospective observational study with median follow-up of 3.5 yr.SETTING: Community-dwelling,   stroke-free   older   men   were studied.PARTICIPANTS: A total of 3443 men at least 70 yr of age participated in the study.MAIN OUTCOME MEASURES: Baseline serum total testosterone, SHBG, and LH were assayed. Free testosterone was calculated using mass action equations. Incident stroke or transient ischemic attack (TIA) was recorded.RESULTS: A first stroke or TIA occurred in 119 men (3.5%). Total and free testosterone concentrations in the lowest quartiles (<11.7 nmol/liter and <222 pmol/liter) were associated with reduced event-free survival (P = 0.014 and P = 0.01, respectively). After adjustment including age, waist-hip ratio, waist circumference, smoking, hypertension, dyslipidemia, and medical comorbidity, lower total testosterone predicted increased incidence of stroke or TIA (hazard ratio = 1.99; 95% confidence interval, 1.33-2.99). Lower free testosterone was also associated (hazard ratio = 1.69; 95% confidence interval, 1.15-2.48), whereas SHBG and LH were not independently associated with incident stroke or TIA.CONCLUSIONS: In older men, lower total testosterone levels predict increased incidence of stroke or TIA after adjusting for conventional risk factors for cardiovascular disease. Men with low-normal testosterone levels had increased risk. Further studies are warranted to determine whether interventions that raise circulating testosterone levels might prevent cerebrovascular disease in men.

Yeap BB et al.   Serum testosterone levels correlate with haemoglobin in middle-aged and older men. Intern Med J. 2008 Aug 16. BACKGROUND: Lower testosterone levels are associated with anaemia in older men and women. The relation between testosterone and haemoglobin (Hb) in younger and middle-aged men is less well defined. The aim of the study was to examine the association between testosterone and Hb levels in men spanning middle to older ages.METHODS: A cross-sectional analysis of 492 men aged 30.7-94.5 years from the Busselton Health Survey, Western Australia, was carried out. Haemoglobin (Hb), early-morning serum total testosterone and sex hormone-binding globulin (SHBG) were measured. Free testosterone was calculated using mass action equations.RESULTS:

Haemoglobin correlated to total and free testosterone concentrations (r= 0.13, P= 0.003 and r= 0.20, P < 0.001, respectively). Hb and SHBG were inversely correlated (r=-0.14, P= 0.001). Hb increased across lowest to highest quartiles of total testosterone (P= 0.02) and free testosterone (P < 0.001), but not SHBG. After adjusting for age, waist circumference, smoking status, alcohol consumption, renal function and ferritin, total testosterone was associated with Hb (beta= 0.037, P= 0.003) as was free testosterone (beta= 2.32, P < 0.001), whereas SHBG was not associated.CONCLUSION: Testosterone concentration modulates Hb levels in community-dwelling men across a wide age range. Further studies are needed to clarify implications of this association between testosterone and Hb in men.

Yeap BB et al. Testosterone and ill-health in aging men. Nat Clin Pract Endocrinol Metab. 2009 Feb; 5(2):113-21. As men age, testosterone levels decline, and decreased testosterone levels are associated with increased risks of osteoporosis, metabolic syndrome, type 2 diabetes mellitus and mortality. Nevertheless, it is still uncertain whether reduced testosterone level is a cause of ill-health or a marker of pre-existing disease, as systemic illness lowers testosterone levels. Most circulating testosterone is bound to sex-hormone-binding globulin (SHBG) and albumin, whereas a small proportion circulates as free testosterone. Decreased SHBG level is associated with increased risks for insulin resistance and metabolic syndrome, although it would also be expected to be associated with increased free testosterone level. During male aging, total and free testosterone levels fall while SHBG level rises. Thus, associations between decreasing androgens and negative health outcomes might differ across men of various ages. Trials of testosterone therapy report benefits for body composition and BMD, but there are limited data on the effect of testosterone supplementation on cardiovascular risk. Whereas men who have androgen deficiency should be considered for testosterone therapy, the role of testosterone supplementation in older men who are not clearly hypogonadal requires further clarification. Further studies are also needed to establish whether the age-related decline in circulating testosterone level in men can be modified or prevented.

Yeap BB et al. Are declining testosterone levels a major risk factor for ill-health in aging men? Int J Impot Res. 2009 Jan-Feb; 21(1):24-36. As men grow older, testosterone levels fall, with a steeper decline in unbound or free testosterone compared with total testosterone concentrations. Lower testosterone levels have been associated with poorer cognitive function, and with impaired general and sexual health in aging men. Recently, lower testosterone levels have been linked with metabolic syndrome and type II diabetes, both conditions associated with cardiovascular disease, and shown to predict higher overall and cardiovascular-related mortality in middle-aged and older men. However, reverse causation has to be considered, as systemic illness may result in reduced testosterone levels. Thus, the strength of these associations and the likely direction of causation need to be carefully considered. Furthermore, these conditions may overlap, for example aging, lower testosterone levels, erectile dysfunction and cardiovascular disease are interrelated. Cross-sectional and longitudinal observational studies may be informative. However, ultimately randomized controlled trials of testosterone therapy are needed to clarify its role in the maintenance of general and sexual health in aging men. Testosterone therapy should be considered in hypogonadal men who meet rigorous criteria for the diagnosis of androgen deficiency. Additional consideration should be given to designing and testing interventions that may prevent or ameliorate the age-related decline in testosterone levels in men.

Yeap BB et al. Healthier lifestyle predicts higher circulating testosterone in older men: the Health In Men Study.   Clin Endocrinol (Oxf). 2009 Mar; 70(3):455-63. OBJECTIVE: Circulating testosterone declines during male ageing, and low testosterone may predispose to ill health. We sought to determine whether greater participation in healthy behaviours predicted reduced risk of subsequent lower circulating testosterone in older men.DESIGN: Cross-sectional analysis of a population-based follow-up study.PARTICIPANTS: A total of 3453 men aged 65-83 years.MEASUREMENTS: Lifestyle score, a tally of eight prudent health-related behaviours, was determined during 1996-99. Early morning sera collected in 2001-04 were assayed for total testosterone, SHBG and LH. Free testosterone was calculated using mass action equations.RESULTS: Mean (+/- SD) time between collection of lifestyle data and blood sampling was 5.7 +/- 0.9 years. Lifestyle score correlated with subsequent total testosterone (r = 0.06, P < 0.001) and SHBG (r = 0.07, P < 0.001), but not free testosterone (r = 0.03, P = 0.08) or LH (r = -0.03, P = 0.12). In multivariate analyses, higher lifestyle scores (4 and above) predicted reduced risk of total testosterone and SHBG in the lowest quartile of values. For the highest category (>or= 7), odds ratio (95% CI) for total testosterone and SHBG in the lowest quartile were 0.37 (0.18-0.77) and 0.26 (0.13-0.54), respectively. Lower lifestyle scores including and excluding body mass index predicted higher risk of total testosterone and SHBG in the lowest quartilesCONCLUSIONS: In men > 65 years old, higher lifestyle score reflecting greater engagement in healthy behaviours predicts higher subsequent total testosterone and SHBG levels. This relationship appears cumulative and may reflect interaction between lifestyle and insulin sensitivity. Successfully promoting healthy behaviours in older men could ameliorate the age-related decline in circulating testosterone.

Yeap BB et al. Luteinizing hormone levels are positively correlated with plasma amyloid-beta protein levels in elderly men. J Alzheimers Dis. 2008 Jun; 14(2):201-8. Dysregulation of the hypothalamic pituitary gonadal (HPG) axis during aging has been associated with increased risk of cognitive decline and developing dementia. Compared to controls, men with Alzheimer's disease (AD) have been shown to have lower serum testosterone levels and higher serum luteinizing hormone (LH) levels. As serum free testosterone concentration is negatively correlated with LH in older men, the independent contributions of these hormones to the pathogenesis of AD warrants further clarification. To explore this notion, we measured plasma amyloid-beta (Abeta), serum testosterone, serum LH and other biochemical parameters in 40 cognitively normal elderly men. Multiple linear regression analysis revealed that serum LH concentration is the only parameter that significantly correlates with plasma Abeta levels in these men (r=0.5, p=0.041). These results suggest that increased serum LH concentration, rather than lower serum free testosterone, is associated with the accumulation of Abeta in plasma. Larger, longitudinal human studies are needed to determine the significance of LH in the pathogenesis of AD.

Yeap BB et al. Lower sex hormone-binding globulin is more strongly associated with metabolic syndrome than lower total testosterone in older men: the Health in Men Study. Eur J Endocrinol. 2008 Jun; 158(6):785-92. BACKGROUND: Reduced circulating testosterone and sex hormone-binding globulin (SHBG) are implicated as risk factors for metabolic syndrome. As SHBG increases with age while testosterone declines, we examined the relative contributions of SHBG and testosterone to the risk of metabolic syndrome in older men.METHODS: We conducted a cross-sectional study of 2502 community-dwelling men aged > or = 70 years without known diabetes. Metabolic syndrome was defined using the National Cholesterol Education Program-Third Adult Treatment Panel (NCEP-ATPIII) criteria. Early morning fasting sera were assayed for total testosterone, SHBG and LH. Free testosterone was calculated using mass action equations.RESULTS: There were 602 men with metabolic syndrome (24.1%). The risk of metabolic syndrome increased for total testosterone < 20 nmol/l, SHBG < 50 nmol/l and free testosterone < 300 pmol/l. In univariate analyses SHBG was associated with all five components of metabolic syndrome, total testosterone was associated with all except hypertension, and free testosterone was associated only with waist circumference and triglycerides. In multivariate analysis, both total testosterone and especially SHBG remained associated with metabolic syndrome, with odds ratios of 1.34 (95% confidence interval (CI): 1.18-1.52) and 1.77 (95% CI: 1.53-2.06) respectively. Men with hypogonadotrophic hypogonadism (total testosterone < 8 nmol/l, LH < or = 12 IU/l) had the highest prevalence of metabolic syndrome (53%, P<0.001).CONCLUSIONS: Lower SHBG is more strongly associated with metabolic syndrome than lower total testosterone in community-dwelling older men. SHBG may be the primary driver of these relationships, possibly reflecting its relationship with insulin sensitivity. Further studies should examine whether measures that raise SHBG protect against the development of metabolic syndrome in older men.

Yeap BB et al Low free testosterone concentration as a potentially treatable cause of depressive symptoms in older men. Arch Gen Psychiatry. 2008 Mar; 65(3):283-9. CONTEXT: Serum concentrations of gonadal hormones have been associated with various measures of well-being, but it is unclear whether their association with mood is confounded by concurrent physical morbidity.OBJECTIVE: To determine whether the association between serum testosterone concentration and mood in older men is independent of physical comorbidity.DESIGN: Cross-sectional study.SETTING: Community of Perth, Western Australia.PARTICIPANTS: A community sample of men aged 71 to 89 years.MAIN OUTCOME MEASURES: We used the 15-item Geriatric Depression Scale (GDS-15) to assess depressed mood. Clinically significant depression was defined a priori as a GDS-15 score of 7 or greater. Physical health was assessed using the weighted Charlson index and the Physical Component Summary score of the 36-Item Short Form Health Survey.RESULTS: Of 3987 men included in the study, 203 (5.1%; 95% confidence interval [CI], 4.4%-5.8%) had depression. Participants with depression had significantly lower total and free testosterone concentrations than nondepressed men (P < .001 for both). However, they were also more likely to smoke and to have low educational attainment, a body mass index categorized as obese, and a Mini-Mental State Examination score less than 24, a history of antidepressant drug treatment, and greater concurrent physical morbidity. After adjusting for these factors and for age, men with depression were 1.55 (95% CI, 0.91-2.63) and 2.71 (95% CI, 1.49-4.93) times more likely to have total and free testosterone concentrations, respectively, in the lowest quintile.CONCLUSIONS: A free testosterone concentration in the lowest quintile is associated with a higher prevalence of depression, and this association cannot be adequately explained by physical comorbidity. A randomized controlled trial is required to determine whether the link between low free testosterone level and depression is causal because older men with depression may benefit from systematic screening of free testosterone concentration and testosterone supplementation.

Yeap BB et al Higher serum free testosterone is associated with better cognitive function in older men, while total testosterone is not. The Health In Men Study. Clin Endocrinol (Oxf). 2008 Mar; 68(3):404-12. OBJECTIVE: To determine the relationship of total and free serum testosterone to cognitive performance in older men.DESIGN: Cross-sectional study of a population-based sample. Participants A total of 2932 men aged 70-89 years.MEASUREMENTS: Cognitive function was assessed using the Standardized Mini-Mental State Examination (SMMSE). Early morning sera were assayed for total testosterone, SHBG and LH. Free testosterone was calculated using the Vermeulen method.RESULTS: There were weak positive correlations between SMMSE score and serum free testosterone (Spearman's rho = 0.06, P = 0.001) and total testosterone (r = 0.04, P = 0.027), and a weak negative correlation with LH (r = -0.07, P < 0.001). Men with SMMSE scores in the top quintile had higher serum free testosterone compared with those in the lowest quintile [median (interquartile range, IQR): 278 (228-335) vs. 262 (212-320) pmol/l, P = 0.003], but similar total testosterone [15.2 (11.9-18.8) vs. 14.8 (11.6-18.3) nmol/l, P = 0.118]. Increasing age, non-English-speaking background, lower educational attainment, presence of clinically significant depressive symptoms, and cardiovascular morbidity were associated with the lowest cognitive performance quintile. After their effects were taken into account in a multivariate analysis, serum free testosterone > or = 210 pmol/l was associated with reduced likelihood of poor cognitive performance on the SMMSE [odds ratio (OR) 0.71, 95% confidence interval (CI) 0.52-0.97].CONCLUSIONS: In community-dwelling older men, serum free testosterone > or = 210 pmol/l is associated with better cognitive performance. In this context, calculated free testosterone seems to be a more informative measure of androgen status than total testosterone. Studies examining the contribution of androgens to age-related cognitive decline should incorporate an assessment of free testosterone concentration.

Yeap BB et al In men older than 70 years, total testosterone remains stable while free testosterone declines with age. The Health in Men Study. Eur J Endocrinol. 2007 May;156(5):585-94OBJECTIVE: An age-related decline in serum total and free testosterone concentration may contribute to ill health in men, but limited data are available for men > 70 years of age. We sought to determine the distribution and associations of reduced testosterone concentrations in older men.DESIGN: The Health in Men Study is a community-representative prospective cohort investigation of 4263 men aged > or = 70 years. Cross-sectional hormone data from 3645 men were analysed.METHODS: Early morning sera were assayed for total testosterone, sex hormone binding globulin (SHBG) and LH. Free testosterone was calculated using the Vermeulen method.RESULTS: Mean (+/- s.d.) serum total testosterone was 15.4 +/- 5.6 nmol/l (444 +/- 162 ng/dl), SHBG 42.4 +/- 16.7 nmol/l and free testosterone 278 +/- 96 pmol/l (8.01 +/- 2.78 ng/dl). Total testosterone correlated with SHBG (Spearman's r = 0.6, P < 0.0001). LH and SHBG increased with age (r = 0.2, P < 0.0001 for both). Instead of declining, total testosterone increased marginally (r = 0.04, P = 0.007) whilst free testosterone declined with age (r = -0.1, P < 0.0001). Free testosterone was inversely correlated with LH (r = -0.1, P < 0.0001). In multivariate analyses, increasing age, body mass index (BMI) and LH were associated with lower free testosterone.CONCLUSIONS: In men aged 70-89 years, modulation of androgen action may occur via an age-related increase in SHBG and reduction in free testosterone without a decline in total testosterone concentration. Increasing age, BMI and LH are independently associated with lower free testosterone. Further investigation would be required to assess the clinical consequences of low serum free testosterone, particularly in older men in whom total testosterone may be preserved.

Zitzmann M Hormone substitution in male hypogonadism Mol Cell Endocrinol 2000 Mar 30; 161(1-2):73-88 Male hypogonadism is characterised by androgen deficiency and infertility. Hypogonadism can be caused by disorders at the hypothalamic or pituitary level (hypogonadotropic forms) or by testicular dysfunction (hypergonadotropic forms). Testosterone substitution is necessary in all hypogonadal patients, because androgen deficiency causes slight anemia, changes in coagulation parameters, decreased bone density, muscle atrophy, regression of sexual function and alterations in mood and cognitive abilities. Androgen replacement comprises injectable forms of testosterone as well as implants, transdermal systems, sublingual, buccal and oral preparations. Transdermal systems provide the pharmacokinetic modality closest to natural diurnal variations in testosterone levels. New injectable forms of testosterone are currently under clinical evaluation (testosterone undecanoate, testosterone buciclate), allowing extended injection intervals. If patients with hypogonadotropic hypogonadism wish to father a child, spermatogenesis can be initiated and maintained by gonadotropin therapy (conventionally in the form of human chorionic gonadotropin (hCG) and human menopausal gonadotropin (hMG) or, more recently, purified or recombinant follicle stimulating hormone (FSH)). Apart from this option, patients with disorders at the hypothalamic level can be stimulated with pulsatile gonadotropin-releasing hormone (GnRH). Both treatment modalities have to be administered on average for 7-10 months until pregnancy is achieved. In individual cases, treatment may be necessary for up to 46 months. Testosterone treatment is interrupted for the time of GnRH of gonadotropin therapy, but resumed after cessation of this therapy.

CHAPTER 5

Estrogen and Progesterone

Today there are more than 45 million women in the United States that are in some stage of menopause and close to 4 million more women will begin to experience some of the signs and symptoms of menopause this year. Menopause causes significant hormone imbalances, which can also lead to severe health problems. Menopause is defined as the cessation of the production of estrogens and progesterone by the ovaries causing one year or more without menstrual bleeding. Estrogen and progesterone levels in the body decrease dramatically in menopause but they do not disappear completely. Women experience a peri-menopausal period, which can start up to fifteen years prior to actual menopause. Current studies consistently conclude that the benefits of estrogen and progesterone replacements are optimized when started early.

Estrogen:

Physiology:
Estrogen receptor sites are found in the bladder, bones, arteries, vagina, heart, liver and the brain. Estrogen is synthesized primarily in the ovaries and other areas of the body via aromatization of testosterone. Estrogen is responsible for regulating the menstrual cycle and the development of secondary female sex characteristics. During the follicular phase of a woman's menstrual cycle, estradiol levels increase, triggering ovulation. Once ovulation has occurred, progesterone levels increase, preparing the uterus for implantation. The mid-luteal phase or around day 21 is the best time to evaluate these levels because both are relatively elevated in normal

fuction. If a woman does not become pregnant, progesterone and estrogen levels decrease and eventually the endometrial lining sheds with the menstrual cycle.

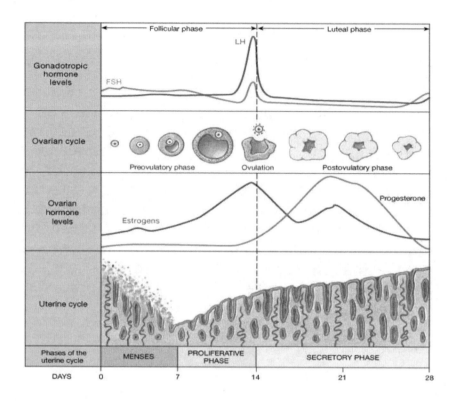

The three major estrogens are estradiol, estriol and estrone. Estra**di**ol (E2) is the strongest estrogen in the body and is necessary for the beneficial effects on the heart and brain to occur. Estr**one** (E1) is transformed to Estradiol by a 17-beta hydroxy steroid dehydrogenase and is elevated relative to Estradiol in menopause. Es**tri**ol (E3), as a weak estrogen, has been shown to have anti-cancer effects by competitively binding estrogen receptors, effectively decreasing the estrogen activity in breast tissue. The usual ratio of E1/E2/E3 is 10/10/80 in a premenopausal female. During menopause the E1 level

136

raises dramatically to about 80 % and the E2 and E3 levels drop leading to a deficiency syndrome.

17β-Estradiol   E2-Estradiol   Estriol   E3- Estriol

E1-Estrone

When a woman transitions into perimenopause, which often can start as early as age 35, hormone levels begin to transiently decline. Hormone deficiencies can have pleiotropic deleterious effects on the cardiovascular, neurocognitive and musculoskeletal system. These hormone deficiencies contribute to an inflammatory state. When hormones are replaced and balanced levels are achieved, inflammation is decreased. Replacing deficient hormones in the body with bio-identical hormones can decrease the onset of heart disease, decrease cholesterol levels, control carbohydrate metabolism, improve memory, reduce the onset of osteoporosis and decrease the incidence of Alzheimer's disease. The symptoms associated with menopause (hot flashes, vaginal dryness, mood swings, night sweats, fatigue and urinary symptoms) are the main indications for physician treatment and patient visits, however the major benefits are found in reduction of cardiovascular and neurological decline.

Atrophic vaginitis results when the walls of the vagina become thinner and vaginal secretions decrease because of low estrogen levels. The vagina actually shrinks and becomes less elastic leading to increased incidence of vaginal infections and dysparenunia. Low estrogen levels can cause the bladder to become thinner, less elastic and the neck of the bladder may actually shrink. The result is urinary frequency and/or painful urination. Because low estrogen levels cause the skin to become thinner and dryer, scalp and body hair become brittle and may fall out more easily.

Symptoms of estrogen deficiency are different for every woman but they may include:

- Anxiety
- Depression
- Night sweats
- Hot flashes
- Dizziness
- Fatigue
- Tearfulness
- Decreased libido
- Vaginal dryness
- Vaginal itching
- Urinary frequency or incontinence
- Headaches
- Burning or discomfort during sexual intercourse
- Dry flaking skin
- Increased wrinkles
- Difficulty sleeping
- Decreased memory
- Decreased attention span

- Shortness of breath
- Heart palpitations
- Increase in weight, especially in abdominal/hip areas
- Increased blood pressure
- Increased cholesterol levels

Literature review:

The benefits of BHRT in improving symptoms of menopause are well known. They include elimination of vasomotor symptoms such as hot flashes and night sweats, reversal of bone loss leading to osteoporosis, improved sleep, emotional stability, libido and quality of life. This review of the current peer reviewed medical literature focuses on safety.

The Fournier study, in the *International Journal of Cancer*, 2005, evaluated 54,000 women who used bio-identical estrogen and either were taking bio-identical progesterone or synthetic progestin. The women taking bio-identical progesterone had a 10% decrease in risk of breast cancer and the women taking artificial progestin had a 40% increase in the risk of breast cancer. Further studies by Fournier et al in 2007 with 80,000 women over 8 years show that those women taking the bio-identical progesterone had no increased risk of breast cancer and the women taking artificial progestin had a 69% increase in the risk of breast cancer. The de Lignieres study from *Climacteric* 2002 concludes that the risk of breast cancer is not increased with bio-identical hormones but is increased with synthetic progestin. These studies are examples of the documented scientific observation that the major problem with synthetic HRT is the synthetic progestin. Several studies document that higher progesterone levels during premenopausal years or during pregnancy are protective against breast cancer. (Campanoli, 2005) The cardiovascular benefits of bio-identical estrogen therapy are reversed by synthetic progestins as documented in the Adams study from *Atherosclerosis Thrombosis and Vascular Biology* in 1997. The Kronos KEEPS study is in progress comparing different hormone replacement therapies and carotid intimal medial thickness and coronary calcium score and we look forward to those results.

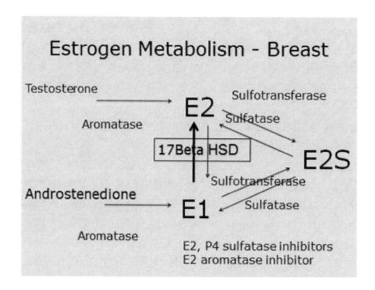

The above diagram explains some of the counter intuitive actions of Bioidentical hormone replacement

in the breast tissue. Women using Bioidentical estrogen and progesterone replacement therapy have the same or slightly less breast cancer rates as the background population. Women with a history of breast cancer have lower mortality when taking Bioidentical estrogen and progesterone. (Durna) Limiting Estradiol actions in the breast occurs through inhibiting the transformation of testosterone to E2 and androstendione to E1 through limiting aromatase. E2 itself causes aromatase inhibition action in the breast. This may explain the anti-cancer benefit of other natural aromatase inhibitors such as melatonin. In addition, E2 and Progesterone inhibit sulfatase, which converts the inactive E2 sulfate to E2. Inhibitors of 17-beta hydroxysteroid dehydrogenase type 1 such as pomegranate decrease the transformation of the less active E1 to the active E2. Hence Estradiol and Progesterone can reduce the risk of breast cancer by intra-breast actions.

Schmitt discusses Estriol (E3 Estrogen) in *Gynecologic Endocrinology* in 2006 and points out that Estriol is protective of brain and heart function and that low levels of Estriol are associated with increased breast cancer. Prior to the Women's Health Initiative study (WHI), many prospective studies showed the benefits of HRT on quality of life, cardiovascular disease and osteoporosis. The WHI study analyzed the outcome of women taking Premarin (conjugated equine estrogen, CEE) and Provera (Medroxyprogesterone Acetate, MPA) and found increased rates of breast cancer and cardiovascular disease. Since the drugs used were not bio-identical hormones the results only apply to CEE and MPA, not BHRT. Problems with this study:

- Wrong Estrogen
  - Premarin is not a human hormone
  - Mostly Equillin
  - Low Estradiol (E2) - cardiovascular benefits are from E2
  - No Estriol (E3) - E3 is protective

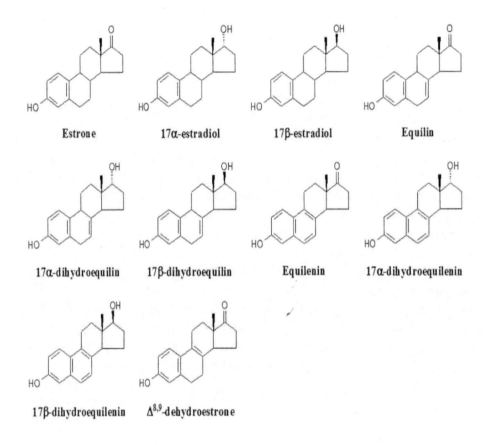

Estrone   17α-estradiol   17β-estradiol   Equilin

17α-dihydroequilin   17β-dihydroequilin   Equilenin   17α-dihydroequilenin

17β-dihydroequilenin $\Delta^{8,9}$-dehydroestrone

- Wrong "Progesterone"
 •MPA blocks progesterone receptors and is not a human hormone. MPA reverses benefits of E2

Progesterone   Medroxyacetateprogesterone

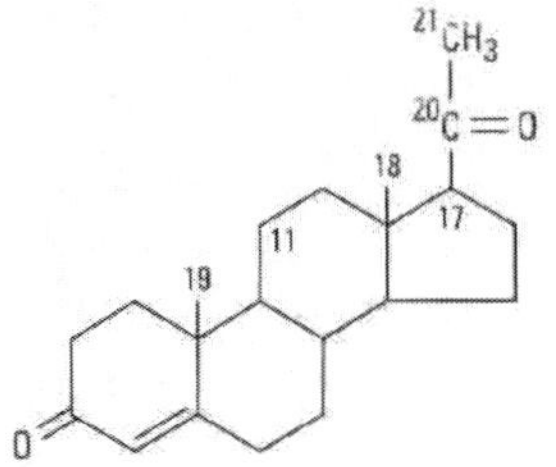

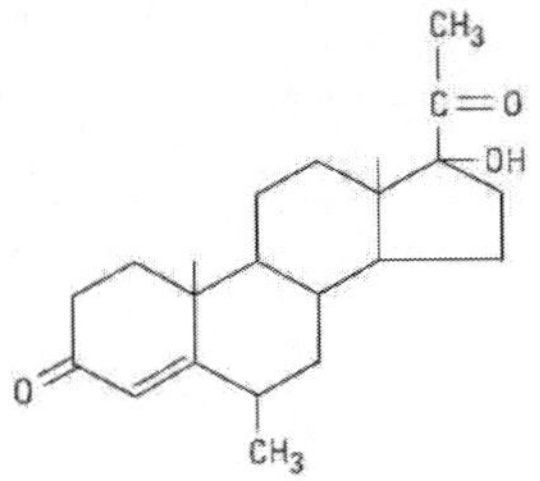

- Wrong route

Oral Estrogens increase inflammation. Estrogens should not be given orally. Oral estrogens, by way of the first pass liver effects, increase the acute phase proteins including CRP and fibrinogen increasing the risk of thrombosis. Transdermal estrogens and bioidentical progesterone instead of progestins do not increase the risk of deep vein thrombosis (DVT) or pulmonaryu emboli (PE). (Archer)

- Wrong women

Most of the women were smokers were already established cardiovascular disease and were 8 or more years out since the onset of menopause. Hodis et al conclude that there is a "window of opportunity" for maximal reduction of CHD and overall mortality, which occurs before age 60 or within 10 years of menopause and continues for 6 years or more. Hodis points out the lipid lowering and aspirin therapy has not been shown to reduce mortality in women. There is a 39% reduction in overall mortality for subjects younger than 60 years of age, that are using "HRT" which is a metaanalysis utilizing data from all types of HRT.

Several articles in current medical literature point out these problems including Clark's analysis in *Nuclear*

Receptors and Signaling, 2006, Descenci in Circulation in 2005 and Dubey in the *Journal of Pharmacology and Experimental Therapeutics* in 2004. Klaiber in *Fertility and Sterility*, 2005, points out the design flaws in this study and that most studies show lower mortality with any form of HRT. Maki et al concludes as well that the MPA is associated with reduced cognitive function in combination therapy. Once again, the main problem is the MPA. When the Women's Health Initiative patients who just received CEE without MPA were analyzed the rate of breast cancer was not increased. (Anderson, *JAMA*, 2004). Recent review of this study, once again years later show that the addition of MPA increased the risk of breast cancer. Grodstein points out in Women*'s Health* in 2006 that beginning any hormone therapy near menopause significantly reduces coronary heart disease and that hormone users have a lower overall risk of death in the New England Journal of Medicine in 1997. Schneider concludes his study in *Maturitas* in 2002, "Cancer mortality is reduced in current or ever HRT users." The editors in chief of Climateric, Fenton and Panay, point out the harm done to women's health, following the misguided recommendations of the WHI study. They further state-

"The guidelines from both the IMS and the North American Menopause Society state, respectively that 'new data and re-analyses of older studies by women's age show that, for most women, the potential benefits of HRT given for a clear indication are many and the risks are few when initiated within a few years of menopause' and 'the absolute risks known to date for use of HT in healthy women ages 50 to 59 years are low."

Pines et al state,"The quality of life of countless menopausal women world-wide has been significantly diminished following the sensationalist reporting of the WHI." The benefits and quality of life far extend past the control of vasomotor symptoms.

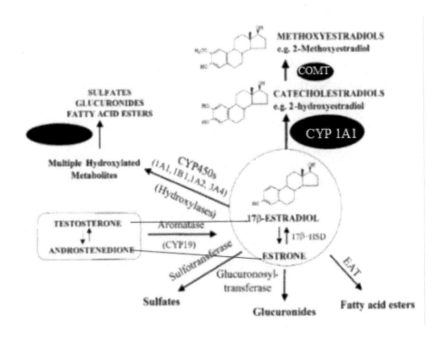

Some of the protective actions of Estradiol may be through conversion to 2-methoxyestradiol, which is thought to be anti cancer and anti atherosclerosis and avoidance of the 4-hydroxy and 16-hydroxy metabolites. 17-beta-Estradiol is transformed to 2-hydroxy-Estradiol via CYP 1A1. 2-hydroxy-Estradiol is converted to 2-methoy-Estradiol via COMT. Cruciferous vegetables and indole-3-carbinol or di-indole-methane can help to maintain a favorable ratio of 2-hydroxy to 16-hydroxy metabolites. The catecholamines induced by mental stress can compete for COMT resulting in less 2-methoxy-estradiol and greater risk for cancer and cardiovascular disease

Management:

If estrogen deficiency is present clinically then replacement is usually indicated. If suboptimal levels are present without clinical symptom, close monitoring and reassement is necessary. For treating estrogen deficiencies we commonly use BiEst. Avoidance of oral estrogens is recommended, since oral estrogens, via the first pass effect, initiate hepatic acute phase response with increased CRP, fibrinogen and serum amyloid A. BiEst is an estrogen transdermal cream, commonly comprised of 20% estradiol and 80% estriol. With compounding pharmacies we can individualize the dose and the percentage of the concentrations to blend a product that is effective for the patient. BiEst 80/20 of 2.5 mg/gm will contain 2 mg of estriol and 0.5 mg of estradiol. BiEst is usually applied in the AM and should be applied over a large area in a thin layer to improve absorption. It is recommended to avoid shower, swimming or heavy workouts immediately after application as this can reduce the amount of hormone absorbed.

There is controversy regarding continuous hormone replacement therapy. Unfortunately there is not sufficient data currently in the medical literature to resolve this issue. Continuous or static means daily treatment of hormones without a break. Cycling is a treatment protocol with cyclical breaks in treatment. A method well accepted by menopausal patient is using a calendar and cyclically skipping treatment on the first 3 days of each month.

We recommend an initial starting dose of estrogen for our patients of 1.25 to 2.5mg/gm if perimenopausal and we try to match her existing cycle. For a "normal" 28 day cycle, treat with biest on days 1-25, with the first day of menses counted as day 1. Individual adjustments may be needed to match her existing cycle.

For menopausal women with mild symptoms, ½ to 1 gm of 2.5 mg /gm of BiEst transdermal cream daily or if using the cycling method needed day 3 to the end of the calendar month. Day 1 being the first day of a calendar month. Doses are titrated up or down depending on a woman's symptoms and side effects and the results of follow-up lab work. If a menopausal woman is having severe symptoms, or trying to wean off of CEE, the higher dosage is often needed. Some women do not want to stop their CEE due to severe vasomotor symptoms, so trying to wean off over 4-6 weeks, with gradual decrease in dosing from daily to every other day to twice a week, etc. works well. CEE has a long half-life and easy to transition this way with gradually increasing the BiEst with the decreasing CEE, until a balance is achieved.

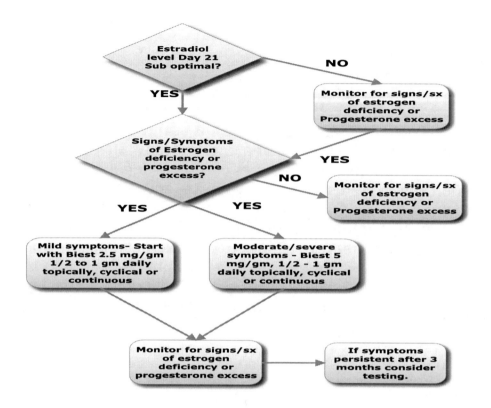

ESTROGEN REPLACEMENT

Estrogen Deficiency/Progesterone Excess
Hot flashes
Night Sweats
Foggy Thinking
Forgetfulness
Fatigue
Palpitations
Depression
Decreased libido
Vaginal Dryness
Excessive daytime sleepiness
Decreased energy
etc.

Progesterone:

Progesterone, primarily a female hormone is produced by the ovaries in the corpus luteum, the adrenal glands and during pregnancy in the placenta. Progesterone helps balance estrogen. If progesterone levels are too low relative to estrogen levels, a woman might experience symptoms of estrogen dominance, such as breast tenderness, poor sleep, and menorrhagia. With an imbalance of excess estrogen and deficient progesterone, the endometrium becomes thicker than normal leading to endometrial hyperplasia, which left untreated, can increase the risk of endometrial cancer. Progesterone reduces this build up and allows the lining to mature and release with the next menstrual cycle. Progesterone protects against breast cancer, decreases fluid retention, helps maintain normal blood sugar levels, assists in lowering LDL cholesterol levels, and has sedative and anxiolytic effects by it's GABA receptor activity.

Like estrogen, progesterone levels decline as we age. Progesterone is commonly the first hormone to become deficient in menopause. Progesterone deficiency is also implicated in premenstrual syndrome and postpartum depression. Synthetic progestins (i.e., MPA and Oral contraceptive) produce unwanted side effects such as fluid retention, weight gain, depression and breast tenderness, as well as increasing the risk of breast cancer with usage.

One controversy that arises is in women who have had a hysterectomy. Traditional medicine doesn't routinely add progesterone or a progestin post hysterectomy. The major concern of unopposed estrogen is endometrial hyperplasia and the development of uterine cancer, and without a uterus this risk doesn't exist. However, there are progesterone receptors widely found throughout the body and in every neural cell and the need to maintain hormonal balance and reduce estrogen dominance in brain, breast tissue, heart, skin is important. It is important to keep progesterone levels in a youthful physiologic range. Bioidentical progesterone replacement therapy has many health benefits and should be part of a female hormone replacement treatment program.

Progesterone deficiency symptoms:

- Anxiety
- Agitation
- Breast swelling
- Breast tenderness
- Bloating
- Fluid retention
- Headaches
- Mood swings
- Sleep disturbances
- Heavy or irregular menstrual bleeding

Management:

Women naturally have a progesterone increase or "surge" after ovulation. Ovulation typically occurs between the 10th to the 14th day of the menstrual cycle. In early perimenopause, progesterone replacement is usually most effective during this "surge" time, which is for most women, day 14 to 28, the luteal phase of a 28-day menstrual cycle. As menopause progresses, a woman may also need to add a small dose of progesterone to treat underlying deficiency during the follicular phase and bump up to the higher dosage during the luteal phase. We prescribe micronized bioidentical progesterone in transdermal cream or gel or capsule form for our female patients. The dosage of progesterone is different for every patient, depending upon the progesterone level and her unique symptoms. We cycle progesterone doses for our female patients according to their natural menstrual cycle or if they are menopausal we may use continuous or cyclical.

For our female patients, we recommend an initial starting dose of 50-100 mg of natural micronized progesterone daily according to the cycle. The progesterone may either be prescribed in capsule form (use the capsule form if the female patient complains of lack of sleep as oral progesterone promotes improved sleep) or in a transdermal gel or cream. The oral form of progesterone has more sedation effects due to greater hepatic biotransformation of progesterone to 5-allo-pregnenolone, which is the more active neurosteroid. There is less 5-allo-pregnenolone effect with the use of transdermal preparations. There is no 5-allo-pregnenolone production with artificial progestins. Unlike estrogens, oral progesterone does not initiate hepatic acute phase response and no increase in inflammation and cardiovascular risks. Doses are titrated up or down according to the symptoms and the results of follow-up lab work.

There are some women who feel uncomfortable on any form of progesterone be it synthetic or bioidentical. Usually a small amount of transdermal progesterone is tolerated, but if not, monitoring for estrogen dominance is an important consideration. If these women still have a uterus, it would be important to perform periodic pelvic ultrasounds to assess the endometrial thickness.

Endometrial biopsies may be required if the endometrial thickness is present.

Progesterone Replacement

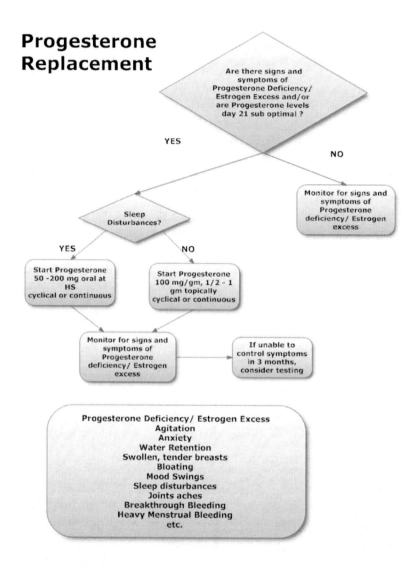

For men who are deficient in progesterone, with lab values in the lower quartile or have symptoms of progesterone deficiency such as insomnia and anxiety, a very low dosage of 10-20 mg/ gm of progesterone cream is usually adequate. It should be applied to thin skin, such as the foream, at night to treat the deficiency. An added benefit for men is improved sleep. It can be effective as an aromatase inhibitor and well as a 5 alpha reductase inhibitor.

Troubleshooting –

1. Continued vasomotor symptoms such as hot flashes and night sweats
   a. Increase the estrogen
   b. Make sure the patient is applying it appropriately
   c. If break through sweats at night only, split the dose in half and have her take a second dose later in the afternoon
   d. Be sure to monitor for other hormone imbalances as well
2. Breakthrough Bleeding or Heavy Menses
   a. If premenopausal and early in treatment, reassure that this is a normal occurrence, if persists may need adjustment
   b. May need to increase progesterone or decrease estrogen especially if estrogen dominance symptoms are present. It is not unusual in perimenopause to have high surges of estrogen and monthly dose changes in progesterone may be needed to achieve the balance.
   c. If persistent, comprehensive management requires a pelvic ultrasound to evaluate the endometrial lining and ovaries for cysts etc. that can lead to bleeding abnormalities.

3. Not Sleeping
    a. Resolving sleep issues may be the highest priority in perimenopausal women. If she is not sleeping, normal adrenal cortisol production is dysregulated. Additional management may include melatonin, increasing progesterone, ashwagandha or other adaptagens, increased exercise, dietary magnesium, etc. to improve this problem.
4. Weight gain
    a. It is not unusual, just like other hormone replacement to see some fluid retention with the addition of BHRT. It is usually transient, but bothersome
    b. Be sure exercise, diet, supplements are in place in life style, along with adequate sleep.
    c. Reassessment of thyroid status and optimization may be required.
    d. Reassurance that this is a process and all will improve as hormones are optimized; energy will return, motivation will improve and weight will come off.

ESTROGEN AND PROGESTERONE ABSTRACTS

Adams MR et al. Medroxyprogesterone Acetate Antagonizes Inhibitory Effects of Conjugated Equine Estrogens on Coronary Artery Atherosclerosis Arteriosclerosis, Thrombosis, and Vascular Biology. Jan1997; 17:217-221
Although estrogen replacement therapy is associated with reduced risk of coronary heart disease and reduced extent of coronary artery atherosclerosis,

the effects of combined (estrogen plus progestin) hormone-replacement therapy are uncertain. Some observational data indicate that users of combined hormone replacement consisting of continuously administered oral conjugated equine estrogens (CEE) and oral sequentially administered (7 to 14 days per month) medroxyprogesterone acetate (MPA) experience a reduction in risk similar to that of users of CEE alone. However, the effects of combined, continuously administered CEE plus MPA (a prescribing pattern that has gained favor) on the risk of coronary heart disease or atherosclerosis are not known. We studied the effects of CEE (monkey equivalent of 0.625 mg/d) and MPA (monkey equivalent of 2.5 mg/d); administered separately or in combination, on the extent of coronary artery atherosclerosis (average plaque size) in surgically postmenopausal cynomolgus monkeys fed atherogenic diets and treated with these hormones for 30 months. Treatment with CEE alone resulted in atherosclerosis extent that was reduced 72% relative to untreated (estrogen-deficient) controls (P < .004). Atherosclerosis extent in animals treated with CEE plus MPA or MPA alone did not differ from that of untreated controls. Although treatment had marked effects on plasma lipoprotein patterns, statistical adjustment for variation in plasma lipoproteins did not alter the between-group relationships in atherosclerotic plaque size, suggesting that these factors do not explain substantially the atheroprotective effect of estrogen or the MPA-associated antagonism. Although the mechanism(s) remains unclear, we conclude that oral CEE inhibits the initiation and progression of coronary artery atherosclerosis and that continuously administered oral MPA antagonizes this atheroprotective effect.

Anderson GL et al. Effects of conjugated equine estrogen in postmenopausal women with hysterectomy: the Women's Health Initiative randomized controlled trial.JAMA. 2004 Apr 4; 291(14):1701-12.CONTEXT: Despite decades of use and considerable research, the role of estrogen alone in preventing chronic diseases in postmenopausal women remains uncertain. OBJECTIVE: To assess the effects on major disease incidence rates of the most commonly used postmenopausal hormone therapy in the United States. DESIGN, SETTING, AND PARTICIPANTS: A randomized, double-blind, placebo-controlled disease prevention trial (the estrogen-alone component of the Women's Health Initiative [WHI]) conducted in 40 US clinical centers beginning in 1993. Enrolled were 10 739 postmenopausal women, aged 50-79 years, with prior hysterectomy, including 23% of minority race/ethnicity. INTERVENTION: Women were randomly assigned to receive either 0.625 mg/d of conjugated equine estrogen (CEE) or placebo. MAIN OUTCOME MEASURES: The primary outcome was coronary heart disease (CHD) incidence (nonfatal myocardial infarction or CHD death). Invasive breast cancer incidence was the primary safety outcome. A global index of risks and benefits, including these primary outcomes plus stroke, pulmonary embolism (PE), colorectal cancer, hip fracture, and deaths from other causes, was used for summarizing overall effects. RESULTS: In February 2004, after reviewing data through November 30, 2003, the National Institutes of Health (NIH) decided to end the intervention phase of the trial early. Estimated hazard ratios (HRs) (95% confidence intervals [CIs]) for CEE vs placebo for the major clinical outcomes available through February 29, 2004 (average follow-up 6.8 years), were: CHD, 0.91 (0.75-1.12) with 376 cases; breast cancer, 0.77 (0.59-1.01) with 218 cases; stroke, 1.39 (1.10-1.77) with 276 cases; PE, 1.34 (0.87-2.06) with 85 cases; colorectal cancer, 1.08 (0.75-1.55) with 119 cases; and hip fracture, 0.61 (0.41-0.91) with 102 cases. Corresponding results for composite outcomes were: total cardiovascular disease, 1.12 (1.01-1.24); total cancer, 0.93 (0.81-1.07); total fractures, 0.70 (0.63-0.79); total mortality, 1.04 (0.88-1.22), and the global index, 1.01 (0.91-1.12). For the outcomes significantly affected by CEE, there was an absolute excess risk of 12 additional strokes per 10 000 person-years and an absolute risk reduction of 6 fewer hip fractures per 10 000 person-years. The estimated excess risk for all monitored events in the global index was a nonsignificant 2 events per 10 000 person-years. CONCLUSIONS: The use of CEE increases the risk of stroke, decreases the risk of hip fracture, and does not affect CHD incidence in postmenopausal women with prior hysterectomy over an average of 6.8 years. A possible reduction in breast cancer risk requires further investigation. The burden of incident disease events was equivalent in the CEE and placebo groups, indicating no overall benefit. Thus, CEE should not be recommended for chronic disease prevention in postmenopausal women

Archer DF et al. Estrogen and progestogen effect on venous thromboemobolism in menopausal women. Climacteric 2012;15:235-240. Prior to 1996, the use of postmenopausal estrogen was not believed to increase the risk of venous thrombosis. Subsequent studies, particularly the prospective, randomized, double-blind, clinical trial of the Women's Health Initiative, have clearly shown an increase in the incidence and risk of venous thrombosis in postmenopausal women using conjugated equine estrogens with or without medroxyprogesterone acetate. The risk of venous thrombosis in postmenopausal women is also increased by obesity and age. Oral hormone therapy has been used principally for management of menopausal symptoms. Transdermal estrogens have not been used as extensively in the United States but have a significant use in Europe. Recent observational studies have indicated no increased risk of venous thrombosis with use of transdermal estrogens. Norpregnane derivatives have been associated with an increased risk of venous thrombosis, suggesting that progestins may contribute to the increased risk in postmenopausal women using estrogen plus progestin therapy.

Barnes SL et al. Colorectal cancer in women: hormone repleacement therpy and chemoprevention. Climacteric 2012;15:250-255. Colorectal cancer (CRC) accounts for 9.4% of new cancer diagnoses among women world-wide. CRC is the third leading cause of incident cancer among women in the United States and has immense impact on morbidity and mortality. We summarize data on CRC pathogenesis and risk in women. We also review the findings from the Women's Health Initiative (WHI) on CRC risk reduction associated with hormone replacement therapy (HRT) use. We then review observational studies since the WHI which evaluated HRT as a chemopreventive agent for CRC among women. The potential mechanisms behind the association between HRT use and CRC are also reviewed. We then discuss the requirements for implementation of chemopreventive agents, and why HRT should not be used for this indication given current knowledge. Further data on the risk-benefit profile of short-term HRT use are needed and will determine whether there is any future role for HRT use in the chemoprevention of CRC.

Batur P et al. Menopausal hormone therapy (HT) in patients with breast cancer. Maturitas. 2006 Jan 20; 53(2):123-32. OBJECTIVES: To assess the effect of menopausal hormone therapy (HT) on reoccurrence, cancer-related mortality, and overall mortality after a diagnosis of breast cancer. METHODS: We performed a quantitative review of all studies reporting experience with menopausal HT for symptomatic use after a diagnosis of breast cancer. Rates of reoccurrence, cancer-related mortality, and overall mortality were calculated in this entire group. A subgroup analysis was performed in studies using a control population to assess the odds ratio of cancer reoccurrence and mortality in hormone users versus non-users. RESULTS: Fifteen studies encompassing 1416 breast cancer survivors using HT were identified. Seven studies included a control group comprised of 1998 patients. Among the 1416 HT users, reoccurrence was noted in 10.0% (95% CI: 8.4-11.6%). Cancer-related mortality occurred at a rate of 2.6% (95% CI: 1.8-3.7%), while overall mortality was 4.5% (95% CI: 3.4-5.8%). Compared to non-users, patients using HT had a decreased chance of reoccurrence and cancer-related mortality with combined odds ratio of 0.5 (95% CI: 0.2-0.7) and 0.3 (95% CI: 0.0-0.6), respectively. CONCLUSIONS: In our review, menopausal HT use in breast cancer survivors was not associated with increased cancer reoccurrence, cancer-related mortality or total mortality. Despite conflicting opinions on this issue, it is important for primary care physicians to feel comfortable medically managing the increasing number of breast cancer survivors. In the subset of women with severe menopausal symptoms, HT options should be reviewed if non-hormonal methods are ineffective. Future trials should focus on better ways to identify breast cancer survivors who may safely benefit from HT versus those who have a substantial risk of reoccurrence with HT use.

Beyer ME et al. Acute gender-specific hemodynamic and inotropic effects of 17beta-estradiol on rats. Hypertension. 2001 Nov; 38(5):1003-10. Estrogen has cardioprotective effects. In addition to beneficial effects on lipid metabolism, estrogen affects the vascular tone and may reduce endothelial dysfunction. In the present study, we examined acute gender-specific hemodynamic and inotropic effects of 17beta-estradiol (17beta-E) versus the control situation in open-chest rats. In addition to measurements in the intact circulation, myocardial function was examined on the basis of isovolumic registration independent of peripheral vascular effects. Regarding the dose-dependent and gender-specific effects of 17beta-E, in female rats, 17beta-E (50, 100, or 200 ng/kg) increased cardiac output (CO) (26%, 43%, and 59% versus control animals) as a result of reduction in total peripheral resistance (TPR) (-13%, -18%, and -24%) without any effect on myocardial contractility (isovolumic left ventricular systolic pressure, -1%, 0%, and -6%). These vascular effects are less pronounced in male rats (for 200 ng/kg 17beta-E: CO, 34%; TPR, -14%). We investigated gender-specific effects of 200 ng/kg 17beta-E after pretreatment with the estrogen receptor (ER) antagonist ICI 182,780. ER blockade reduced the effects of estrogen in female rats (CO, 29%; TPR, -17%) and male rats (CO, 19%; TPR, -11%). Regarding the effects of 200 ng/kg 17beta-E after pretreatment with N(G)-nitro-L-arginine methyl ester, NO synthesis inhibition completely prevented the acute vascular effects of estrogen in female rats (CO, -4%; TPR, 1%). In addition, immunohistochemical staining revealed no gender-specific differences of the vascular ER distribution. 17beta-E caused an acute dose-dependent and gender-specific reduction in the afterload. ERs are involved in both genders in this vasodilative effect that is mediated by NO. This NO-mediated effect may explain in part the cardioprotective effect of estrogen.

Booth EA et al. 17Beta-estradiol as a receptor-mediated cardioprotective agent. J Pharmacol Exp Ther. 2003 Oct; 307(1):395-401. Cardiac tissue that undergoes an ischemic episode exhibits irreversible alterations that become more extensive upon reperfusion. Estrogen treatment has been reported to protect against reperfusion injury, but the mechanism remains unknown. The cardioprotective effects of 17beta-estradiol, a biologically active form of the hormone, and 17alpha-estradiol were assessed in an in vivo occlusion-reperfusion model. Anesthetized, ovariectomized rabbits were administered 17beta-estradiol (20 microg), 17alpha-estradiol (1 mg), or vehicle intravenously 30 min before a 30-min occlusion of the left anterior descending (LAD) coronary artery followed by 4 h of reperfusion. Infarct size as a percentage of area at risk decreased in the 17beta-estradiol-treated group (18.8 +/- 1.7) compared with 17alpha-estradiol (41.9 +/- 4.8; P < 0.01) or vehicle groups (48 +/- 5.5; P < 0.001). Similar results were obtained when infarct size was expressed as a percentage of total left ventricle. The second objective of the study was to assess fulvestrant (Faslodex, ICI 182,780), an estrogen receptor antagonist, for its effects on infarct size in ovariectomized female rabbits treated with 17beta-estradiol. ICI 182,780 was administered intravenously 1 h before the administration of 17beta-estradiol (20 microg) or vehicle. The hearts were subjected to 30-min LAD coronary artery occlusion and 4 h of reperfusion. Pretreatment with ICI 182,780 significantly limited the infarct size sparing effect of 17beta-estradiol when expressed as a percentage of the risk region (53.0 +/- 5.0). The results indicate that 17beta-estradiol protects the heart against ischemia-reperfusion injury and that the observed cardioprotection is mediated by the estrogen receptor.

Brown, S. Shock, terror and controversy: how the media reacted to the Women's Health Initiative. Climacteric 2012;15:275-280. Results from the first publication of the Women's Health Initiative trial were announced by press release and press conference in July 2002. The announcement explained that the combined hormone trial had been terminated early because of 'increased breast cancer risk'. The dramatic nature of the announcement set the tone for the early news reporting from the study and introduced a note of confusion into the media's perception of hormone replacement therapy (HRT). Such a tone persisted until July 2007, when the trial revised its findings on cardiovascular risk. Despite investigators' protests to the contrary, the results were perceived by the press as a U-turn, and reinforced the media's confused interpretation of the safety and benefits of HRT. We argue that the WHI's melodramatic presentation of its results explains the media response.

Campagnoli C et al. Pregnancy progesterone and progestins in relation to breast cancer risk. Journal of Steroid Biochemistry and Molecular Biology 97 (2005, Dec) 441-450. In the last two decades the prevailing opinion, supported by the "estrogen augmented by progesterone" hypothesis, has been that progesterone contributes to the development of breast cancer (BC). Support for this opinion was provided by the finding that some synthetic progestins, when added to estrogen in hormone replacement therapy (HRT) for menopausal complaints, increase the BC risk more than estrogen alone. However, recent findings suggest that both the production of progesterone during pregnancy and the progesterone endogenously produced or exogenously administered outside pregnancy, does not increase BC risk, and could even be protective. The increased BC risk found with the addition of synthetic progestins to estrogen in HRT seems in all likelihood due to the fact that these progestins (medroxyprogesterone acetate and 19-nortestosterone-derivatives) are endowed with some non-progesterone-like effects which can potentiate the proliferative action of estrogens. The use of progestational agents in pregnancy, for example to prevent preterm birth, does not cause concern in relation to BC risk.

Chang KJ et al. Influences of percutaneous administration of estradiol and progesterone on human breast epithelial cell cycle in vivo.Fertil Steril. 1995 Apr; 63(4):785-91.OBJECTIVE: To study the effect of E2 and P on the epithelial cell cycle of normal human breast in vivo. DESIGN: Double-blind, randomized study. Topical application to the breast of a gel containing either a placebo, E2, P, or a combination of E2 and P, daily, during the 10 to 13 days preceding breast surgery. PATIENTS: Forty premenopausal women undergoing breast surgery for the removal of a lump. MAIN OUTCOME MEASURES. Plasma and breast tissue concentrations of E2 and P. Epithelial cell cycle evaluated in normal breast tissue areas by counting mitoses and proliferating cell nuclear antigen immunostaining quantitative analyses. RESULTS: Increased E2 concentration increases the number of cycling epithelial cells. Increased P

159

concentration significantly decreases the number of cycling epithelial cells. CONCLUSION: Exposure to P for 10 to 13 days reduces E2-induced proliferation of normal breast epithelial cells in vivo.

Clark JH. A critique of Women's Health Initiative Studies (2002-2006). Nucl Recept Signal. 2006 Oct.The Women's Health Initiative Studies (WHI) were designed to examine the effects of estrogen and progestin (E+P; Prempro) and estrogen alone (Premarin) in post-menopausal women. The authors of the WHI studies and the National Heart Lung and Blood Institute (NHLBI) concluded that E+P treatment increased the risks of coronary heart disease, invasive breast cancer, stroke and venous thromboembolism. The following paper contains a reevaluation of these studies based on the graphic analysis of their tabulated data. In contrast to the conclusions reached by the WHI and the NHLBI, I conclude that treatment of post-menopausal women with estrogen and progestin (Prempro) does not increase the risks of cardiovascular disease, invasive breast cancer, stroke or venous thromboembolism. I also disagree with the claim that an increased risk of stroke existed in women treated with estrogen alone.

Dalessandri KM et al. Pilot study: effect of 3, 3'-diindolylmethane supplements on urinary hormone metabolites in postmenopausal women with a history of early-stage breast cancer. Nutr Cancer. 2004; 50(2):161-7. Dietary indoles, present in Brassica plants such as cabbage, broccoli, and Brussels sprouts, have been shown to provide potential protection against hormone-dependent cancers. 3, 3'-Diindolylmethane (DIM) is under study as one of the main protective indole metabolites. Postmenopausal women aged 50-70 yr from Marin County, California, with a history of early-stage breast cancer, were screened for interest and eligibility in this pilot study on the effect of absorbable DIM (BioResponse-DIM) supplements on urinary hormone metabolites. The treatment group received daily DIM (108 mg DIM/day) supplements for 30 days, and the control group received a placebo capsule daily for 30 days. Urinary metabolite analysis included 2-hydroxyestrone (2-OHE1), 16-alpha hydroxyestrone (16alpha-OHE1), DIM, estrone (EI), estradiol(E2), estriol (E3), 6beta-hydroxycortisol (6beta-OHC), and cortisol in the first morning urine sample before intervention and 31 days after intervention. Nineteen women completed the study, for a total of 10 in the treatment group and 9 in the placebo group. DIM-treated subjects, relative to placebo, showed a significant increase in levels of2-OHE1 (P=0. 020), DIM (P =0. 045), and cortisol (P = 0.039), and a nonsignificant increase of 47% in the 2-OHE1/16alpha-OHE1 ratio from 1.46 to 2.14 (P=0.059). In this pilot study, DIM increased the 2-hydroxylation of estrogen urinary metabolites.

Decensi A et al. Effect of transdermal estradiol and oral conjugated estrogen on C-reactive protein in retinoid-placebo trial in healthy women Circulation 2002 Sep 3;106(10):1224-

8BACKGROUND: The increase in C-reactive protein (CRP) during oral conjugated equine estrogen (CEE) may explain the initial excess of cardiovascular disease observed in clinical studies. Because the effect of transdermal estradiol (E2) on CRP is unclear, we compared CRP changes after 6 and 12 months of transdermal E2 and oral CEE in a randomized 2x2 retinoid-placebo trial. METHODS AND RESULTS: A total of 189 postmenopausal women were randomized to 50 microg/d transdermal E2 and 100 mg BID of the retinoid fenretinide (n=45), 50 microg/d transdermal E2 and placebo (n=49), 0.625 mg/d oral CEE and 100 mg BID fenretinide (n=46), or 0.625 mg/d oral CEE and placebo (n=49) for 1 year. Sequential medroxyprogesterone acetate was added in each group. Relative to baseline, CRP increased by 10% (95% CI -9% to 33%) and by 48% (95% CI 22% to 78%) after 6 months of transdermal E2 and oral CEE, respectively. The corresponding figures at 12 months were 3% (95% CI -14% to 23%) for transdermal E2 and 64% (95% CI 38% to 96%) for oral CEE. Fenretinide did not change CRP levels at 6 and 12 months relative to placebo. Relative to oral CEE, the mean change in CRP after 12 months of transdermal E2 was -48% (95% CI -85% to -7%, P=0.012), whereas fenretinide was associated with a mean change of -1% (95% CI -34% to 40%, P=0.79) compared with placebo. CONCLUSIONS: In contrast to oral CEE, transdermal E2 does not elevate CRP levels up to 12 months of treatment. The implications for early risk of coronary heart disease require further studies.

de Lignieres B et al. Combined hormone replacement therapy and risk of breast cancer in a French cohort study of 3175 women.Climacteric. 2002 Dec; 5(4):332-40. The largest-to-date randomized trial (Women's Health Initiative) comparing the effects of hormone replacement therapy (HRT) and a placebo concluded that the continuous use of an oral combination of conjugated equine estrogens (CEE) and medroxy-progesterone acetate (MPA) increases the risk of breast cancer. This conclusion may not apply to women taking other estrogen and progestin formulations, as suggested by discrepancies in the findings of in vitro studies, epidemiological surveys and, mostly, in vivo studies of human breast epithelial cell proliferation showing opposite effects of HRT combining CEE plus MPA or estradiol plus progesterone. To evaluate the risk of breast cancer associated with the use of the latter combination, commonly prescribed in France, a cohort including 3175 postmenopausal women was followed for a mean of 8.9 years (28 367 woman-years). In total, 1739 (55%) of these women were users of one type of estrogen replacement with systemic effect during at least 12 months, any time after the menopause, and were classified as HRT users. Among them, 83% were receiving exclusively or mostly a combination of a transdermal estradiol gel and a progestin other than MPA. Some 105 cases of breast cancer occurred during the follow-up period, corresponding to a mean of 37 new cases per 10 000 women/year. Using multivariate analysis adjusted for the calendar period of treatment, date of birth and age at menopause, we were unable to detect an increase in the relative risk (RR) of breast cancer (RR 0.98, 95% confidence interval (CI): 0.65-1.5) in the HRT users. The RR of breast cancer per year of use of HRT was 1.005 (95% CI 0.97-1.05). These results do not justify early interruption of such a type of HRT, which is beneficial for quality of life, prevention of bone loss and cardiovascular risk profile, without the activation of coagulation and inflammatory protein synthesis measured in users of oral estrogens.

Dessoli S et al. Efficacy of low-dose intravaginal estriol on urogenital aging in postmenopausal women. Menopause. 11(1):49-56, January/February 2004.OBJECTIVE: To assess the efficacy and safety of intravaginal estriol administration on urinary incontinence, urogenital atrophy, and recurrent urinary tract infections in postmenopausal women. DESIGN: Eighty-eight postmenopausal women with urogenital aging symptoms were enrolled in this prospective, randomized, placebo-controlled study. Participants were randomly divided into two groups, with each group consisting of 44 women. Women in the treatment group received intravaginal estriol ovules: 1 ovule (1 mg) once daily for 2 weeks and then 2 ovules once weekly for a total of 6 months as maintenance therapy. Women in the control group received inert placebo vaginal suppositories in a similar regimen. We evaluated urogenital symptomatology, urine cultures, colposcopic findings, urethral cytologic findings, urethral pressure profiles, and urethrocystometry before as well as after 6 months of treatment. RESULTS: After therapy, the symptoms and signs of urogenital atrophy significantly improved in the treatment group in comparison with the control group. Thirty (68%) of the treated participants, and only seven (16%) of the control participants registered a subjective improvement of their incontinence. In the treated participants, we observed significant improvements of colposcopic findings, and there were statistically significant increases in mean maximum urethral pressure, in mean urethral closure pressure as well as in the abdominal pressure transmission ratio to the proximal urethra. Urethrocystometry showed positive but not statistically significant modifications. CONCLUSIONS: Our results show that intravaginal administration of estriol may represent a satisfactory therapeutic choice for those postmenopausal women with urogenital tract disturbances who have contraindications or refuse to undergo standard hormone therapy.

Dubey RK et al. CYP450- and COMT-derived estradiol metabolites inhibit activity of human coronary artery SMCs. Hypertension. 2003 Mar; 41(3 Pt 2):807-13. The purpose of this study is to test the hypothesis that the inhibitory effects of estradiol in human coronary vascular smooth muscle cells are mediated via local conversion to methoxyestradiols via specific cytochrome P450s (CYP450s) and catechol-O-methyltransferase (COMT). The inhibitory effects of estradiol on serum-induced cell activity (DNA synthesis, cell number, collagen synthesis, and cell migration) were enhanced by 3-methylcholantherene, phenobarbital (broad-spectrum CYP450 inducers), and beta-naphthoflavone (CYP1A1/1A2 inducer) and were blocked by 1-aminobenzotriazole (broad-spectrum CYP450 inhibitor). Ellipticine, alpha-naphthoflavone (selective CYP1A1 inhibitors), and pyrene (selective CYP1B1 inhibitor), but not ketoconazole (selective CYP3A4 inhibitor) or furafylline (selective CYP1A2 inhibitor), abrogated the inhibitor effects of estradiol on cell activity, a profile consistent with a CYP1A1/CYP1B1-mediated mechanism. The inhibitory effects of estradiol were blocked by the COMT inhibitors OR486 and quercetin. The estrogen receptor antagonist ICI 182,780 blocked the inhibitory effects of estradiol, but only at concentrations that also blocked the metabolism of estradiol to hydroxyestradiols (precursors of methoxyestradiols). Western blot analysis revealed that coronary smooth muscle cells expressed CYP1A1 and CYP1B1. Moreover, these cells metabolized estradiol to hydroxyestradiols and methoxyestradiols, and the conversion of 2-hydroxyestradiol to 2-methoxyestradiol was blocked by OR486 and quercetin. These findings provide evidence that the inhibitory effects of estradiol on coronary smooth muscle cells are largely mediated via CYP1A1- and CYP1B1-derived hydroxyestradiols that are converted to methoxyestradiols by COMT.

Dubey R. et al. Cardiovascular Pharmacology of Estradiol Metabolites. The Journal of Pharmacology and Experimental Therapeutics. 308:403–409, 2004A discussion of the role of endogenous estradiol metabolites in mediating important biological actions of estradiol is essentially nonexistent in standard textbooks of pharmacology and endocrinology. Indeed, the prevailing view is that all biological effects of estradiol are initiated by binding of estradiol per se to estrogen receptors and that estradiol metabolites are more or less irrelevant. This orthodox view, which is most likely incorrect, is the fundamental premise (an estrogen is an estrogen is an estrogen) underlying the design of important clinical trials such as the Heart and Estrogen/Progestin Replacement Study and the Women's Health Initiative Study. Accumulating data provide convincing evidence that some metabolites of estradiol, the major estrogen secreted by human ovaries, are biologically active and mediate multiple effects on the cardiovascular and renal systems that are largely independent of estrogen receptors. More specifically, metabolites of estradiol, particularly catecholestradiols and methoxyestradiols, induce multiple estrogen receptor-independent actions that protect the heart, blood vessels, and kidneys from disease. These protective effects are mediated in part by the inhibition of the ability of vascular smooth muscle cells, cardiac fibroblasts, and glomerular mesangial cells to migrate, proliferate, and secrete extracellular matrix proteins, as well as by an improvement in vascular endothelial cell function. The purpose of this review is to highlight the cardiovascular and renal pharmacology of catecholestradiols and methoxyestradiols. The take home message is simple: that when it comes to cardiovascular and renal protection, the concept that all estrogenic compounds are created equal may not be true.

Dubey RK et al. Catecholamines block the antimitogenic effect of estradiol on human coronary artery smooth muscle cells.J Clin Endocrinol Metab. 2004 Aug; 89(8):3922-31. Sequential conversion of estradiol to catecholestradiols and methoxyestradiols by cytochrome-P(450) (CYP450) and catechol-O-methyltransferase (COMT), respectively, contributes to the antimitogenic effects of estradiol on vascular smooth muscle cell (SMC) growth via estrogen receptor-independent mechanisms. Because catecholamines are also substrates for COMT, we hypothesize that catecholamines may abrogate the vasoprotective effects of estradiol by competing for COMT and inhibiting methoxyestradiol formation. To test this hypothesis, we investigated the antimitogenic/inhibitory effects of estradiol on human coronary artery SMC growth (cell number, DNA synthesis, collagen synthesis, and SMC migration) and ERK1/2 phosphorylation in the presence and absence of catecholamines. Norepinephrine, epinephrine, isoproterenol, and OR486 (COMT inhibitor) abrogated the inhibitory effects of estradiol on SMC growth and ERK1/2 phosphorylation. The interaction of catecholamines with estradiol was not affected by phentolamine or propanolol, alpha- and beta-adrenoceptor antagonists, respectively. The antimitogenic effects of 2-hydroxy-estradiol, but not 2-methoxyestradiol, were abrogated by epinephrine, isoproterenol, and OR486. Catecholamines inhibited the conversion of both estradiol and 2-hydroxy-estradiol to 2-methoxyestradiol, and SMCs expressed CYP1A1 and CYP1B1. Our findings suggest that catecholamines within the coronary arteries may abrogate the antivasoocclusive effects of estradiol by blocking the conversion of catecholestradiols to methoxyestradiols. The interaction between catecholamines and estradiol metabolism may importantly define the cardiovascular effects of estradiol therapy in postmenopausal women.

Duckles SP et al. Estrogen and Mitochondria: A New Paradigm for Vascular Protection? Molecular Interventions 6:26-35, (2006) Mitochondrial dysfunction has been implicated as a cause of age-related disorders, and the mitochondrial theory of aging links aging, exercise, and diet. Endothelial dysfunction is a key paradigm for vascular disease and aging, and there is considerable evidence that exercise and dietary restriction protect against cardiovascular disease. Recent studies demonstrate that estrogen receptors are present in mitochondria and that estrogen promotes mitochondrial efficiency and decreases oxidative stress in the cerebral vasculature. Chronic estrogen treatment increases mitochondrial capacity for oxidative phosphorylation while decreasing production of reactive oxygen species. The effectiveness of estrogen against age-related cardiovascular disorders, including stroke, may thus arise in part from hormonal effects on mitochondrial function. Estrogen-mediated mitochondrial efficiency may also be a contributing factor to the longer lifespan of women.

Durna EM et al. Hormone replacement therapy after a diagnosis of breast cancer: cancer recurrence and mortality. Med J Aust. 2002 Oct 7;177(7):347-51.OBJECTIVE: To determine whether hormone replacement therapy (HRT) after treatment for breast cancer is associated with increased risk of recurrence and mortality.DESIGN: Retrospective observational study.PARTICIPANTS AND SETTING: Postmenopausal women diagnosed with breast cancer and treated by five Sydney doctors between

1964 and 1999.OUTCOME MEASURES: Times from diagnosis to cancer recurrence or new breast cancer, to death from all causes and to death from primary tumour were compared between women who used HRT for menopausal symptoms after diagnosis and those who did not. Relative risks (RRs) were determined from Cox regression analyses, adjusted for patient and tumour characteristics.RESULTS: 1122 women were followed up for 0-36 years (median, 6.08 years); 154 were lost to follow-up. 286 women used HRT for menopausal symptoms for up to 26 years (median, 1.75 years). Compared with non-users, HRT users had reduced risk of cancer recurrence (adjusted relative risk [RR], 0.62; 95% CI, 0.43-0.87), all-cause mortality (RR, 0.34; 95% CI, 0.19-0.59) and death from primary tumour (RR, 0.40; 95% CI, 0.22-0.72). Continuous combined HRT was associated with a reduced risk of death from primary tumour (RR, 0.32; 95% CI, 0.12-0.88) and all-cause mortality (RR, 0.27; 95% CI, 0.10-0.73).CONCLUSION: HRT use for menopausal symptoms by women treated for primary invasive breast cancer is not associated with an increased risk of breast cancer recurrence or shortened life expectancy.

Fenton A et al.   Editorial- the Women's health Initiative—a decade of progress. Climacteric 2012;15:205. July 2002 marks an important milestone in our understandingof the risks and benefi ts of using hormone therapy to managesymptoms of menopause. Prior to that date, hormone replacementtherapy (HRT) had been widely prescribed for womenon the understanding that it improved quality of life and reduced the incidence of fractures. Research also supported reductions in the risks of coronary artery disease, bowel cancer and dementia 1 . These benefi ts appeared to be counterbalanced by increased risks of breast cancer and venous thromboembolic events (VTE). The Women ' s Health Initiative (WHI) set out to examinethe effects of HRT in a much older, largely asymptomatic population of women. The premature cessation of the WHI in mid-2002 was accompanied by reports that HRT not only worsened quality of life but lead to increases in the incidence of coronary heart disease, stroke, dementia, breast cancer and VTE 2 . Benefi ts related to bowel cancer, fracture incidence and overall mortality, as well as risk stratifi cation based on age,received substantially less attention.Over the past decade, there has been much critical appraisal.

Finset A. Musculo-skeletal pain, psychological distress, and hormones during the menopausal transition Psychoneuroendocrinology. 2004 Jan; 29(1):49-64. OBJECTIVE: To investigate the relationship between sex hormones (estradiol, testosterone, androstendione, DHEA-S) and prolactin on one hand and musculo-skeletal pain and psychological distress on the other during the menopausal transition. METHOD: Fifty-seven regularly menstruating women, who were studied over five consecutive years, who reached menopause before the fifth assessment, and did not use hormone replacement therapy were included in the study. Hormones were sampled and a questionnaire including questions on psychological distress and musculo-skeletal pain were administered at the five points of assessment. Data on last year before menopause (T1), first (T2) and second (T3) year after menopause are reported. RESULTS: DHEA-S, but neither testosterone nor androstendione, was inversely related to distress and pain. Pain contributed to the variance of DHEA-S over the menopausal transition, whereas DHEA-S levels did not predict pain or distress when baseline levels were controlled for. Prolactin was at T1 and T2 positively associated with distress and at T2 positively associated with musculo-skeletal pain. Musculo-skeletal pain pre-menopause was significantly related to estradiol. CONCLUSION: DHEA-S was negatively associated, and prolactin positively associated with musculo-skeletal pain and psychological distress. Whereas post-menopause DHEA-S levels were influenced by pain scores, no significant effect of pre-menopause hormones on post-menopause pain and distress was found.

Fournier A et al. Breast cancer risk in relation to different types of hormone replacement therapy in the E3N-EPIC cohort. Int J Cancer. 2005 Apr 10; 114(3):448-54. Most epidemiological studies have shown an increase in breast cancer risk related to hormone replacement therapy (HRT) use. A recent large cohort study showed effects of similar magnitude for different types of progestogens and for different routes of administration of estrogens evaluated. Further investigation of these issues is of importance. We assessed the risk of breast cancer associated with HRT use in 54,548 postmenopausal women who had never taken any HRT 1 year before entering the E3N-EPIC cohort study (mean age at inclusion: 52.8 years); 948 primary invasive breast cancers were diagnosed during follow-up (mean duration: 5.8 years). Data were analyzed using multivariate Cox proportional hazards models. In this cohort where the mean duration of HRT use was 2.8 years, an increased risk in HRT users compared to nonusers was found (relative risk (RR) 1.2 [95% confidence interval 1.1-1.4]). The RR was 1.1 [0.8-1.6] for estrogens used alone and 1.3 [1.1-1.5] when used in combination with oral progestogens. The risk was significantly greater (p <0.001) with HRT containing synthetic progestins than with HRT containing micronized progesterone, the RRs being 1.4 [1.2-1.7] and 0.9 [0.7-1.2], respectively. When combined with synthetic progestins, both oral and transdermal/percutaneous estrogens use were associated with a significantly increased risk; for transdermal/percutaneous estrogens, this was the case even when exposure was less than 2 years. Our results suggest that, when combined with synthetic progestins, even short-term use of estrogens may increase breast cancer risk. Micronized progesterone may be preferred to synthetic progestins in short-term HRT. This finding needs further investigation.

166

Fournier A et al. Unequal risks for breast cancer associated with different hormone replacement therapies: results from the E3N cohort study. Breast Cancer Res Treat. 2008 Jan; 107(1):103-11. Large numbers of hormone replacement therapies (HRTs) are available for the treatment of menopausal symptoms. It is still unclear whether some are more deleterious than others regarding breast cancer risk. The goal of this study was to assess and compare the association between different HRTs and breast cancer risk, using data from the French E3N cohort study. Invasive breast cancer cases were identified through biennial self-administered questionnaires completed from 1990 to 2002. During follow-up (mean duration 8.1 postmenopausal years), 2,354 cases of invasive breast cancer occurred among 80,377 postmenopausal women. Compared with HRT never-use, use of estrogen alone was associated with a significant 1.29-fold increased risk (95% confidence interval 1.02-1.65). The association of estrogen-progestagen combinations with breast cancer risk varied significantly according to the type of progestagen: the relative risk was 1.00 (0.83-1.22) for estrogen-progesterone, 1.16 (0.94-1.43) for estrogen-dydrogesterone and 1.69 (1.50-1.91) for estrogen combined with other progestagens. This latter category involves progestins with different physiologic activities (androgenic, nonandrogenic, antiandrogenic), but their associations with breast cancer risk did not differ significantly from one another. This study found no evidence of an association with risk according to the route of estrogen administration (oral or transdermal/percutaneous). These findings suggest that the choice of the progestagen component in combined HRT is of importance regarding breast cancer risk; it could be preferable to use progesterone or dydrogesterone.

Grodstein F et al. Postmenopausal hormone therapy and mortality.N Engl J Med. 1997 Jun 19; 336(25):1769-75.BACKGROUND: Postmenopausal hormone therapy has both benefits and hazards, including decreased risks of osteoporosis and cardiovascular disease and an increased risk of breast cancer. METHODS: We examined the relation between the use of postmenopausal hormones and mortality among participants in the Nurses' Health Study, who were 30 to 55 years of age at base line in 1976. Data were collected by biennial questionnaires beginning in 1976 and continuing through 1992. We documented 3637 deaths from 1976 to 1994. Each participant who died was matched with 10 controls alive at the time of her death. For each death, we defined the subject's hormone status according to the last biennial questionnaire before her death or before the diagnosis of the fatal disease; this reduced bias caused by the discontinuation of hormone use between the time of diagnosis of a potentially fatal disease and death. RESULTS: After adjustment for confounding variables, current hormone users had a lower risk of death (relative risk, 0.63; 95 percent confidence interval, 0.56 to 0.70) than subjects who had never taken hormones; however, the apparent benefit decreased with long-term use (relative risk, 0.80; 0.67 to 0.96, after 10 or more years) because of an increase in mortality from breast cancer among long-term hormone users. Current hormone users with coronary risk factors (69 percent of the women) had the largest reduction in mortality (relative risk, 0.51; 95 percent confidence interval, 0.45 to 0.57), with substantially less benefit for those at low risk (13 percent of the women; relative risk, 0.89; 95 percent confidence interval, 0.62 to 1.28). CONCLUSIONS: On average, mortality among women who use postmenopausal hormones is lower than among nonusers; however, the survival benefit diminishes with longer duration of use and is lower for women at low risk for coronary disease.

Grodstein F, Manson JE, Stampfer MJ The Role of Time since Menopause and Age at Hormone Initiation.Womens Health J Hormone Therapy and Coronary Heart Disease: 2006 January/February;15(1BACKGROUND: Apparently discrepant findings have been reported by the Women's Health Initiative (WHI) trial compared with observational studies of postmenopausal hormone therapy (HT) and coronary heart disease (CHD). METHODS: We prospectively examined the relation of HT to CHD, according to timing of hormone initiation relative to age and time since menopause. Participants were postmenopausal women in the Nurses' Health Study, with follow-up from 1976 to 2000. Information on hormone use was ascertained in biennial, mailed questionnaires. We used proportional hazards models to calculate multivariable adjusted relative risks (RR) and 95% confidence intervals (CI). We also conducted sensitivity analyses to determine the possible influence of incomplete capture of coronary events occurring shortly after initiation of HT. RESULTS: Women beginning HT near menopause had a significantly reduced risk of CHD (RR = 0.66, 95% CI 0.54-0.80 for estrogen alone; RR = 0.72, 95% CI 0.56-0.92 for estrogen with progestin). In the subgroup of women demographically similar to those in the WHI, we found no significant relation between HT and CHD among women who initiated therapy at least 10 years after menopause (RR = 0.87, 95% CI 0.69-1.10 for estrogen alone; RR = 0.90, 95% CI 0.62-1.29 for estrogen with progestin). Among women who began taking hormones at older ages, we also found no relation between current use of estrogen alone and CHD (for women aged 60+ years, RR = 1.07, 95% CI 0.65-1.78), although there was a suggestion of possible reduced risk for combined HT (RR = 0.65, 95% CI 0.31-1.38). In sensitivity analyses, we found that the incomplete capture of coronary events occurring shortly after initiation of HT could not explain our observation of a reduced risk of coronary disease for current users of HT. CONCLUSIONS: These data support the possibility that timing of HT initiation in relation to menopause onset or to age might influence coronary risk.

Harman et al. KEEPS: Kronos Early Estrogen Prevention Study. Climacteric 2005:8:3-12. Observational studies have indicated that hormone therapy given at or after menopause is linked to substantial reduction in cardiovascular disease and its risk factors. Recent findings from the Women's Health Initiative (WHI) clinical trial, however, indicate that combined estrogen plus progestin hormone therapy, as well as estrogen-alone hormone therapy (given to women without a uterus), is ineffective in preventing the new onset of cardiac events in previously healthy late menopausal women. Further, the secondary prevention trial, the Heart and Estrogen/progestin Replacement Study (HERS), also failed to demonstrate any benefit of initiation of hormone therapy in women with established coronary heart disease. In light of these results, a hypothesis has arisen that early initiation of hormone therapy, in women who are at the inception of their menopause, will delay the onset of subclinical cardiovascular disease in women. The rationale that earlier intervention than that performed in the WHI and HERS trials will provide cardiovascular benefit to women is the driving force behind the Kronos Early Estrogen Prevention Study, or KEEPS. KEEPS is a multicenter, 5-year clinical trial that will evaluate the effectiveness of 0.45 mg of conjugated equine estrogens, 50 microg weekly transdermal estradiol (both in combination with cyclic oral, micronized progesterone, 200 mg for 12 days each month), and placebo in preventing progression of carotid intimal medial thickness and the accrual of coronary calcium in women aged 42-58 years who are within 36 months of their final menstrual period. A total of 720 women are planned to be enrolled in 2005, with an anticipated close-out of the trial in 2010. This overview summarizes the recruitment and methodology of the KEEPS trial.

Henderson VW et al. Hormone therapy and the risk of stroke: perspectives 10 years after the Women's Health Initiative trials. Climacteric 2012;15:229-234. Principal findings on stroke from the Women's Health Initiative (WHI) clinical trials of hormone therapy indicate that estrogen, alone or with a progestogen, increases a woman's risk of stroke. These results were not unexpected, and research during the past decade has tended to support these findings. Consistent evidence from clinical trials and observational research indicates that standard-dose hormone therapy increases stroke risk for postmenopausal women by about one-third; increased risk may be limited to ischemic stroke. Risk is not modified by age of hormone initiation or use, or by temporal proximity to menopause, and risk is similar for estrogen plus progestogen and for unopposed estrogen. Limited evidence implies that lower doses of transdermal estradiol (≤50 μg/day) may not alter stroke risk. For women less than 60 years of age, the absolute risk of stroke from standard-dose hormone therapy is rare, about two additional strokes per 10 000 person-years of use; the absolute risk is considerably greater for older women. Other hormonally active compounds - including raloxifene, tamoxifen, and tibolone - can also affect stroke risk.

Hermsmeyer RK et al. Prevention of coronary hyperreactivity in preatherogenic menopausal rhesus monkeys by transdermal progesterone. Arterioscler Thromb Vasc Biol. 2004 May; 24(5):955-61. OBJECTIVE: To test if transdermal progesterone (P) confers coronary vascular protection in surgically menopausal preatherosclerotic rhesus monkeys. METHODS AND RESULTS: Ovariectomized rhesus monkeys fed an atherogenic diet (AD) for 19 months were treated with an investigational transdermal P cream (n=7) or identical placebo cream (n=5) for 4 weeks. Aorta and carotids showed fatty streaks and Oil Red O staining demonstrated lipid deposition. Serum P levels in P-treated rhesus monkeys (0.6 ng/mL) were significantly greater than placebo (0.2 ng/mL). Significant elevation of cholesterol, LDL cholesterol, and HDL cholesterol, was noted in all animals. Lp (a) was significantly attenuated in the AD-fed P-treated monkeys. Coronary angiographic experiments stimulating vasoconstriction by intracoronary injections of serotonin plus U46619 showed exaggerated prolonged actions amplified by AD, but significant protection against severe prolonged vasoconstriction in P-treated monkeys. Immunocytochemistry confirmed co-expression of P and thromboxane prostanoid (TP) receptors in coronaries and aorta. Western blotting demonstrated TP receptor attenuation in vascular muscle after P treatment. CONCLUSIONS: Coronary hyperreactivity, a putative component of coronary artery disease mediated via increased vascular muscle thromboxane prostanoid receptors, can be prevented by subphysiological levels of P, not only in nonatherosclerotic (previously shown) but also in preatherosclerotic primates.

Hodis HN et al. The timing hypothesis for coronary heart disease prevention with hormone therapy: past, present and futre in perspective. Climacteric 2012;15:217-228.

Over the past decade, two informative events in primary prevention of coronary heart disease (CHD) have occurred for women's health. The first concerns hormone replacement therapy (HRT) where data have come full circle from presumed harm to consistency with observational data that HRT initiation in close proximity to menopause significantly reduces CHD and overall mortality. The other concerns sex-specific efficacy of CHD primary prevention therapies where lipid-lowering and aspirin therapy have not been conclusively shown to significantly reduce CHD and, more importantly, where there is lack of evidence that either therapy reduces overall mortality in women. Cumulated data support a 'window-of-opportunity' for maximal reduction of CHD and overall mortality and minimization of risks with HRT initiation before 60 years of age and/or within 10 years of menopause and continued for 6 years or more. There is a substantial increase in quality-adjusted life-years over a 5-30-year period in women who initiate HRT in close proximity to menopause, supporting HRT as a highly cost-effective strategy for improving quality-adjusted life. Although primary prevention therapies and HRT contrast in their efficacy to significantly reduce CHD and especially overall mortality in postmenopausal women, the magnitude and types of risks associated with HRT are similar to those associated with other medications commonly used in women's health. The cumulated data highlight the importance of studying the HRT cardioprotective hypothesis in women representative of those from whom the hypothesis was generated.

Hugel S et al. Multiple mechanisms are involved in the acute vasodilatory effect of 17beta-estradiol in the isolated perfused rat heart. J Cardiovasc Pharmacol. 1999 Jun; 33(6):852-8. The purpose of this study was to define the dose-dependent effects of 17beta-estradiol on coronary flow and cardiac function in isolated rat hearts and to identify the mechanisms involved in its vasodilator action. Hearts from female and male Wistar rats were perfused at constant pressure (100 mm Hg). Stereoisomer specificity and the mechanism of vasodilation by 17beta-estradiol were examined in female rat hearts. Function was measured by a left ventricular (LV) balloon and coronary flow (CF) with an ultrasonic flowmeter. 17Beta-estradiol at 10(-6), 5 x 10(-6), and 10(-5) M increased CF in female hearts by 5 +/- 2, 27 +/- 4 (p < 0.05 vs. baseline), and 40 +/- 4% (p < 0.05 vs. baseline), respectively. The effect of 17beta-estradiol in hearts from male rats was similar but less pronounced compared with females [deltaCF 8 +/- 3, 19 +/- 3 (p < 0.05 vs. baseline)] and 25 +/- 7% (p < 0.05 vs. baseline; p < 0.05 vs. female 17beta-estradiol). Maximum vasodilation by the stereoisomer 17alpha-estradiol was significantly smaller [deltaCF 5 +/- 3, 4 +/- 3 (p < 0.05 vs. female 17beta-estradiol) and 14 +/- 1% (p < 0.05 vs. baseline; p < 0.05 vs. female 17beta-estradiol)] for 10(-6), 5 x 10(-6), and 10(-5) M. Pretreatment with the NO-synthesis inhibitor Nomega-methyl-L-arginine (10(-4) M) had no effect on the maximal vasodilator response to 17beta-estradiol (10(-5) M) [deltaCF 36 +/- 6% (p < 0.05 vs. baseline)]. When hearts were pretreated with the prostaglandin-synthesis inhibitor diclofenac (10(-6) M), the maximal vasodilator effect of 17beta-estradiol was partially attenuated [deltaCF 12 +/- 7% (p < 0.05 vs. female 17beta-estradiol)]. Similarly, pretreatment with the K+ATP-blocker glibenclamide (10(-6) M) partially inhibited the maximal vasodilator effect of 17beta-estradiol [deltaCF 22 +/- 6% (p < 0.05 vs. baseline; p < 0.05 vs. female 17beta-estradiol)]. Pretreatment with the Ca2+ channel antagonist nifedipine (7.2 x 10(-8) M) completely blocked the vasodilator effect. In isolated perfused rat hearts, 17beta-estradiol induced marked acute coronary vasodilation; this effect is in part gender specific, and in female hearts, largely stereoisomer specific. The dilator effect is mediated predominantly by calcium channel blockade, but prostaglandin release and K+ATP channel activation also are involved. In the isolated perfused rat heart, NO production does not contribute to the acute vasodilator effect of 17beta-estradiol.

Klaiber EL, Vogel W, Rako S A critique of the Women's Health Initiative hormone therapy study. Fertil Steril. 2005 Dec; 84(6):1589-601. OBJECTIVE: This review critiques The Women's Health Initiative (WHI) study, focusing on aspects of the study design contributing to the adverse events resulting in the study's discontinuation. CONCLUSION(S): Two aspects of the design contributed to the adverse events: [1] The decision to administer continuous combined conjugated equine estrogen (CEE)/medroxyprogesterone acetate (MPA) or E alone as a standard regimen to a population with little previous hormonal treatment, ranging in age from 50-79 years, who, because of their age, were predisposed to coronary and cerebral atherosclerosis. [2] Selection of an untested regimen of continuous combined CEE plus MPA, which we hypothesize, negated the protective effect of E on the cardiovascular and cerebrovascular systems. Multiple observational studies that preceded the WHI study concluded that the use of E alone and E plus cyclic (not daily) progestin combination treatments initiated in early menopause had beneficial effects. The therapeutic regimens resulted in prevention of atherosclerosis and reductions in coronary artery disease mortality. It is our conclusion that the WHI hormonal replacement study had major design flaws that led to adverse conclusions about the positive effects of hormone therapy. An alternative hormonal regimen is proposed that, on the basis of data supporting its beneficial cardiovascular effects, when initiated appropriately in a population of younger, more recently menopausal women, has promise to yield a more favorable risk/benefit outcome.

Koh KK et al. Should progestins be blamed for the failure of hormone replacement therapy to reduce cardiovascular events in randomized controlled trials? Arterioscler Thromb Vasc Biol. 2004 Jul; 24(7):1171-9. Many observational studies and experimental and animal studies have demonstrated that estrogen replacement therapy (ERT) or hormone replacement therapy (HRT) (estrogen plus progestin) significantly reduces the risk of coronary heart disease. Nonetheless, recent randomized controlled trials demonstrated some trends toward an increased risk of cardiovascular events rather than a reduction of risk. Recently, both the HRT and ERT arms of the Women's Health Initiative (WHI) study were terminated early because of an increased/no incidence of invasive breast cancer, increased incidence of stroke, and increased trend/no protective effects of cardiovascular disease. We discuss the controversial effects of HRT and ERT on cardiovascular system and provide a hypothesis that the failure of HRT and ERT in reducing the risk of cardiovascular events in postmenopausal women might be because of the stage of their atherosclerosis at the time of initiation of HRT or ERT.

Liu ZJ et al. Selective insensitivity of ZR-75-1 human breast cancer cells to 2-methoxyestradiol: evidence for type II 17beta-hydroxysteroid dehydrogenase as the underlying cause. Cancer Res. 2005 Jul 1; 65(13):5802-11. 2-Methoxyestradiol (2-MeO-E2), a nonpolar endogenous metabolite of 17beta-estradiol, has strong antiproliferative, apoptotic, and antiangiogenic actions. Among the four human breast cancer cell lines tested (MCF-7, T-47D, ZR-75-1, and MDA-MB-435s), the ZR-75-1 cells were selectively insensitive to the antiproliferative actions of 2-MeO-E2, although these cells had a similar sensitivity as other cell lines to several other anticancer agents (5-fluorouracil, mitomycin C, doxorubicin, colchicine, vinorelbine, and paclitaxel). Mechanistically, this insensitivity is largely attributable to the presence of high levels of a steroid-selective metabolizing enzyme, the type II 17beta-hydroxysteroid dehydrogenase (17beta-HSD), in the ZR-75-1 cells, which rapidly converts 2-MeO-E2 to the inactive 2-methoxyestrone, but this enzyme does not metabolically inactivate other nonsteroidal anticancer agents. The type II 17beta-HSD-mediated conversion of 2-MeO-E2 to 2-methoxyestrone in

ZR-75-1 cells followed the first-order kinetics, with a very short half-life (approximately 2 hours). In comparison, the T-47D, MCF-7, and MDA-MB-435s human breast cancer cells, which were highly sensitive to 2-MeO-E2, had very low or undetectable catalytic activity for the conversion of 2-MeO-E2 to 2-methoxyestrone. Reverse transcription-PCR analysis of the mRNA levels of three known oxidative 17beta-HSD isozymes (types II, IV, and VIII) revealed that only the type II isozyme was selectively expressed in the ZR-75-1 cells, whereas the other two isozymes were expressed in all four cell lines. Taken together, our results showed, for the first time, that the high levels of type II 17beta-HSD present in ZR-75-1 cells were largely responsible for the facile conversion of 2-MeO-E2 to 2-methoxyestrone and also for the selective insensitivity to the antiproliferative actions of 2-MeO-E2.

Maki, P et al. Hormone therapy, dementia, and cognition: The Women's Helath Initiative 10 years on. Climacteric 2012:15:256-262 Principal findings on dementia from the Women's Health Initiative Memory Study (WHIMS) showed that conjugated equine estrogens plus medroxyprogesterone acetate (CEE/MPA) increase dementia risk in women aged 65 years and above, but not risk of mild cognitive impairment. The dementia finding was unexpected, given consistent observational evidence that associates use of estrogen-containing hormone therapy with reduced risk of Alzheimer's disease. It remains controversial whether hormone use by younger postmenopausal women near the time of menopause reduces dementia risk or whether WHIMS findings should be generalized to younger women. Given the challenges of conducting a primary prevention trial to address that question, it is helpful to consider the impact of hormone therapy on cognitive test performance, particularly verbal memory, for its own sake and as a proxy for dementia risk. The WHI Study of Cognitive Aging (WHISCA) showed that CEE/MPA worsened verbal memory, whereas CEE alone had no influence on cognition. These findings have been replicated in several randomized, clinical trials. The apparent negative effect of CEE/MPA on verbal memory does not appear to be age-dependent. Additional investigations are needed to understand the impact of other hormonally active compounds on dementia and cognitive outcomes.

Menon DV et al. Effects of transdermal estrogen replacement therapy on cardiovascular risk factors.Treat Endocrinol. 2006; 5(1):37-51. The prevalence of hypertension and cardiovascular disease increases dramatically after menopause in women, implicating estrogen as having a protective role in the cardiovascular system. However, recent large clinical trials have failed to show cardiovascular benefit, and have even demonstrated possible harmful effects, of opposed and unopposed estrogen in postmenopausal women. While these findings have led to a revision of guidelines such that they discourage the use of estrogen for primary or secondary prevention of heart disease in postmenopausal women, many investigators have attributed the negative results in clinical trials to several flaws in study design, including the older age of study participants and the initiation of estrogen late after menopause.Because almost all clinical trials use oral estrogen as the primary form of hormone supplementation, another question that has arisen is the importance of the route of estrogen administration with regards to the cardiovascular outcomes. During oral estrogen administration, the concentration of estradiol in the liver sinusoids is four to five times higher than that in the systemic circulation. This supraphysiologic concentration of estrogen in the liver can modulate the expression of many hepatic-derived proteins, which are not observed in premenopausal women. In contrast, transdermal estrogen delivers the hormone directly into the systemic circulation and, thus, avoids the first-pass hepatic effect.Although oral estrogen exerts a more favorable influence than transdermal estrogen on traditional cardiovascular risk factors such as high- and low-density lipoprotein-cholesterol levels, recent studies have indicated that oral estrogen adversely influences many emerging risk factors in ways that are not seen with transdermal estrogen. Oral estrogen significantly increases levels of acute-phase proteins such as C-reactive protein and serum amyloid A; procoagulant factors such as prothrombin fragments 1+2; and several key enzymes involved in plaque disruption, while transdermal estrogen does not have these adverse effects.Whether the advantages of transdermal estrogen with regards to these risk factors will translate into improved clinical outcomes remains to be determined. Two ongoing clinical trials, KEEPS (Kronos Early Estrogen Prevention Study) and ELITE (Early versus Late Intervention Trial with Estradiol) are likely to provide invaluable information regarding the role of oral versus transdermal estrogen in younger postmenopausal women.

Mishra RG et al. Metabolite ligands of estrogen receptor-beta reduce primate coronary hyperreactivity Am J Physiol Heart Circ Physiol. 2006 Jan; 290(1):H295-303. Previous reports showed that 17beta-estradiol implants attenuate in vivo coronary hyperreactivity (CH), characterized by long-duration vasoconstrictions (in coronary angiographic experiments), in menopausal rhesus monkeys. Prolonged Ca2+ contraction signals that correspond with CH in coronary vascular muscle cells (VMC) to the same dual-constrictor stimulus, serotonin + the thromboxane analog U-46619, in estrogen-deprived VMC were suppressed by >72 h in 17beta-estradiol. The purpose of this study was to test whether an endogenous estrogen metabolite with estrogen receptor-beta (ER-beta) binding activity, estriol (E3), suppresses in vivo and in vitro CH. E3 treatment in vivo for 4 wk significantly attenuated the angiographically evaluated vasoconstrictor response to intracoronary serotonin + U-46619 challenge. In vitro treatment of rhesus coronary VMC for >72 h with nanomolar E3 attenuated late Ca2+ signals. This reduction of late Ca2+ signals also appeared after >72 h of treatment with subnanomolar 5alpha-androstane-3beta, 17beta-diol (3beta-Adiol), an endogenous dihydrotestosterone metabolite with ER-beta binding activity. R, R-tetrahydrochrysene, a selective ER-beta antagonist, significantly blocked the E3- and 3beta-Adiol-mediated attenuation of late Ca2+ signal increases. ER-beta and thromboxane-prostanoid receptor (TPR) were coexpressed in coronary arteries and aorta. In vivo E3 treatment attenuated aortic TPR expression. Furthermore, in vitro treatment with E3 or 3beta-Adiol downregulated TPR expression in VMC, which was blocked for both agonists by pretreatment with R, R-tetrahydrochrysene. E3- and 3beta-Adiol-mediated reduction in persistent $Ca2+$ signals is associated with ER-beta-mediated attenuation of TPR expression and may partly explain estrogen benefits in coronary vascular muscle.

Ouyang P et al. Hormone replacement therapy and the cardiovascular system lessons learned and unanswered questions. J Am Coll Cardiol. 2006 May 2; 47(9):1741-53. Cardiovascular disease is the leading cause of death among women in the U.S., exceeding breast cancer mortality in women of all ages. Women present with cardiovascular disease a decade after men and this has been attributed to the protective effect of female ovarian sex hormones that is lost after menopause. Animal and observational studies have shown beneficial effects of hormone therapy when it is initiated early in the perimenopausal period or before the development of significant atherosclerosis. However, randomized, placebo-controlled trials in older women have not shown any benefit in either primary prevention or secondary prevention of cardiovascular events, with a concerning trend toward harm. This review outlines the lessons learned from the basic science, animal, observational, and randomized trials, and then summarizes yet-unanswered questions of hormone therapy and cardiovascular risk.

Philp KL et al. Greater antiarrhythmic activity of acute 17beta-estradiol in female than male anaesthetized rats: correlation with Ca (2+) channel blockade. Br J Pharmacol. 2006 Aug 29 BACKGROUND AND PURPOSE: Female sex hormones may protect pre-menopausal women from sudden cardiac death. We therefore investigated the effects of the main female sex hormone, 17beta-estradiol, on ischaemia-induced cardiac arrhythmias and on the L-type $Ca2+$ current (ICaL). EXPERIMENTAL APPROACH: In vivo experiments were performed in pentobarbital-anaesthetized rats subjected to acute coronary artery occlusion. ICaL was measured by the whole-cell patch-clamp technique, in rat isolated ventricular myocytes. KEY RESULTS: Acute intravenous administration of 17beta-estradiol as a bolus dose followed by a continuous infusion, commencing 10 min before coronary artery occlusion, had dose-dependent antiarrhythmic activity. In female rats 300 ng kg (-1) + 30 ng kg (-1) min (-1) 17beta-estradiol significantly reduced the number of ventricular premature beats (VPBs) and the incidence of ventricular fibrillation (VF). A ten fold higher dose of 17beta-estradiol was required to cause similar effects in male rats. In vitro 17beta-estradiol reduced peak ICaL in a concentration-dependent manner. The EC50 was ten-fold higher in male myocytes (0.66 microM) than in females (0.06 microM). CONCLUSIONS AND IMPLICATIONS: These results indicate that 17beta-estradiol has marked dose-dependent antiarrhythmic activity that is greater in female rats than in males. A similar differential potency in blocking ICaL in myocytes from female and male rats can account for this effect. This provides an explanation for the antiarrhythmic activity of 17beta-estradiol and gender-selective protection against sudden cardiac death.

Patten RD et al. 17beta-estradiol reduces cardiomyocyte apoptosis in vivo and in vitro via activation of phospho-inositide-3 kinase/Akt signaling. Circ Res. 2004 Oct 1; 95(7):692-9. Female gender and estrogen-replacement therapy in postmenopausal women are associated with improved heart failure survival, and physiological replacement of 17beta-estradiol (E2) reduces infarct size and cardiomyocyte apoptosis in animal models of myocardial infarction (MI). Here, we characterize the molecular mechanisms of E2 effects on cardiomyocyte survival in vivo and in vitro. Ovariectomized female mice were treated with placebo or physiological E2 replacement, followed by coronary artery ligation (placebo-MI or E2-MI) or sham operation (sham) and hearts were harvested 6, 24, and 72 hours later. After MI, E2 replacement significantly increased activation of the prosurvival kinase, Akt, and decreased cardiomyocyte apoptosis assessed by terminal deoxynucleotidyltransferase dUTP nick-end labeling (TUNEL) staining and caspase 3 activation. In vitro, E2 at 1 or 10 nmol/L caused a rapid 2.7-fold increase in Akt phosphorylation and a decrease in apoptosis as measured by TUNEL staining, caspase 3 activation, and DNA laddering in cultured neonatal rat cardiomyocytes. The E2-mediated reduction in apoptosis was reversed by an estrogen receptor (ER) antagonist, ICI 182,780, and by phospho-inositide-3 kinase inhibitors, LY294002 and Wortmannin. Overexpression of a dominant negative-Akt construct also blocked E2-mediated reduction in cardiomyocyte apoptosis. These data show that E2 reduces cardiomyocyte apoptosis in vivo and in vitro by ER- and phospho-inositide-3 kinase-Akt-dependent pathways and support the relevance of these pathways in the observed estrogen-mediated reduction in myocardial injury.

Pines A et al. Quality of life and the role of menopausal hormone therapy. Climacteric 2012;15:213-216. The quality of life of countless menopausal women world-wide has been significantly diminished following the sensationalist reporting of the Women's Health Initiative (WHI) and the resulting 50% or more decline in the use of hormone replacement therapy (HRT) over the subsequent 10 years. Quality of life is difficult to measure as there are so many contributing factors and a large number of different instruments, some of which assess general health and only a few which specifically include symptoms related to menopause. HRT improves quality of life of symptomatic menopausal women and some studies of the effects of HRT provide reliable evidence on quality of life other than reduction in vasomotor symptoms. Until there is a better understanding of the minimal risks of HRT for the majority of women, too many will continue to suffer a reduced quality of life unnecessarily.

Plu-Bureau G et al. Percutaneous progesterone use and risk of breast cancer: results from a French cohort study of premenopausal women with benign breast disease. Cancer Detect Prev. 1999; 23(4):290-6. Percutaneous progesterone topically applied on the breast has been proposed and widely used in the relief of mastalgia and benign breast disease by numerous gynecologists and general practitioners. However, its chronic use has never been evaluated in relation to breast cancer risk. The association between percutaneous progesterone use and the risk of breast cancer was evaluated in a cohort study of 1150 premenopausal French women with benign breast disease diagnosed in two breast clinics between 1976 and 1979. The follow-up accumulated 12,462 person-years. Percutaneous progesterone had been prescribed to 58% of the women. There was no association between breast cancer risk and the use of percutaneous progesterone (RR = 0.8; 95% confidence interval 0.4-1.6). Although the combined treatment of oral progestogens with percutaneous progesterone significantly decreased the risk of breast cancer (RR = 0.5; 95% confidence interval 0.2-0.9) as compared with nonusers, there was no significant difference in the risk of breast cancer in percutaneous progesterone users versus nonusers among oral progestogen users. Taken together, these results suggest at least an absence of deleterious effects caused by percutaneous progesterone use in women with benign breast disease.

Puder JJ et al. Estrogen modulates the hypothalamic-pituitary-adrenal and inflammatory cytokine responses to endotoxin in women.Clin Endocrinol Metab. 2001 Jun; 86(6):2403-8 Endotoxin stimulates the release of the inflammatory cytokines interleukin (IL)-1, IL-6, and tumor necrosis factor (TNF)-alpha, which are potent activators of the hypothalamic-pituitary-adrenal (HPA) axis. Recent studies in the rodent and in the primate have shown that the HPA responses to endotoxin and IL-1 were enhanced by gonadectomy and attenuated by estradiol (E2) replacement. In addition, there is some evidence, in the rodent, that estrogen modulates inflammatory cytokine responses to endotoxin. To determine whether estrogen has similar effects in humans, we studied the cytokine and HPA responses to a low dose of endotoxin (2--3 ng/kg) in six postmenopausal women with and without transdermal E2 (0.1 mg) replacement. Mean E2 levels were 7.3 +/- 0.8 pg/mL in the unreplaced subjects and increased to 102 +/- 13 pg/mL after estrogen replacement. Blood was sampled every 20 min for 1--2 h before, and for 7 h after, iv endotoxin administration. Endotoxin stimulated ACTH, cortisol, and cytokine release in women with and without E2 replacement. E2 significantly attenuated the release of ACTH (P < 0.0001) and of cortisol (P = 0.02). Mean ACTH levels peaked at 190 +/- 91 pg/mL in the E2-replaced group vs. 411 +/- 144 pg/mL in the unreplaced women, whereas the corresponding mean cortisol levels peaked at 27 +/- 2.9 microg/dL with E2 vs.

31 +/- 3.2 microg/dL without E2. Estrogen also attenuated the endotoxin-induced release of IL-6 (P = 0.02), IL-1 receptor antagonist (P = 0.003), and TNF-alpha (P = 0.04). Mean cytokine levels with and without E2 replacement peaked at 341 +/- 94 pg/mL vs. 936 +/- 620 pg/mL for IL-6, 82 +/- 14 ng/mL vs. 133 +/- 24 ng/mL for IL-1 receptor antagonist, and 77 +/- 46 pg/mL vs. 214 +/- 87 pg/mL for TNF-alpha, respectively. We conclude that inflammatory cytokine and HPA responses to a low dose of endotoxin are attenuated in postmenopausal women receiving E2 replacement. These data show, for the first time in the human, that a physiological dose of estrogen can restrain cytokine and neuroendocrine responses to an inflammatory challenge.

Purbrick B et al. Future long-term trials of postmenopausal hormone replacement therapy—what is possible and what is the optimal protocol and regimen? Climacteric 2012;15:288-293. The ideal long-term, randomized, placebo-controlled trial of hormone replacement therapy (HRT) from near menopause for up to 30 years to assess major morbidity and mortality is impractical because of high cost, participant retention, therapy compliance, and continuity of research staff and funding. Also the trial regimen may become outdated. It is nihilistic to demand such a long-term trial before endorsing HRT. However, medium-term trials using surrogate measures for long-term morbidity and mortality are possible and two are near completion. If these studies have been able to maintain reasonable participant retention, therapy compliance and minimal breach of protocol, they will set standards for trials of new HRT regimens. This paper discusses lessons learnt from past attempts at long-term trials and suggests the currently optimal protocol and cost of assessing new HRT regimens to optimize potential benefits and minimize adverse effects. A 5-7-year randomized, placebo-controlled trial of a flexible transdermal estrogen regimen ± either a selective estrogen receptor modulator, e.g. bazedoxifene, or micronized progesterone is discussed. Mild to moderately symptomatic women, 1-4 years post menopause, can be recruited via general practice and group meetings. Future trials should be funded by independent agencies and are high priority in women's health.

Ridker PM et al. Hormone replacement therapy and increased plasma concentration of C-reactive protein Circulation. 1999 Aug 17;100(7)BACKGROUND: It has been hypothesized that postmenopausal hormone replacement therapy (HRT) may increase levels of C-reactive protein (CRP), a marker of inflammation associated with increased risk of future cardiovascular events. However, data evaluating this hypothesis are sparse and limited to older women. METHODS AND RESULTS: CRP levels were evaluated in a cross-sectional survey of 493 healthy postmenopausal women; mean age was 51 years. Overall, median CRP levels were 2 times higher among women taking HRT than among women not taking HRT (0.27

versus 0.14 mg/dL; P=0.001). This difference was present in all subgroups evaluated, including those with no history of hypertension, hyperlipidemia, obesity, diabetes, or cigarette consumption or a family history of premature coronary artery disease (all P< 0.01). Compared with nonusers of HRT, median CRP levels were higher among women using estrogen alone (P=0.003) and women using estrogen plus progesterone (P=0.03); however, there was no significant difference in CRP levels between users of different HRT preparations. In multivariate analysis, the relationship between HRT use and CRP remained significant after control for body mass index, age, diabetes, hypertension, hyperlipidemia, alcohol use, and cigarette consumption (P=0.001). CONCLUSIONS: In this cross-sectional survey, CRP levels were increased among apparently healthy postmenopausal women taking HRT. The potential impact of HRT on inflammatory parameters should be investigated in ongoing clinical trials.

Schairer C et al. Cause-specific mortality in women receiving hormone replacement therapy. Epidemiology. 1997 Jan; 8(1):59-65. To assess the risks and benefits of menopausal hormone replacement therapy, we followed a 23,346-member, population-based cohort of Swedish women who were prescribed menopausal estrogens for an average of 8.6 years for mortality. Compared with the general population, the standardized mortality ratio for all-cause mortality in this cohort was 0.77 (95% confidence limits = 0.73, 0.81). Deaths in each of the 12 major categories of causes of death except for injuries occurred 12% to 86% less frequently than expected. We examined in detail four specific causes of death according to the type of hormone prescribed, namely weak estrogens (primarily estriol), more potent estrogens (primarily estradiol and conjugated estrogens) in combination with a progestin, and more potent estrogens without a progestin. Mortality from endometrial cancer was not related to the prescription of weak estrogens or an estrogen-progestin combination, but mortality was 40% higher in women prescribed more potent estrogens without a progestin. Women prescribed weak estrogens, more potent estrogens, and the combined estrogen-progestin regimen were at reduced risk of death from ischemic heart disease (standardized mortality ratios of 0.7, 0.6, and 0.4, respectively). The more potent estrogens and the estrogen-progestin combination were associated with a marked reduction in risk of intracerebral hemorrhage (standardize mortality ratios of 0.4 and 0.6, respectively) and "other" cerebrovascular disease, but not other types of stroke. The concern that use of progestins would lead to psychic disorders related to suicide received no support from our results. Breast cancer results are described elsewhere. These data provide little evidence of an adverse effect of the combined estrogen-progestin regimen as compared with estrogens alone on mortality. They do indicate, however, that both selection factors and biology may contribute to the almost across-the-board-reduction in mortality associated with hormone replacement therapy.

Schmidt M et al. Inflammation and sex hormone metabolism. Ann N Y Acad Sci. 2006 Jun; 1069:236-46. The incidence of autoimmune diseases is higher in females than in males. In both sexes, adrenal hormones, that is, glucocorticoids, dehydroepiandrosterone (DHEA), and androgens, are inadequately low in patients when compared to healthy controls. Hormonally active androgens are anti-inflammatory, whereas estrogens are pro-inflammatory. Therefore, the mechanisms responsible for the alterations of steroid profiles in inflammation are of major interest. The local metabolism of androgens and estrogens may determine whether a given steroid profile found in a subject's blood results in suppression or promotion of inflammation. The steroid metabolism in mixed synovial cells, fibroblasts, macrophages, and monocytes was assessed. Major focus was on cells from patients with rheumatoid arthritis (RA), while cells from patients with osteoarthritis served as controls. Enzymes directly or indirectly involved in local sex steroid metabolism in RA are: DHEA-sulfatase, 3beta-hydroxysteroid dehydrogenase, 17beta-hydroxysteroid dehydrogenase, and aromatase (CYP19), which are required for the synthesis of sex steroids from precursors, 5alpha-reductase and 16alpha-hydroxylase, which can be involved either in the generation of more active steroids or in the pathways leading to depletion of active hormones, and 3alpha-reductase and 7alpha-hydroxylase (CYP7B), which unidirectionally are involved in the depletion of active hormones. Androgens inhibit aromatization in synovial cells when their concentration is sufficiently high. As large amounts of estrogens are formed in synovial tissue, there may be a relative lack of androgens. Production of 5alpha-reduced androgens should increase the local anti-inflammatory activity; however, it also opens a pathway for the inactivation of androgens. The data discussed here suggest that therapy of RA patients may benefit from the use of nonaromatizable androgens and/or the use of aromatase inhibitors.

Schmidt JW et al. Hormone replacement therapy in menopausal women: Past problems and future possibilities. Gynecol Endocrinol. 2006 Oct; 22(10):564-77 Oral administration of conjugated equine estrogens (CEE) with and without the synthetic progestin medroxyprogesterone acetate (MPA) in postmenopausal women is associated with side-effects that include increased risk of stroke and breast cancer. The current evidence that transdermal administration of estradiol may provide a safer alternative to orally administered CEE is reviewed. Transdermally administered estradiol has been shown to be an efficacious treatment for hot flushes possibly without the increase in blood clotting that is associated with administration of oral CEE. Further, natural progesterone may have a more beneficial spectrum of physiological effects than synthetic progestins. The substantial differences between CEE compared with estradiol and estriol, as well as the differences between synthetic MPA and natural progesterone, are detailed. Estriol is an increasingly popular alternative hormone therapy used for menopausal symptoms. There is evidence that estriol, by binding preferentially to estrogen receptor-beta, may inhibit some of the unwanted effects of estradiol. New clinical trials are needed to evaluate the safety and efficacy of topically or transdermally administered combinations of estradiol, estriol and progesterone. Future studies should focus on relatively young women who begin estrogen supplement use near the start of menopause.

Tengstrand B et al. Abnormal levels of serum dehydroepiandrosterone, estrone, and estradiol in men with rheumatoid arthritis: high correlation between serum estradiol and current degree of inflammation.J Rheumatol. 2003 Nov; 30(11):2338-43.OBJECTIVE: Men with rheumatoid arthritis (RA) have a higher than normal frequency of low testosterone levels, but not much is known about other sex hormones. We investigated serum levels of estradiol, estrone, and the adrenal androgen dehydroepiandrosterone (DHEAS) in men with RA and evaluated the association of various disease variables with these sex hormones. METHODS: Inflammatory activity, measured as disease activity score including 28 joints (Disease Activity Score 28), and degree of disability, measured with the Health Assessment Questionnaire, was estimated in 101 men with RA. Presence of erosions, rheumatoid factor (RF), smoking habits, and body mass index were recorded. DHEAS (not measured in patients taking glucocorticoids), estradiol, and estrone were measured in patients and in healthy controls. RESULTS: DHEAS and estrone concentrations were lower and estradiol was higher in patients compared with healthy controls. DHEAS differed between RF positive and RF negative patients. Estrone did not correlate with any disease variable, whereas estradiol correlated strongly and positively with all measured indices of inflammation. CONCLUSION: Men with RA had aberrations in all sex hormones analyzed, although only estradiol consistently correlated with inflammation. The high levels of estradiol may have positive implications for bone health. The low levels of estrone and DHEAS may depend on a shift in the adrenal steroidogenesis towards the glucocorticoid pathway, whereas increased conversion of estrone to estradiol seemed to be the cause of the high estradiol levels.

Tivesten A et al. Circulating Estradiol is an Independent Predictor of Progression of Carotid Artery Intima-Media Thickness in Middle-Aged Men Journal of Clinical Endocrinology & Metabolism, 2006 Nov;91(11):4433-7. CONTEXT: Estrogen treatment of men with prostate cancer is associated with increased cardiovascular morbidity and mortality; however, the role of endogenous estrogen levels for atherosclerotic disease in men is unknown. OBJECTIVE: The objective of the study was to determine whether endogenous serum estradiol (E2) levels predict the progression of carotid artery intima-media thickness in men. DESIGN, SETTING AND PARTICIPANTS: This was a population-based, prospective cohort study (the Atherosclerosis and Insulin Resistance study) conducted in Goteborg, Sweden, among 313 Caucasian men without cardiovascular or other clinically overt diseases. Carotid artery intima-media thickness, an index of preclinical atherosclerosis, was measured by ultrasound at baseline (58 yr of age) and after 3 yr of follow-up. Serum sex hormone levels and cardiovascular risk factors (body mass index, waist to hip ratio, systolic blood pressure, serum triglycerides, plasma c-peptide, and smoking status) were assessed at study entry. INTERVENTION: There was no intervention. MAIN OUTCOME MEASURES: Association between baseline total and free E2 levels and progression of carotid intima-media thickness over 3 yr with adjustments for cardiovascular risk factors was measured. RESULTS: In univariate analyses, both total and free E2 levels at baseline were positively associated with the annual change in intima-media thickness. In linear regression models including E2 and cardiovascular risk factors, low-density lipoprotein and high-density lipoprotein cholesterol and E2 were identified as independent predictors of progression of carotid artery intima-media thickness (total E2 beta = 0.187, P = 0.001; and free E2 beta = 0.183, P = 0.003). CONCLUSIONS: Circulating E2 is a predictor of progression of carotid artery intima-media thickness in middle-aged men. Further studies are needed to investigate the role of endogenous E2 for incident cardiovascular disease events.

Villiers TJ et al. The WHI:the effect of hormone replacement therapy on fracture prevention. Climacteric 2012;15:263-266.
The Women's Health Initiative (WHI) randomized, controlled trial was the first study to prove that hormone replacement therapy (HRT) reduces the incidence of all osteoporosis-related fractures in postmenopausal women, even those at low risk of fracture. The study authors concluded that the bone-friendly aspect of HRT was limited in clinical practice as possible adverse effects outweighed possible benefit. On the strength of these publications, regulatory authorities downgraded the use of HRT for the prevention of fracture to second-line therapy. This article examines the original and subsequent evidence presented by the WHI study and concludes that the restrictions placed on HRT as a bone-specific drug by regulatory bodies have not withstood the test of time and are not supported by the data of the WHI.

CHAPTER 6

DHEA

DHEA (dehydroepiandrosterone) is a precursor to the sex steroids in both males and females. Treating women with DHEA will usually assist in raising their serum testosterone levels to a youthful range and may make the need for testosterone replacement unnecessary. DHEA can improve mood, improve cognitive function, improve immune system response, improve bone density, increase energy and improve the sense of well-being.

There is not that much in the way of clinical studies to document the benefits of DHEA replacement therapy. However, multiple adverse clinical outcomes are associated with low DHEA levels, such as cognitive and immune dysfunction, some cancers, inflammatory diseases, type II diabetes and cardiovascular disorders. Most people over 40 have DHEAS levels lower than youthful range. When ordering serum lab testing it is necessary to order DHEA Sulfate since this is the storage form that gives an accurate assessment of DHEA status. Unsulfated DHEA levels vary widely throughout the day and serum levels are not useful.

DHEA levels can decline as much as 90% by 70 years of age. DHEA is synthesized in the brain and in the adrenal cortex and is the most plentiful steroid hormone in the human body. However, a specific DHEA receptor has not been identified. It has been suggested that the hormonal environment may influence the receptor type with which DHEA interacts. DHEA and DHEA-S appear to have the capacity to bind to several different receptor types. There are no specific symptoms of DHEA deficiency, just health conditions associated with low levels of DHEA. The steroid metabolic pathway shown below indicates that Pregnenolone and DHEA are at the top of the pyramid. However just replacing DHEA or Pregnenolone will not necessarily go downstream and replace the hormones below.

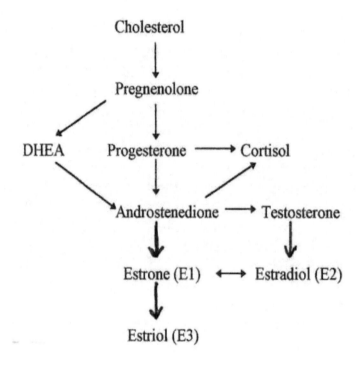

Literature Review

Adequate levels of DHEA can improve sexual function, increase muscle mass, decrease body fat, improve memory, improve mental acuity, decrease depression and improve the immune system response by controlling cortisol levels and adrenaline levels. However in the DAWN study by Kritz-Silverstein, even though there were increased testosterone levels in women, not men, with 50 mg daily there was no improvement in cognitive or sexual function, including life satisfaction scores. There was also no adverse effect of treatment. Shikaitas found that in rats, DHEA increased immune system response and may confer protection against cancer. Yang found that sufficient levels of DHEA decrease systemic inflammation by decreasing inflammatory cytokines such as interleukin-6 (IL-6), nfkb and tumor necrosis factor alpha (TNF-alpha). It has common usage in rheumatology with autoimmune disease. (Sawatha) A meta-analysis by Crosby et al. there may be mild clinical benefits in treatment of SLE.

When DHEA levels are in an optimal range, there can be less risk of developing atherosclerosis. Rabijewski found that DHEA could lower insulin levels and decrease the risk for developing type II diabetes. DHEA also decreases the risk of cancer because it enhances the immune system response. DHEA is thought to be neuroprotective. It assists in improving symptoms associated with learning disabilities, impaired memory, HIV infection, obesity and autoimmune diseases such as chronic fatigue syndrome, arthritis, lupus, herpes and Epstein-Barr.

Jankowski found that DHEA might also play a role in treating and/or preventing osteoporosis. DHEA is manufactured in the adrenal glands but DHEA, along with testosterone, estrogen and progesterone is produced in the ovaries in females. Testosterone and progesterone stimulate bone formation and estrogen inhibits bone resorption, DHEA, like estrogen, may also inhibit bone resorption. Further, because DHEA, like testosterone, is an androgenic hormone, DHEA may additionally play a role in bone formation. Therefore, DHEA may have a dual role in preventing osteoporosis because it is capable of stimulating bone formation and inhibiting bone resorption.

In some animal studies, DHEA slowed the aging process. Mice treated with DHEA had glossier coats, less gray hair and looked and acted younger than mice not treated with DHEA. Chariampopoulos found that DHEA turned on neuronal stem cells to maintin population of neurons and glia. Alhaj found using the LORETA scan there was improved mood and memory and reduction of evening salivary cortisol.

Management:

Maintaining DHEA Sulfate serum levels to that of a 25-30 year old is optimal.

The male dose of DHEA varies from 25-100 mg. The female dose varies from 5-25 mg. Monitor serum levels to see that DHEAS is in the physiological range but we do aim for a precise numerical value.

Since DHEA can produce androgenic side effects in women (but not in men) decrease dose for oily skin, acne or facial hair growth. If there are androgenic side effects in women they may be due to DHEA, testosterone or the combination.

7-oxo-DHEA = 7-keto DHEA is a metabolite that rarely has androgenic side effects. Hampl and Ihler found that another benefit is that there may be thermogenesis and fat loss with its use. If side effects are a concern women can be treated with 7-keto DHEA with a dose of 25 mg. Men can be treated with 100 mg. The serum level of DHEAS does not usually change with this treatment.

DHEA MEN

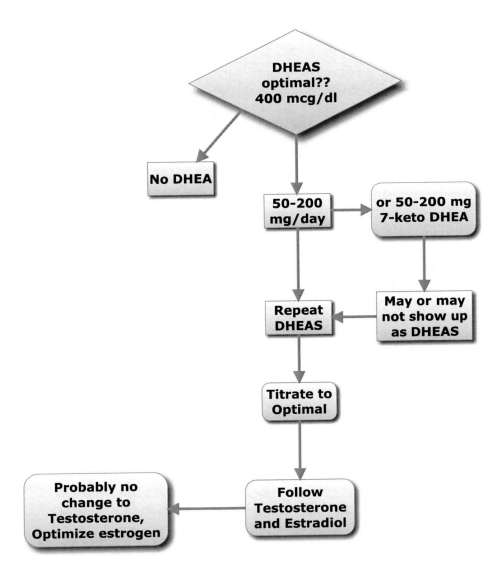

DHEA WOMEN

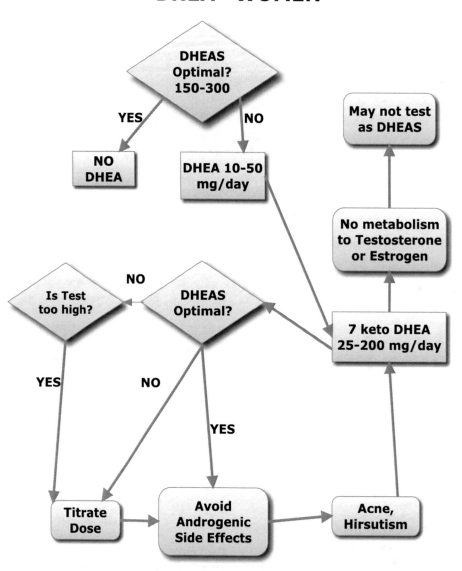

Cortisol:

Cortisol is produced in the Zona fasciculata of the adrenal gland. The secretion of the corticotropin releasing hormone (CRH) from the hypothalamus causes adrenocorticotropic hormone, ACTH, to be released triggering cortisol release. Cortisol stimulates glucose neogenesis and activates anti stress and anti-inflammatory pathways. In our ancestors, this fight or flight mechanism was important to our survival and was intended as a short release of energy to combat danger. High levels of cortisol over long periods of time can have detrimental effects interfering with normal metabolic processes by muscle wasting, osteoporosis, decreasing the effectiveness of DHEA, and decreasing the immune response. Elevated cortisol levels over any lengthened period of time may cause the adrenal glands to become fatigued. Adrenal fatigue is associated with autoimmune diseases, chronic fatigue syndrome and fibromyalgia. Elevated glucocorticoids increase glucose and can exacerbate subclinical diabetes. Adrenal fatigue can also worsen hypothyroidism. Cushing's disease is the effect of prolonged elevation of cortisol and Addison's disease is an example of severe cortisol deficiency. These two extremes are presented in traditional medicine as the possible adrenal conditions to consider. However, as the case with many of the hormones to be optimized most patients fall into the vast middle range. We can make a major impact in our patient's quality of life by recognizing mild to moderate deficiencies when they exist and treating them with lifestyle, nutraceuticals and hormonal therapies. We can identify adrenal fatigue by the clinical picture along with salivary cortisol profiles.

Symptoms:

- o Tired for no reason
- o Trouble getting up in the morning
- o Crave caffeine, sugar or salty foods
- o Feeling run down and stressed
- o Difficulty keeping up with daily routine
- o Hard to bounce back after illness or stressful experience
- o Decreased libido

Management:

The first step of management of cortisol dysregulation is lifestyle modification. The adrenals secrete cortisol in the middle of the night, so sleep is important. If REM sleep is disrupted, cortisol secretion will be decreased. Stress reduction, healthy diet, moderate exercise all contribute to improving adrenal health. However excessive dieting and overexercise can deplete reserves. Maintaining optimal hormones such as thyroid, progesterone and DHEA is important. Low levels of any of these will decrease the available cortisol.

Treatment

- High
  - ✓ Lifestyle
  - ✓ Eliminate stress
  - ✓ Meditation
- Low
  - ✓ Adrenal support
    - Vitamins
    - Glandular
  - ✓ Bio-identical cortisol
  - ✓ Compounded cortisol
    - 2.5-20 mg divided BID

Nutraceutical supplements such as phosphatidyl serine, the B-vitamins, vitamin C, magnesium, omega 3 fatty acids can support adrenal function. An adaptogen is a natural herb product that normalizes the body's response to stresses. Common adaptogens used for the adrenals include rhodiola, licorice, ashwagandha and ginseng. A glandular extract is desiccated adrenal gland from bovine sources. This is considered in early replacement therapy for adrenal fatigue. With the additional support of comprehensive hormone optimization, adrenal fatigue can be managed. If the symptoms persist despite lifestyle changes and adaptogens and glandular extract, then a low dose compounded hydrocortisone to replace the deficient adrenal hormone may be needed. When cortisol replacement is indicated, we usually start patients on 2.5mg of compounded extended release hydrocortisone twice daily and monitor the patient's symptoms and follow-up lab testing results. An important patient education item for treatment with adrenal fatigue is inform the patient that it is possible that they may feel worse before they feel better. Adrenal fatigue is a continuum and a patient will need to back up thru the levels which they have experienced until they reach adrenal health. With life style changes and intervention and patience, adrenal health can be restored, and bioidentical cortisol replacement can be tapered off.

ADRENAL IMBALANCE
A CONTINUUM OF CARE

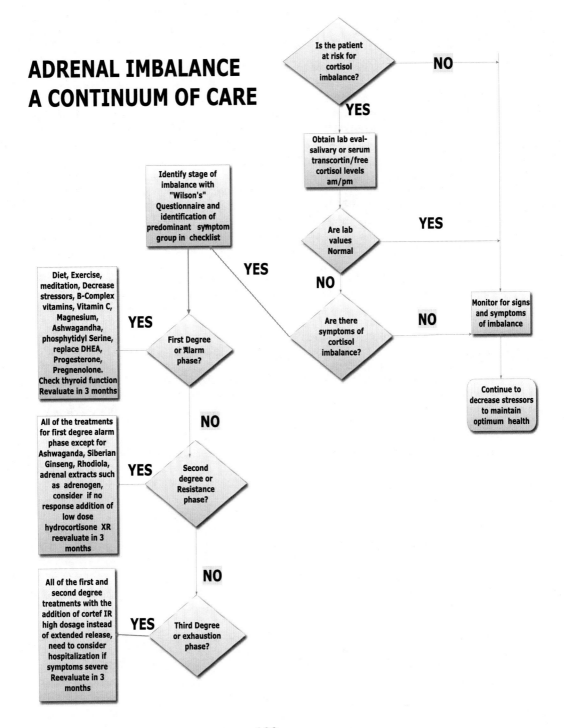

193

DHEA AND CORTISOL ABSTRACTS

Alhaj HA et al. Effects of DHEA administration on episodic memory, cortisol and mood in healthy young men: a double-blind, placebo-controlled study. Psychopharmacology (Berl) 2005Oct18; 1-11 Rationale: Dehydroepiandrosterone (DHEA) has been reported to enhance cognition in rodents, although there are inconsistent findings in humans. OBJECTIVES: The aim of this study was to investigate the effects of DHEA administration in healthy young men on episodic memory and its neural correlates utilising an event-related potential (ERP) technique. METHODS: Twenty-four healthy young men were treated with a 7-day course of oral DHEA (150 mg b.d.) or placebo in a double blind, random, crossover and balanced order design. Subjective mood and memory were measured using visual analogue scales (VASs). Cortisol concentrations were measured in saliva samples. ERPs were recorded during retrieval in an episodic memory test. Low-resolution brain electromagnetic tomography (LORETA) was used to identify brain regions involved in the cognitive task. RESULTS: DHEA administration led to a reduction in evening cortisol concentrations and improved VAS mood and memory. Recollection accuracy in the episodic memory test was significantly improved following DHEA administration. LORETA revealed significant hippocampal activation associated with successful episodic memory retrieval following placebo. DHEA modified ERPs associated with retrieval and led to a trend towards an early differential activation of the anterior cingulate cortex (ACC). CONCLUSIONS: DHEA treatment improved memory recollection and mood and decreased trough cortisol levels. The effect of DHEA appears to be via neuronal recruitment of the steroid sensitive ACC that may be involved in pre-hippocampal memory processing. These findings are distinctive, being the first to show such beneficial effects of DHEA on memory in healthy young men.

Arlt W et al. DHEA replacement in women with adrenal insufficiency--pharmacokinetics, bioconversion and clinical effects on well-being, sexuality and cognition. Endocr Res 2000 Nov; 26(4):505-11. Standard replacement for adrenal insufficiency (AI) consists of glucocorticoids and mineralocorticoids while DHEA deficiency is routinely ignored. Thus, AI represents the ideal pathophysiological model of isolated DHEA deficiency. We investigated the effects of DHEA replacement in 24 women with primary and secondary AI employing a double blind, placebo-controlled, randomized crossover design. A DHEA dose of 50 mg/d was chosen based on preceding single-dose pharmacokinetics and bioconversion studies. Each patient received four months of treatment with DHEA and four months placebo, with a one-month washout period. Measurements included serum steroid hormones, somatotropic parameters and psychometric assessment of well-being, mood, cognition and sexuality. Treatment with DHEA raised the initially low serum concentrations of DHEA, DHEAS, androstenedione, and testosterone into the normal range. DHEA induced a slight increase in serum IGF-I, but only in patients with primary AI, suggesting a growth hormone-mediated effect. DHEA treatment significantly improved overall wellbeing as well as scores for depression, anxiety, and their physical correlates. Furthermore, DHEA significantly increased both sexual interest and the level of satisfaction with sex. DHEA replacement had no influence on the cognitive performance, which was already on a high level at baseline. In conclusion, DHEA replacement improves well-being and sexuality in women with adrenal insufficiency. If this is due to a direct effect of DHEA on the brain, an indirect effect via increased androgen synthesis, or both, remains to be elucidated. Long-term studies in patients of both sexes are needed to further define the role of DHEA in standard replacement for adrenal insufficiency.

Arlt W, Dehydroepiandrosterone Replacement in Women with Adrenal Insufficiency The New England Journal of Medicine -- September 30, 1999 -- Vol. 341, No. 14.BACKGROUND: The physiologic role of dehydroepiandrosterone in humans is still unclear. Adrenal insufficiency leads to a deficiency of dehydroepiandrosterone; we therefore, investigated the effects of dehydroepiandrosterone replacement, in patients with adrenal insufficiency. METHODS: In a double-blind study, 24 women with adrenal insufficiency received in random order 50 mg of dehydroepiandrosterone orally each morning for four months and placebo daily for four months, with a one-month washout period. We measured serum steroid hormones, insulin-like growth factor I, lipids, and sex hormone-binding globulin, and we evaluated well-being and sexuality with the use of validated psychological questionnaires and visual-analogue scales, respectively. The women were assessed before treatment, after one and four months of treatment with dehydroepiandrosterone, after one and four months of placebo, and one month after the end of the second treatment period. RESULTS: Treatment with dehydroepiandrosterone raised the initially low serum concentrations of dehydroepiandrosterone, dehydroepiandrosterone sulfate, androstenedione, and testosterone into the normal range; serum concentrations of sex hormone-binding globulin, total cholesterol, and high-density lipoprotein cholesterol decreased significantly. Dehydroepiandrosterone significantly improved overall well-being as well as scores for depression and anxiety. For the global severity index, the mean (+/-SD) change from base line was -0.18+/-0.29 after four months of dehydroepiandrosterone therapy, as compared with 0.03+/-0.29 after four months of placebo (P=0.02). As compared with placebo, dehydroepiandrosterone significantly increased the frequency of sexual thoughts (P=0.006), sexual interest (P=0.002), and satisfaction with both mental and physical aspects of sexuality (P=0.009 and P=0.02, respectively). CONCLUSIONS: Dehydroepiandrosterone improves well-being and sexuality in women with adrenal insufficiency

Barrett-Connor E et al. Dehydroepiandrosterone sulfate and breast cancer risk. Cancer Res 1990 Oct 15; 50(20):6571-4 It has been suggested that dehydroepiandrosterone (DHEA) and its sulfate ester, dehydroepiandrosterone sulfate (DHEAS), have a protective effect against breast cancer. In our investigation, DHEAS levels were measured in plasma obtained and frozen in 1972-1974 from 534 women aged 50-79 yr. This group, which has been followed for 15 yr, included 21 incident cases of breast cancer, 20 cases with earlier diagnosis, and ten cases with unknown date of onset who were identified from death certificates only. Two sets of analyses were done: one using all women and one which excluded women using estrogen. No significant differences in age-adjusted DHEAS levels were found between any case type and noncases. Age-adjusted rates of breast cancer by DHEAS tertile also showed no significant trends or differences among tertiles for any case type. A multivariate model in which the DHEAS level was adjusted for age, body mass index, estrogen use, and cigarette smoking status also showed no significant association between DHEAS and risk of breast cancer. These results do not support a protective role for plasma DHEAS in breast cancer risk in postmenopausal women.

Barry NN, McGuire JL, van Vollenhoven RF. Dehydroepiandrosterone in systemic lupus erythematosus: relationship between dosage, serum levels, and clinical response. J Rheumatol 1998 Dec;25(12):2352-6. OBJECTIVE: To examine in women with systemic lupus erythematosus (SLE) who participated in a clinical trial the relationship between daily dose of dehydroepiandrosterone (DHEA), serum levels of DHEA and DHEA sulfate (DHEAS), clinical effectiveness, and side effects. METHODS: Twenty-three women with mild to moderate SLE were treated with DHEA for a 6 month period. The starting dose was 50 mg/day, and monthly stepwise increases were allowed. Subjects were assessed monthly by the Systemic Lupus Erythematosus Disease Activity Index, Systemic Lupus Activity Measure (SLAM), Health Assessment Questionnaire, and other outcomes. Serum testosterone, DHEA, and DHEAS levels were obtained and side effects noted monthly. RESULTS: Statistically significant improvements were found in all lupus outcomes over 6 months. Serum DHEA and DHEAS levels correlated with the dose of DHEA. Serum DHEA and DHEAS correlated negatively with SLAM score. A second order regression analysis of serum DHEAS level versus SLAM score suggested that the optimal serum level of DHEAS was 1000 microg/dl. The most common side effect was acne. CONCLUSION: The clinical response to DHEA was not clearly dose dependent. Serum levels of DHEA and DHEAS correlated only weakly with lupus outcomes, but suggested an optimum serum DHEAS of 1000 microg/dl. Monitoring these serum levels appears to have limited clinical utility.

Bastianetto S Dehydroepiandrosterone (DHEA) protects hippocampal cells from oxidative stress-induced damage.Brain

Res Mol Brain Res 1999 Mar 20; 66(1-2):35-41 It has been postulated that decreases in plasma levels of dehydroepiandrosterone (DHEA) may contribute to the development of some age-related disorders. Along with neuroprotective and memory enhancing effects, DHEA has been shown to display antioxidant properties. Moreover, oxidative stress is known to cause lipid peroxidation and degenerative changes in the hippocampus, an area involved in memory processes and especially afflicted in Alzheimer's disease (AD). Accordingly, we investigated the antioxidant effects of DHEA in models of oxidative stress using rat primary hippocampal cells and human hippocampal tissue from AD patients and age-matched controls. A pre-treatment of rat primary mixed hippocampal cell cultures with DHEA (10-100 microM) protected against the toxicity induced by H_2O_2 and sodium nitroprusside. Moreover, DHEA (10-100 microM) was also able to prevent $H_2O_2/FeSO_4$-stimulated lipid oxidation in both control and AD hippocampal tissues. Taken together, these data suggest that DHEA may be useful in treating age-related central nervous system diseases based on its protective effects in the hippocampus.

Bauer ME et al. Stress, glucocorticoids and ageing of the immune system.Stress. 2005 Mar; 8(1):69-83. Ageing has been associated with immunological changes (immunosenescence) that resemble those observed following chronic stress or glucocorticoid (GC) treatment. These changes include thymic involution, lower number of naive T cells, reduced cell-mediated immunity, and poor vaccination response to new antigens. It follows that immunosenescence could be associated with changes of peripheral GC levels. Indeed, when compared with young subjects, healthy elders are more stressed and show activation of the hypothalamus-pituitary-adrenal (HPA) axis. However, both beneficial and undesirable effects of GCs ultimately depend on the target tissue sensitivity to these steroids. Recent data indicate that peripheral lymphocytes from elders respond poorly to GC treatment in vitro. The present review summarizes recent findings which suggest that immunosenescence may be closely related to both psychological distress and stress hormones. Furthermore, chronically stressed elderly subjects may be particularly at risk of stress-related pathology because of further alterations in GC-immune signalling. Finally, the neuroendocrine hypothesis of immunosenescence is finally reconsidered in which the age-related increase in the cortisol/DHEA ratio is major determinant of immunological changes observed during ageing.

Baulieu EE et al. Dehydroepiandrosterone (DHEA), DHEA sulfate, and aging: contribution of the DHEAge Study to a sociobiomedical issue. Proc Natl Acad Sci U S A 2000 Apr 11;97(8):4279-84. The secretion and the blood levels of the adrenal steroid dehydroepiandrosterone (DHEA) and its sulfate ester (DHEAS) decrease profoundly with age, and the question is posed whether administration of the steroid to compensate for the decline counteracts defects associated with aging. The commercial availability of DHEA outside the regular pharmaceutical-medical network in the United States creates a real public health problem that may be resolved only by appropriate long-term clinical trials in elderly men and women. Two hundred and eighty healthy individuals (women and men 60-79 years old) were given DHEA, 50 mg, or placebo, orally, daily for a year in a double-blind, placebo-controlled study. No potentially harmful accumulation of DHEAS and active steroids was recorded. Besides the reestablishment of a "young" concentration of DHEAS, a small increase of testosterone and estradiol was noted, particularly in women, and may be involved in the significantly demonstrated physiological-clinical manifestations here reported. Bone turnover improved selectively in women >70 years old, as assessed by the dual-energy x-ray absorptiometry (DEXA) technique and the decrease of osteoclastic activity. A significant increase in most libido parameters was also found in these older women. Improvement of the skin status was observed, particularly in women, in terms of hydration, epidermal thickness, sebum production, and pigmentation. A number of biological indices confirmed the lack of harmful consequences of this 50 mg/day DHEA administration over one year, also indicating that this kind of replacement therapy normalized ome effects of aging, but does not create "supermen/women" (doping).

Canning MO et al. Opposing effects of dehydroepiandrosterone and dexamethasone on the generation of monocyte-derived dendritic cells. Eur J Endocrinol 2000 Nov; 143(5):687-95BACKGROUND: Dehydroepiandrosterone (DHEA) has been suggested as an immunostimulating steroid hormone, of which the effects on the development of dendritic cells (DC) are unknown. The effects of DHEA often oppose those of the other adrenal glucocorticoid, cortisol. Glucocorticoids (GC) are known to suppress the immune response at different levels and have recently been shown to modulate the development of DC, thereby influencing the initiation of the immune response. Variations in the duration of exposure to, and doses of, GC (particularly dexamethasone (DEX)) however, have resulted in conflicting effects on DC development. AIM: In this study, we describe the effects of a continuous high level of exposure to the adrenal steroid DHEA (10 M) on the generation of immature DC from monocytes, as well as the effects of the opposing steroid DEX on this development. RESULTS: The continuous presence of DHEA (10 M) in GM-CSF/IL-4-induced monocyte-derived DC cultures resulted in immature DC with a morphology and functional capabilities similar to those of typical immature DC (T cell stimulation, IL-12/IL-10 production), but with a slightly altered phenotype of increased CD80 and decreased CD43 expression (markers of maturity). The continuous presence of DEX at a concentration of 10 M in the monocyte/DC cultures resulted in the generation of plastic-adherent macrophage-like cells in place of typical immature DC, with increased CD14 expression, but decreased expression of the typical DC markers CD1a, CD40 and CD80. These cells were strongly reactive to acid phosphatase, but equally capable of stimulating T cell proliferation as immature DC. The production of IL-12 by these macrophage-like cells was virtually shut down; whereas the production of IL-10 was significantly higher than that of control immature DC. CONCLUSION: The continuous presence of a high level of GC during the generation of immature DC from monocytes can modulate this development away from DC towards a macrophage-like cell. The combination of a low CD80 expression and a shutdown of IL-12 production suggests the possibility of DEX-generated cells initiating a Th2-biased response. These effects by DEX on DC development contrast with those by DHEA, which resulted in a more typical DC although possessing a phenotype possibly indicating a more mature state of the cell.

Davidson M, Marwah A, Sawchuk RJ, et al. Safety and pharmacokinetic study with escalating doses of 3-acetyl-7-oxo-dehydroepiandrosterone in healthy male volunteers. Clin Invest Med. 2000 Oct; 23(5):300-10. OBJECTIVES: To evaluate the safety and pharmacokinetics of 3-acetyl-7-oxo-DHEA (3beta-acetoxyandrost-5-ene-7, 17-dione) given orally. DESIGN: A randomized, double blind, placebo-controlled, escalating dose study. SETTING: The Chicago Center for Clinical Research. PARTICIPANTS: Twenty-two healthy men. STUDY METHOD: The participants received placebo (n = 6) or 3-acetyl-7-oxo-DHEA (n = 16) at 50 mg/d for 7 days followed by a 7-day washout; 100 mg/d for 7 days followed by a 7-day washout; and 200 mg/d for 28 days. OUTCOME MEASURES: Safety parameters, evaluated at each dose level, included measurement of total testosterone, free testosterone, dihydrotestosterone, estradiol, cortisol, thyroxin and insulin levels. Analyses for 7-oxo-DHEA-3beta-sulfate (DHEA-S), the only detectable metabolic product of the administered steroid, were conducted on plasma drawn from all subjects at 0.25, 0.5, 1, 2, 4, 6 and 12 hours after the final 100 mg dose of 3beta-acetyl-7-oxo-DHEA. RESULTS: There were no differences in the clinical laboratory values or in reported minor adverse experiences, between treatment and placebo groups. In general, blood hormone concentrations were unaffected by the treatment with 3beta-acetyl-7-oxo-DHEA and remained within the normal range. No changes in vital signs, blood chemistry or urinalysis occurred during treatment with 3beta-acetyl-7-oxo-DHEA compared to placebo. The administered steroid was not detected in the blood but was rapidly converted to 7-oxo-DHEA-S, the concentrations of which were proportional to dose. This steroid sulfate did not accumulate; plasma concentrations 12 hours after the 3beta-acetyl-7-oxo-DHEA dose at 7 and 28 days on the 200 mg/d dose were 15.8 and 16.3 microg/L respectively. The mean time to peak plasma level of 7-oxo-DHEA-S was 2.2 hours; the mean half-life was 2.17 hours. The apparent clearance averaged 172 L/h, and the apparent mean volume of distribution was 540 L. CONCLUSION: These results indicate that 3beta-acetyl-7-oxo-DHEA is safe and well tolerated in normal healthy men at doses up to 200 mg/d for 4 weeks.

Dessein PH et al. Hyposecretion of the adrenal androgen dehydroepiandrosterone sulfate and its relation to clinical

variables in inflammatory arthritis. Arthritis Res 2001; 3(3):183-8 Hypothalamic-pituitary-adrenal underactivity has been reported in rheumatoid arthritis (RA). This phenomenon has implications with regard to the pathogenesis and treatment of the disease. The present study was designed to evaluate the secretion of the adrenal androgen dehydroepiandrosterone sulfate (DHEAS) and its relation to clinical variables in RA, spondyloarthropathy (Spa), and undifferentiated inflammatory arthritis (UIA). Eighty-seven patients (38 with RA, 29 with Spa, and 20 with UIA) were studied, of whom 54 were women. Only 12 patients (14%) had taken glucocorticoids previously. Age-matched, healthy women (134) and men (149) served as controls. Fasting blood samples were taken for determination of the erythrocyte sedimentation rate (ESR), serum DHEAS and insulin, and plasma glucose. Insulin resistance was estimated by the homeostasis-model assessment (HOMAIR). DHEAS concentrations were significantly decreased in both women and men with inflammatory arthritis (IA) ($P < 0.001$). In 24 patients (28%), DHEAS levels were below the lower extreme ranges found for controls. Multiple intergroup comparisons revealed similarly decreased concentrations in each disease subset in both women and men. After the ESR, previous glucocorticoid usage, current treatment with nonsteroidal anti-inflammatory drugs, duration of disease and HOMAIR were controlled for, the differences in DHEAS levels between patients and controls were markedly attenuated in women ($P = 0.050$) and were no longer present in men ($P = 0.133$). We concluded that low DHEAS concentrations are commonly encountered in IA and, in women; this may not be fully explainable by disease-related parameters. The role of hypoadrenalism in the pathophysiology of IA deserves further elucidation. DHEA replacement may be indicated in many patients with IA, even in those not taking glucocorticoids.

Du C Administration of dehydroepiandrosterone suppresses experimental allergic encephalomyelitis in SJL/J mice. J Immunol. 2001 Dec 15; 167(12):7094-101. Experimental allergic encephalomyelitis (EAE) is a Th1-mediated inflammatory demyelinating disease in the CNS, an animal model of multiple sclerosis. We have examined the effect of dehydroepiandrosterone (DHEA) on the development of EAE in mice. The addition of DHEA to cultures of myelin basic protein-primed splenocytes resulted in a significant decrease in T cell proliferation and secretion of (pro) inflammatory cytokines (IFN-gamma, IL-12 p40, and TNF-alpha) and NO in response to myelin basic protein. These effects were associated with a decrease in activation and translocation of NF-kappaB. In vivo administration of DHEA significantly reduced the severity and incidence of acute EAE, along with a decrease in demyelination/inflammation and expressions of (pro) inflammatory cytokines in the CNS. These studies suggest that DHEA has potent anti-inflammatory properties, which at least are in part mediated by its inhibition of NF-kappaB activation.

Feldman HA et al. Low dehydroepiandrosterone and ischemic heart disease in middle-aged men: prospective results from the Massachusetts Male Aging Study. Am J Epidemiol 2001 Jan 1;153(1):79-89. The adrenal steroid dehydroepiandrosterone (DHEA) and its sulfate (DHEAS) have been characterized as "protective" against ischemic heart disease (IHD), especially in men, on the basis of sparse epidemiologic evidence. The authors used data from the Massachusetts Male Aging Study, a random sample prospective study of 1,709 men aged 40-70 years at baseline, to test whether serum levels of DHEA or DHEAS could predict incident IHD over a 9-year interval. At baseline (1987-1989) and follow-up (1995-1997), an interviewer-phlebotomist visited each subject in his home to obtain comprehensive health information, body measurements, and blood samples for hormone and lipid analysis. Incident IHD between baseline and follow-up was ascertained from hospital records and death registries, supplemented by self-report and evidence of medication. In the analysis sample of 1,167 men, those with serum DHEAS in the lowest quartile at baseline (<1.6 microg/ml) were significantly more likely to incur IHD by follow-up (adjusted odds ratio = 1.60, 95 percent confidence interval: 1.07, 2.39; p = 0.02), independently of a comprehensive set of known risk factors including age, obesity, diabetes, hypertension, smoking, serum lipids, alcohol intake, and physical activity. Low serum DHEA was similarly predictive. These results confirm prior evidence that low DHEA and DHEAS can predict IHD in men.

Flood JF Dehydroepiandrosterone sulfate improves memory in aging mice. Brain Res 1988 May 10; 448(1):178-81. Middle-aged (18 month old) and old (24 month old) mice showed poorer retention of footshock active avoidance training (FAAT) than young mice (2 month old). Immediate post-training subcutaneous injection of dehydroepiandrosterone sulfate (DHEAS) improved retention of FAAT in middle-aged and old mice to the high levels observed in young mice. DHEAS, a major naturally occurring adrenal steroid that decreases in blood serum with age, could be rate-limiting in achievement of retention of learning.

Hampl et al. Steroids and thermogenesis. Physiol Res. 2005 May 24. Apart from thyroid hormones, as the main hormonal regulators of obligatory thermogenesis, and catecholamines, as major hormonal regulators of facultative thermogenesis, production of heat in homeotherms can also be influenced by steroids. Generally, hormones can influence heat production by regulating the activity of various enzymes of oxidative metabolism, by modulating membrane protein carriers and other membrane or nuclear protein factors. Proton carriers in the inner mitochondrial membrane, known as uncoupling proteins, play the key role in heat dissipation to the detriment of the formation of energy-rich phosphates. In this minireview we have focused on the effects of steroids and thyroid hormones on heat production in brown adipose tissues and in skeletal muscles, with particular respect to their effect on uncoupling protein expression. Apart from hormonal steroids, dehydroepiandrosterone, an important precursor in the metabolic pathway leading to hormonal steroids which possess many, mostly beneficial effects on human health, modulates metabolic pathways which may lead to increased heat production. Recent studies demonstrate that 7-oxo-dehydroepiandrosterone, one of its 7-oxygenated metabolites, is even more effective than dehydroepiandrosterone. Recent findings of various actions of these steroids support the view that they may also participate in modulating thermogenic effects.

Ihler G et al. 7-oxo-DHEA and Raynaud's phenomenon. Med Hypotheses. 2003 Mar; 60(3):391-7. Patients with Raynaud's phenomenon have abnormal digital vasoconstriction in response to cold. The pathogenesis remains unknown but may involve a local neurovascular defect leading to vasoconstriction. Diagnosis of primary Raynaud's phenomenon is based on typical symptomatology coupled with normal physical examination, normal laboratory studies and lack of observable pathology by nail fold capillaroscopy. Secondary Raynaud's phenomenon is known to occur associated with several connective tissue diseases, vascular injury due to repeated vibrational trauma, and other causes which produce demonstrable vascular and microcirculatory damage. Treatment of Raynaud's symptoms is conservative and aimed at prevention of attacks. Patients are advised to remain warm and, if possible, to live in warm climates. We suggest that an ergogenic (thermogenic) steroid, 7-oxo-DHEA (3-acetoxyandrost-5-ene-7, 17-dione), which is available without prescription as the trademarked 7-keto DHEA, may be very helpful in prevention of primary Raynaud's attacks by increasing the basal metabolic rate and inhibiting vasospasm.

Iwasaki Y et al. Dehydroepiandrosterone-sulfate inhibits nuclear factor-kappaB-dependent transcription in hepatocytes, possibly through antioxidant effect.J Clin Endocrinol Metab. 2004 Jul; 89(7):3449-54. Dehydroepiandrosterone (DHEA) and DHEA-sulfate (DHEAS), the representative sex steroid precursors, are postulated to have antiinflammatory effects, although the molecular background remains unknown. In this study, we examined the effects of these sex steroid precursors on cytokine-induced, nuclear factor-kappaB (NF-kappaB)-mediated transcription. The HuH7 human hepatocyte cell line was stably transfected with an NF-kappaB-luciferase reporter gene or transiently transfected with other representative response elements-luciferase fusion genes, and the effects of DHEA/DHEAS on proinflammatory cytokine-induced transcription were estimated by luciferase assay. The results showed that DHEA/DHEAS potently inhibited TNF-alpha-induced NF-kappaB-dependent transcription in a time- and dose-dependent manner. The effect was more obvious for DHEAS than for DHEA, and both steroids preferentially inhibited the cytokine-stimulated rather than basal NF-kappaB-mediated transcription. Similar effects were observed in activator protein-1-dependent but not constitutive Rous sarcoma virus promoter-dependent transcription. Two major downstream products of the sex steroid precursors, estradiol and testosterone, had no effect, indicating that the observed suppressive effect is not mediated by these metabolites. In contrast, glucocorticoids showed inhibitory effects on both basal and stimulated transcription and had an additive effect with DHEAS, suggesting the independent mechanisms of action of these steroid hormones. Finally, DHEAS eliminated hydroxyradical-induced activation of NF-kappaB-dependent transcription as well. Altogether, these results suggest that DHEA/DHEAS have an antiinflammatory effect in such a way that they inhibit proinflammatory cytokine-stimulated, NF-kappaB-mediated transcription, at least partly through their antioxidant properties.

Jankowski CM et al. Effects of DHEA Replacement Therapy on Bone Mineral Density in Older Adults: A Randomized, Controlled Trial. J Clin Endocrinol Metab. 2006 May 30 CONTEXT: Dehydroepiandrosterone (DHEA) and its sulfate (DHEAS) decrease with aging and are important androgen and estrogen precursors in older adults. Declines in DHEAS with aging may contribute to physiological changes that are sex hormone dependent. OBJECTIVE: The aim was to determine whether DHEA replacement increases bone mineral density (BMD) and fat-free mass. DESIGN, SETTING, AND PARTICIPANTS: A randomized, double-blinded, controlled trial was conducted at an academic research institution. Participants were 70 women and 70 men, aged 60-88 yr, with low serum DHEAS levels. INTERVENTION: The intervention was oral DHEA 50 mg/d or placebo for 12 months. MEASUREMENTS: BMD, fat mass and fat-free mass were measured before and after intervention. RESULTS: Intent-to-treat analyses revealed trends for DHEA to increase BMD more than placebo at the total hip (1.0%, P = 0.05), trochanter (1.2%, P = 0.06), and shaft (1.2%, P = 0.05). In women only, DHEA increased lumbar spine BMD (2.2%, P = 0.04; sex-by-treatment interaction, P = 0.05). In secondary compliance analyses, BMD increases in hip regions were significant (1.2-1.6%; all P < 0.02) in the DHEA group. There were no significant effects of DHEA on fat or fat-free mass in intent-to-treat or compliance analyses. CONCLUSIONS: DHEA replacement therapy for 1 yr improved hip BMD in older adults and spine BMD in older women. Because there have been few randomized, controlled trials of the effects of DHEA therapy, these findings support the need for further investigations of the benefits and risks of DHEA replacement and the mechanisms for its actions.

Jo H et al. Effects of dehydroepiandrosterone on articular cartilage during the development of osteoarthritis. Arthritis Rheum. 2004 Aug; 50(8):2531-8.OBJECTIVE: To investigate the in vivo effects of dehydroepiandrosterone (DHEA) on knee joints during the development of experimentally induced osteoarthritis (OA). METHODS: Twenty-two mature NZW rabbits underwent bilateral anterior cruciate ligament transection (ACLT) and received 0.3-ml intraarticular injections of DHEA (at a concentration of 100 microM in phosphate buffered saline) and control solution in the right and left knees, respectively, beginning 4 weeks after ACLT and continuing once weekly for 5 weeks. All animals were killed 9 weeks after surgery, and the knee joints were assessed by gross morphologic, histologic, histomorphometric, and biochemical methods. RESULTS: Gross morphologic inspection following India ink application showed that the right femoral condyles, which received DHEA, demonstrated less severe cartilage damage than did the contralateral condyles. The thickness, area, and roughness of the DHEA-treated femoral condyles provided evidence of a cartilage-protecting effect of DHEA following ACLT. These results were supported by gene expression analysis. Messenger RNA expression of a proinflammatory cytokine, interleukin-1beta, and catabolic enzymes, matrix metalloproteinases 1 and 3, was reduced in the cartilage of the DHEA-treated knee joints, and expression of tissue inhibitor of metalloproteinase 1 was increased. CONCLUSION: Results of the present study demonstrate a cartilage-protecting effect of DHEA during the development of OA following ACLT in a rabbit model.

Kaiman DS, Colker CM, Swain MA, Torina GC, Shi Q. A randomized, double-blind, placebo-controlled study of 3-acetyl-7-oxo-dehydroepiandrosterone in healthy overweight adults. Curr Therap Res. 2000; 61(7):435-42. Objective:The purpose of this study was to determine the effects of 3-acetyl-7-oxo-dehydroepiandrosterone (7-oxo-DHEA) in healthy overweight adults.Methods:In a double-blind, placebo-controlled protocol, 30 adults (28 women and 2 men; mean age, 44.5 ± 11.5 years) with a mean body mass index of 31.9 ± 6.2 kg/m2 were randomly divided into 2 groups of 15: Group 1 received 7-oxo-DHEA 100 mg twice daily and Group 2 received placebo for 8 weeks. All subjects participated in an exercise training program 3 times per week. Each exercise session consisted of 60 minutes of cross-training (aerobic and anaerobic exercise) under the supervision of an exercise physiologist. In addition, each subject was instructed to follow a diet of ~1800 kcal/d (20 kcal/ [kg • d]) by a registered dietitian. Subjects received biweekly dietary counseling to encourage compliance. Study participants underwent serum multiple-assay chemistry testing, as well as body composition, blood pressure, and dietary analysis at baseline, week 4, and week 8.Results: Of the 30 subjects who entered the study, 23 completed the 8-week protocol. Seven subjects dropped out for personal reasons unrelated to the study. Group 1 lost a significant amount of body weight compared with Group 2 (−2.88 kg vs −0.97 kg; P = 0.01) over the 8 weeks. Group 1 also achieved a significant reduction in body fat compared with Group 2 (−1.8% vs −0.57%; P = 0.02). The rate of change in body fat per 4-week interval in Group 1 was 3.1 times that in Group 2 (−0.88% vs −0.28%; P < 0.01). Group 1 also experienced a significant increase in triiodothyronine (T3) levels compared with Group 2 over the 8-week study period (+17.88 ng/dL vs 2.75 ng/dL; P = 0.04). There were no significant changes in levels of thyroid-stimulating hormone (TSH) or thyroxine (T4) in either group. In addition, no significant changes were observed in vital signs, blood sugar, testosterone and estradiol levels, liver and renal function, or overall caloric intake during the study. No subjective adverse effects were reported throughout the study. Conclusions: The results of the study suggest that 7-oxo-DHEA combined with moderate exercise and a reduced-calorie diet significantly reduces body weight and body fat compared with exercise and a reduced-calorie diet alone. In addition, 7-oxo-DHEA significantly elevated T3 levels but did not affect TSH or T4 levels, indicating that it does not adversely affect thyroid function in the short term.

Kurzman ID The effect of dehydroepiandrosterone combined with a low-fat diet in spontaneously obese dogs: a clinical trial. Obes Res 1998 Jan; 6(1):20-8 Dehydroepiandrosterone (DHEA) has been shown to have antiobesity activity in rodents and spontaneously obese dogs. This study evaluated the effect of DHEA or placebo combined with a low-fat/high-fiber diet in spontaneously obese dogs in a clinical trial. Spontaneously obese, euthyroid dogs, referred to the University of Wisconsin School of Veterinary Medicine for treatment of their obesity, were evaluated for percent overweight, rate of weight loss, serum cholesterol, plasma lipoprotein and serum biochemistry profiles, complete blood count, and endocrine profiles (T4, T3, cortisol, insulin, and DHEA-sulfate). DHEA-treated dogs had a significantly increased rate of actual and percent excess weight loss compared with placebo-treated dogs. Serum cholesterol decreased in both treatment groups; however, DHEA-treated dogs had a significantly greater reduction than placebo-treated dogs. DHEA-treated dogs had a significant 32% reduction in total plasma cholesterol, which was due to a 27% reduction in the lipoprotein fraction containing the high-density lipoprotein (HDL) and a 50% reduction in the lipoprotein fraction containing the low-density lipoprotein (LDL). Placebo-treated dogs did not have a significant reduction in total plasma cholesterol or in the fraction containing LDL; however, they did have a significant 11% reduction in the fraction containing HDL. Significant decreases in serum T4 and T3 observed in dogs receiving DHEA were not noted in dogs receiving placebo. DHEA in combination with caloric restriction results in a faster rate of weight loss than does caloric restriction alone. In addition, DHEA has hypocholesterolemic activity, particularly affecting the lipoprotein fraction containing the LDL cholesterol.

Leowattana W DHEA(S): the fountain of youth. J Med Assoc Thai 2001 Oct; 84 Suppl 2:S605-12. Dehydroepiandrosterone (DHEA) and its sulfate ester (DHEAS) are weak androgens produced primarily by the adrenal gland. Although their plasma concentrations by far exceed those of any other adrenal product, their physiological roles have not yet been determined. In plasma, where the major portion of these hormones is present in the sulfate form, it is possible that DHEAS serves as a reservoir for DHEA. Since various tissues have been shown to contain steroid sulfatases. The peak plasma levels of DHEA and DHEAS occur at approximately age 25 years, decrease progressively thereafter, and diminish by 95 per cent around the age of 85 years. The decline of DHEAS concentrations with aging has led to the suggestion that DHEAS could play a role in itself and be implicated in longevity. Moreover, the epidemiological evidence has shown that adult men with high plasma DHEAS levels are less likely to die of cardiovascular disease.

DHEA has also been shown to increase the body's ability to transform food into energy and burn off excess fat. Another recent finding involves the anti-inflammatory properties of DHEA. It has been known that DHEA can lower the levels of interleukin-6 (IL-6) and tumor necrosis factor alpha (TNF-alpha). It should be pointed out that chronic inflammation is known to play a critical role in the development of the killer diseases of aging: heart disease, Alzheimer's disease and certain types of cancer. In conclusion, DHEA or DHEAS administration combined with conventional treatment may be implicated in particular conditions to improve the quality of life.

Marenich LP. Excretion of testosterone, epitestosterone, androstenedione and 7-ketodehydroepiandrostenedione in healthy men of different ages Probl Endokrinol (Mosk). 1979 Jul-Aug; 25(4):28-31. Urinary excretion of testosterone, epitestosterone, androstendion, and 7-keto-dehydroepistendion was studied in 34 healthy men, aged from 20 to 72 years. The maximal excretion of these steroids and observed in men, aged between 20 and 30 years; their reduction was noted with the advance of age.

Martina V et al. Short-term dehydroepiandrosterone treatment increases platelet cGMP production in elderly male subjects. Clin Endocrinol (Oxf). 2006 Mar; 64(3):260-4. OBJECTIVE: Several clinical and population-based studies suggest that dehydroepiandrosterone (DHEA) and its sulphate (DHEA-S) play a protective role against atherosclerosis and coronary artery disease in human. However, the mechanisms underlying this action are still unknown. It has recently been suggested that DHEA-S could delay atheroma formation through an increase in nitric oxide (NO) production. STUDY DESIGN AND METHODS: Twenty-four aged male subjects [age (mean +/- SEM): 65.4 +/- 0.7 year; range: 58.2-67.6 years] underwent a blinded placebo controlled study receiving DHEA (50 mg p.o. daily at bedtime) or placebo for 2 months. Platelet cyclic guanosine-monophosphate (cGMP) concentration (as marker of NO production) and serum levels of DHEA-S, DHEA, IGF-I, insulin, glucose, oestradiol (E(2)), testosterone, plasminogen activator inhibitor (PAI)-1 antigen (PAI-1 Ag), homocysteine and lipid profile were evaluated before and after the 2-month treatment with DHEA or placebo. RESULTS: At the baseline, all variables in the two groups were overlapping. All parameters were unchanged after treatment with placebo. Conversely, treatment with DHEA (a) increased (P < 0.001 vs. baseline) platelet cGMP (111.9 +/- 7.1 vs. 50.1 +/- 4.1 fmol/10(6) plts), DHEA-S (13.6 +/- 0.8 vs. 3.0 +/- 0.3 micromol/l), DHEA (23.6 +/- 1.7 vs. 15.3 +/- 1.4 nmol/l), testosterone (23.6 +/- 1.0 vs. 17.7 +/- 1.0 nmol/l) and E(2) (72.0 +/- 5.0 vs. 60.0 +/- 4.0 pmol/l); and (b) decreased (P < 0.05 vs. baseline) PAI-1 Ag (27.4 +/- 3.8 vs. 21.5 +/- 2.5 ng/ml) and low-density lipoprotein (LDL) cholesterol (3.4 +/- 0.2 vs. 3.0 +/- 0.2 mmol/l). IGF-I, insulin, glucose, triglycerides, total cholesterol, HDL cholesterol, HDL2 cholesterol, HDL3 cholesterol, apolipoprotein A1 (ApoA1), apolipoprotein B

(ApoB) and homocysteine levels were not modified by DHEA treatment. CONCLUSIONS: This study shows that short-term treatment with DHEA increased platelet cGMP production, a marker of NO production, in healthy elderly subjects. This effect is coupled with a decrease in PAI-1 and LDL cholesterol levels as well as an increase in testosterone and E (2) levels. These findings, therefore, suggest that chronic DHEA supplementation would exert antiatherogenic effects, particularly in elderly subjects who display low circulating levels of this hormone.

Morales AJ, Haubrich RH, Hwang JY, Asakura H, Yen SS. The effect of six months treatment with a 100 mg daily dose of dehydroepiandrosterone (DHEA) on circulating sex steroids, body composition and muscle strength in age-advanced men and women. Clin Endocrinol (Oxf) 1998 Oct; 49(4):421-32.OBJECTIVE: The biological role of the adrenal sex steroid precursors--DHEA and DHEA sulphate (DS) and their decline with ageing remains undefined. We observed previously that administration of a 50 daily dose of DHEA for 3 months to age-advanced men and women resulted in an elevation (10%) of serum levels of insulin-like growth factor-I (IGF-I) accompanied by improvement of self-reported physical and psychological well-being. These findings led us to assess the effect of a larger dose (100 mg) of DHEA for a longer duration (6 months) on circulating sex steroids, body composition (DEXA) and muscle strength (MedX). SUBJECTS AND DESIGN: Healthy non-obese age-advanced (50-65 yrs of age) men (n = 9) and women (n = 10) were randomized into a double-blind placebo-controlled cross-over trial. Sixteen subjects completed the one-year study of six months of placebo and six months of 100 mg oral DHEA daily. MEASUREMENTS: Fasting early morning blood samples were obtained. Serum DHEA, DS, sex steroids, IGF-I, IGFBP-1, IGFBP-3, growth hormone binding protein (GHBP) levels and lipid profiles as well as body composition (by DEXA) and muscle strength (by MedX testing) were measured at baseline and after each treatment. RESULTS: Basal serum levels of DHEA, DS, androsternedione (A), testosterone (T) and dihydrotestosterone (DHT) were at or below the lower range of young adult levels. In both sexes, a 100 mg daily dose of DHEA restored serum DHEA levels to those of young adults and serum DS to levels at or slightly above the young adult range. Serum cortisol levels were unaltered; consequently the DS/cortisol ratio was increased to pubertal (10:1) levels. In women, but not in men, serum A, T and DHT were increased to levels above gender-specific young adult ranges. Basal SHBG levels were in the normal range for men and elevated in women, of whom 7 of 8 were on oestrogen replacement therapy. While on DHEA, serum SHBG levels declined with a greater (P < 0.02) response in women (-40 +/- 8%; P = 0.002) than in men (-5 +/- 4%; P = 0.02). Relative to baseline, DHEA administration resulted in an elevation of serum IGF-I levels in men (16 +/- 6%, P = 0.04) and in women (31 +/- 12%, P = 0.02). Serum levels of IGFBP-1 and IGFBP-3 were unaltered but GHBP levels declined in women (28 +/- 6%; P = 0.02) not in men. In men, but not in women, fat body mass decreased 1.0 +/- 0.4 kg (6.1 +/- 2.6%, P = 0.02) and knee muscle strength 15.0 +/- 3.3% (P = 0.02) as well as lumbar back strength 13.9 +/- 5.4% (P = 0.01) increased. In women, but not in men, an increase in total body mass of 1.4 +/- 0.4 kg (2.1 +/- 0.7%; P = 0.02) was noted. Neither gender had changes in basal metabolic rate, bone mineral density, urinary pyridinoline cross-links, fasting insulin, glucose, cortisol levels or lipid profiles. No significant adverse effects were observed. CONCLUSIONS: A daily oral 100 mg dose of DHEA for 6 months resulted in elevation of circulating DHEA and DS concentrations and the DS/cortisol ratio. Biotransformation to potent androgens near and slightly above the range of their younger counterparts occurred in women with no detectable change in men. Given this hormonal milieu, an increase in serum IGF-I levels was observed in both genders but dimorphic responses were evident in fat body mass and muscle strength in favour of men. These differences in response to DHEA administration may reflect a gender specific response to DHEA and/or the presence of confounding factor(s) in women such as oestrogen replacement therapy.

Nawata H et al. Mechanism of action of anti-aging DHEA-S and the replacement of DHEA-S. Mech Ageing Dev 2002 Apr 30; 123(8):1101-6. The plasma ACTH and cortisol levels do not change during aging. On the other hand, the plasma dehydroepiandrosterone sulfate (DHEA-S) changes remarkably during aging. Before puberty, the plasma DHEA-S level both in males and females is very low; however, it rapidly increases at puberty, and thereafter significantly decreases both linearly and age-dependently. Cytochrome P450c17 has two enzyme activities, 17-alpha-hydroxylase and 17, 20-lyase. Cortisol is synthesized by 17-alpha-hydroxylase, and DHEA is synthesized by 17, 20-lyase. The mechanism of dissociation of cortisol and DHEA synthesis in aging depends on another regulator of 17, 20-lyase of cytochrome P450c17 such as cytochrome P450 reductase. We demonstrated significant decrease in cytochrome P450 reductase activity in bovine aged adrenal glands. We clarified the beneficial effects of DHEA as an anti-aging steroid based on both in vitro and in vivo experiments, such as the stimulatory effect of immune system, anti-diabetes mellitus, anti-atherosclerosis, anti-dementia (neurosteroid), anti-obesity and anti-osteoporosis. It is very important to identify the mechanism of action of DHEA. We clarified the conversion of DHEA to estrone by cytochrome P450 aromatase in primary cultured human osteoblasts. We indentified high affinity of DHEA binding with K (d) =6.6 nM in antigen and DHEA stimulated human T lymphocytes. We searched for the target genes that are specifically induced in activated T lymphocytes in the presence of DHEA by subtractive hybridization screening for differentially expressed transcripts. The double blind, randomized human replacement therapies utilizing DHEA are also reviewed.

Nordmark G et al. Effects of dehydroepiandrosterone supplement on health-related quality of life in glucocorticoid treated female patients with systemic lupus erythematosus.

Autoimmunity. 2005 Nov; 38(7):531-40. The objective of this study was to evaluate the efficacy of low dose dehydroepiandrosterone (DHEA) on health-related quality of life (HRQOL) in glucocorticoid treated female patients with systemic lupus erythematosus (SLE). Forty one women (>or= 5 mg prednisolone/day) were included in a double-blind, randomized, placebo-controlled study for 6 months where DHEA was given at 30 mg/20 mg (<or= 45/ >or= 46 years) daily, or placebo, followed by 6 months open DHEA treatment to all patients. HRQOL was assessed at baseline, 6 and 12 months, using four validated questionnaires and the patients' partners completed a questionnaire assessing mood and behaviour at 6 months. DHEA treatment increased serum levels of sulphated DHEA from subnormal to normal. The DHEA group improved in SF-36 "role emotional" and HSCL-56 total score (both $p<0.05$). During open DHEA treatment, the former placebo group improved in SF-36 "mental health" ($p<0.05$) with a tendency for improvement in HSCL-56 total score ($p=0.10$). Both groups improved in McCoy's Sex Scale during active treatment ($p<0.05$). DHEA replacement decreased high-density lipoprotein (HDL) cholesterol and increased insulin-like growth factor I (IGF-I) and haematocrit. There were no effects on bone density or disease activity and no serious adverse events. Side effects were mild. We conclude that low dose DHEA treatment improves HRQOL with regard to mental well-being and sexuality and can be offered to women with SLE where mental distress and/or impaired sexuality constitutes a problem.

Rabijewski M et al. Positive effects of DHEA therapy on insulin resistance and lipids in men with angiographically verified coronary heart disease - preliminary study.Endokrynol Pol. 2005;56(6):904-910OBJECTIVES: The aim of this study was to analyze the influence of DHEA therapy on insulin resistance (FIRI, FG/FI) and serum lipids in men with angiographically verified coronary heart disease (CHD). MATERIAL AND METHODS: The study included thirty men aged 41-60 years (mean age 52+/-0.90 yr) with serum DHEA-S concentration<2000 microg/l, who were randomized into a double-blind, placebo-controlled, cross-over trial. Subjects completed the 80 days study of 40 days of 150 mg oral DHEA daily or placebo, and next groups were changed after 30 days of wash-out. Fasting early morning blood samples were obtained at baseline and after each treatment to determine serum hormones levels (testosterone, DHEA-S, LH, FSH estradiol and IGF-1) and also metabolic profile (total cholesterol, LDL-cholesterol, triglicerides, HDL-cholesterol, insulin, glucose, fasting insulin resistance index--FIRI and FG/FI ratio). RESULTS: Administration of DHEA was associated with 4.5-fold increase in DHEA-S levels. Relative to baseline DHEA administration resulted in a decrease in insulin levels by 40% ($p<0.005$) and fasting insulin resistance index (FIRI) by 47% ($p<0.004$). Also total cholesterol levels and LDL-cholesterol levels decreased significantly (from 222.9+/-6.6 mg/dL to 207.4+/-6.6 mg/dL and from 143.9+/-6.9 mg/dL to 130.5+/-6.0 mg/dL respectively; $p<0.05$). Glucose levels dropped significant below baseline values after DHEA ($p<0.001$). Estrogen levels significantly increased after DHEA ($p<0.05$). While changes of serum concentrations of testosterone,

LH, FSH, IGF-I, HDL-cholesterol, triglycerides were not statistical significant. Tolerance of the treatment was good and no adverse effects were observed. CONCLUSIONS: DHEA therapy in dose of 150 mg daily during 40 days in men with DHEA levels<2000 microg/l decreased total cholesterol concentration, insulin and glucose levels and fasting insulin resistance index (FIRI). This therapy may be a beneficial against CHD risk factors.

Rao KV et al. Chemoprevention of rat prostate carcinogenesis by early and delayed administration of dehydroepiandrosterone. Cancer Res 1999 Jul 1; 59(13):3084-9 Two in vivo bioassays were conducted to evaluate the efficacy of dehydroepiandrosterone (DHEA) as an inhibitor of prostate carcinogenesis in rats. Prostate adenocarcinomas were induced in male Wistar-Unilever rats by a sequential regimen of cyproterone acetate and testosterone propionate, followed by a single i.v. injection of N-methyl-N-nitrosourea (MNU) and chronic androgen stimulation. In the first experiment, DHEA (1000 or 2000 mg/kg diet) was administered continuously to rats beginning 1 week before MNU exposure. In the second experiment, continuous administration of DHEA (2000 mg/kg diet) was begun either 1 week before, 20 weeks after, or 40 weeks after MNU exposure. Controls received basal diet without added DHEA. Studies were terminated at 13 months after MNU administration, and prostate cancer incidence was determined by histopathological evaluation of step sections of accessory sex glands. In the first study, continuous dietary administration of DHEA beginning 1 week before MNU resulted in a dose-related inhibition of prostate cancer induction. In the second experiment, comparable reductions in prostate cancer incidence were observed in groups exposed to DHEA beginning 1 week before, 20 weeks after, and 40 weeks after carcinogen exposure. These data demonstrate that nontoxic doses of DHEA confer significant protection against prostate carcinogenesis in rats. The efficacy of delayed administration of DHEA suggests that the compound confers protection against later stages of prostate cancer induction and can suppress the progression of existing preneoplastic lesions to invasive disease.

Rudman D Plasma dehydroepiandrosterone sulfate in nursing home men.J Am Geriatr Soc 1990 Apr; 38(4):421-7. Previous studies have shown the normal range of plasma dehydroepiandrosterone sulfate (DHEAS) for independent community men over 60 years old to be 30-200 micrograms/dL. In human adults, low levels of plasma DHEAS have been correlated with a high mortality rate. In rodents, dehydroepiandrosterone, the precursor of DHEAS, has exhibited antidiabetic, anticarcinogenic, neurotropic, and memory-enhancing effects. We have now measured plasma DHEAS in 50 independent community men age 55-94 and in 61 nursing home men age 57-104. Mean DHEAS was significantly lower in the nursing home men than in the community men. Plasma DHEAS was subnormal (less than 30 micrograms/dL) in 40% of the nursing home residents and in only 6% of the community subjects. In both groups, DHEAS was inversely related to age. In the nursing home men, additionally, plasma DHEAS was inversely related to the presence of an organic brain syndrome and to the degree of dependence in activities of daily living. Plasma DHEAS was subnormal in 80% of the nursing home men who required total care. There was no significant correlation between the plasma concentrations of DHEAS and testosterone, or between plasma DHEAS and one-year mortality rate.

Severi G et al. Circulating steroid hormones and the risk of prostate cancer.Cancer Epidemiol Biomarkers Prev. 2006 Jan; 15(1):86-91. Epidemiologic studies have failed to support the hypothesis that circulating androgens are positively associated with prostate cancer risk and some recent studies have even suggested that high testosterone levels might be protective particularly against aggressive cancer. We tested this hypothesis by measuring total testosterone, androstanediol glucuronide, androstenedione, DHEA sulfate, estradiol, and sex hormone-binding globulin in plasma collected at baseline in a prospective cohort study of 17,049 men. We used a case-cohort design, including 524 cases diagnosed during a mean 8.7 years follow-up and a randomly sampled sub-cohort of 1,859 men. The association between each hormone level and prostate cancer risk was tested using Cox models adjusted for country of birth. The risk of prostate cancer was approximately 30% lower for a doubling of the concentration of estradiol but the evidence was weak (P (trend) =0.07). None of the other hormones was associated with overall prostate cancer (P (trend) >or= 0.3). None of the hormones was associated with nonaggressive prostate cancer (all P (trend) >or= 0.2). The hazard ratio [HR; 95% confidence interval (95% CI)] for aggressive cancer almost halved for a doubling of the concentration of testosterone (HR, 0.55; 95% CI, 0.32-0.95) and androstenedione (HR, 0.51; 95% CI, 0.31-0.83), and was 37% lower for a doubling of the concentration of DHEA sulfate (HR, 0.63; 95% CI, 0.46-0.87). Similar negative but nonsignificant linear trends in risk for aggressive cancer were obtained for free testosterone, estradiol, and sex hormone-binding globulin (P (trend) =0.06, 0.2, and 0.1, respectively). High levels of testosterone and adrenal androgens are thus associated with reduced risk of aggressive prostate cancer but not with nonaggressive disease.

Shi J, Schulze S, Lardy HA. The effect of 7-oxo-DHEA acetate on memory in young and old C57BL/6 mice. Steroids. 2000 Mar; 65(3):124-9. 7-Oxo-dehydroepiandrosterone, which can be formed from dehydroepiandrosterone (DHEA) by several mammalian tissues, is more effective than its parent steroid as an inducer of thermogenic enzymes when administered to rats. Using the Morris water maze procedure, we tested DHEA and its 7-oxo-derivative for their ability to reverse the memory abolition induced by scopolamine in young C57BL/6 mice, and for their effect on memory in old mice. A single dose of 7-oxo-DHEA-acetate at 24 mg/kg b.w. completely reversed the impairment caused by 1 mg of scopolamine per kg b.w. (P < 0.001). DHEA (20 mg/kg) was also effective (P < 0.01). In old mice given the same single doses followed by feeding 0.05% of the respective steroid in the diet, memory of the water maze training was retained through a four week test period in mice receiving 7-oxo-DHEA-acetate (P < 0.05) but not in the control or DHEA-treated groups. When old mice were not tested until five weeks after being trained 7-oxo-DHEA exerted a slight, but statistically insignificant, improvement in memory retention. The possible effect of 7-oxo-DHEA in human memory problems deserves investigation.

Shilkaitis A et al. Dehydroepiandrosterone inhibits the progression phase of mammary carcinogenesis by inducing cellular senescence via a p16-dependent but p53-independent mechanism. Breast Cancer Res. 2005; 7(6):R1132-40. INTRODUCTION: Dehydroepiandrosterone (DHEA), an adrenal 17-ketosteroid, is a precursor of testosterone and 17beta-estradiol. Studies have shown that DHEA inhibits carcinogenesis in mammary gland and prostate as well as other organs, a process that is not hormone dependent. Little is known about the molecular mechanisms of DHEA-mediated inhibition of the neoplastic process. Here we examine whether DHEA and its analog DHEA 8354 can suppress the progression of hyperplastic and premalignant (carcinoma in situ) lesions in mammary gland toward malignant tumors and the cellular mechanisms involved. METHODS: Rats were treated with N-nitroso-N-methylurea and allowed to develop mammary hyperplastic and premalignant lesions with a maximum frequency 6 weeks after carcinogen administration. The animals were then given DHEA or DHEA 8354 in the diet at 125 or 1,000 mg/kg diet for 6 weeks. The effect of these agents on induction of apoptosis, senescence, cell proliferation, tumor burden and various effectors of cellular signaling were determined. RESULTS: Both agents induced a dose-dependent decrease in tumor multiplicity and in tumor burden. In addition they induced a senescent phenotype in tumor cells, inhibited cell proliferation and increased the number of apoptotic cells. The DHEA-induced cellular effects were associated with increased expression of p16 and p21, but not p53 expression, implicating a p53-independent mechanism in their action. CONCLUSION: We provide evidence that DHEA and DHEA 8354 can suppress mammary carcinogenesis by altering various cellular functions, inducing cellular senescence, in tumor cells with the potential involvement of p16 and p21 in mediating these effects.

Williams MR et al. Dehydroepiandrosterone increases endothelial cell proliferation in vitro and improves endothelial function in vivo by mechanisms independent of androgen and estrogen receptors. J Clin Endocrinol Metab. 2004 Sep; 89(9):4708-15. Dehydroepiandrosterone (DHEA) may be beneficial in cardiovascular health, but mechanisms of DHEA action in the cardiovascular system are unclear. We have therefore 1) determined DHEA effects on the proliferation of cultured endothelial cells (EC), 2) compared effects of DHEA with estradiol (E) and testosterone (T), and 3) examined DHEA effects on subcellular messengers. We have in addition examined effects of DHEA (100 mg/d, 3 months) in 36 healthy postmenopausal women on blood pressure, lipids, and endothelial function, assessed noninvasively in large vessels by flow-mediated dilation of the brachial artery during reactive hyperemia, and in small vessels by laser Doppler velocimetry with iontophoresis of acetylcholine. DHEA, E, and T all increased EC proliferation; the effect of E was abolished by the estrogen receptor antagonist ICI 182,780, and that of T was abolished by the androgen receptor antagonist flutamide; neither blocked the effect of DHEA. In vitro, DHEA increased EC expression of endothelial nitric oxide synthase and activity of extracellular signal-regulated kinase 1/2. In vivo, DHEA increased flow-mediated dilation and laser Doppler velocimetry and reduced total plasma cholesterol. Thus, DHEA increases EC proliferation in vitro by mechanism(s) independently of either androgen receptor or estrogen receptor and in vivo enhances large and small vessel EC function in postmenopausal women.

Wilson, James ND, DC, PHD. Adrenal Fatigue: The 21st Century Stress Syndrome. Adrenal Fatigue: the 21st Century Stress Syndrome™ is a self-help lifesaver for everyone who regularly experiences any of the above or any of the many other signs of stress described in the book. Stress related adrenal fatigue often plays a role in many health conditions, such as frequent infections, chemical sensitivities, allergies, autoimmune diseases like fibromyalgia and rheumatoid arthritis, menopause and PMS, thyroid function imbalances, chronic fatigue syndrome, low libido, chronic anxiety, and mild depression. Smart Publications; (January 25, 2002)

Wolkowitz et al, Double-blind treatment of major depression with dehydroepiandrosterone. AmJPsychiatry. 1999 Apr; 156(4):646-9.OBJECTIVE: This study was designed to assess possible antidepressant effects of dehydroepiandrosterone (DHEA), an abundant adrenocortical hormone in humans. METHOD: Twenty-two patients with major depression, either medication-free or on stabilized antidepressant regimens, received either DHEA (maximum dose = 90 mg/day) or placebo for 6 weeks in a double-blind manner and were rated at baseline and at the end of the 6 weeks with the Hamilton Depression Rating Scale. Patients previously stabilized with antidepressants had the study medication added to that regimen; others received DHEA or placebo alone. RESULTS: DHEA was associated with a significantly greater decrease in Hamilton depression scale ratings than was placebo. Five of the 11 patients treated with DHEA, compared with none of the 11 given placebo, showed a 50% decrease or greater in depressive symptoms. CONCLUSIONS: These results suggest that DHEA treatment may have significant antidepressant effects in some patients with major depression. Further, larger-scale trials are warranted.

Von Muhlen et al. The Dehydroepiandrosterone And WellNess (DAWN) study: research design and methods. Contemp Clin Trials 2007 Feb;28(2):153-68.Levels of dehydroepiandrosterone (DHEA) and DHEA-sulfate (DHEAS), the major secretory products of the adrenal gland, decline dramatically with age, concurrent with the onset of degenerative changes and chronic diseases associated with aging. Epidemiological evidences in humans and animal studies suggest that DHEA(S) may have cardioprotective, antiobesity, antidiabetic, and immuno-enhancing properties. These observations led to the proposal that restoration of DHEA to young adult levels may have beneficial effects on age-related conditions. Most clinical trials of DHEA replacement have been limited due to small samples and short duration, restriction to one sex, failure to adjust for baseline endogenous hormone level and age, or lack of placebo comparison groups. We designed a double blind, placebo-controlled randomized trial to determine the acceptability, benefits, and adverse effects of 50 mg daily oral DHEA replacement for one year in 110 men and 115 women, aged 55 to 85, who were healthy and not currently using hormone therapy. A wide range of biological outcomes were studied including bone mineral density and metabolism, body composition and muscle strength, immune function, and cardiovascular risk factors. Steroid hormone levels, bone markers, cytokines, and the IGF-I, IGF binding protein system were measured at baseline and at 3 follow-up clinic visits. Changes in mood and well-being, cognitive function, and sexuality were assessed. Information on potentially confounding covariates such as smoking, alcohol consumption, exercise, diet and dietary supplements were obtained, and potential adverse effects of DHEA administration were monitored. This study enables an examination of the benefits of DHEA administration on the health of older men and women, and the influence of gender, age, and baseline endogenous DHEA level on each outcome variable. Potential mechanisms of DHEA action, including the biotransformation of DHEA to active steroids and steroid metabolites, enhancement of IGF-I bioavailability, and inhibition of IL-6 production can also be evaluated.

Yang SC et al. Interactive effect of an acute bout of resistance exercise and dehydroepiandrosterone administration on glucose tolerance and serum lipids in middle-aged women. Chin J Physiol. 2005 Mar 31; 48(1):23-9. The present study determined the interactive effect of an acute bout of resistance exercise and dehydroepiandrosterone (DHEA) administration on glucose tolerance and serum lipids. Twenty middle-aged female subjects performed an acute bout of resistance exercise and were subsequently divided into two groups: placebo (age 40.7 +/- 2.0) and DHEA administered (age 39.0 +/- 2.7). Ten subjects who received DHEA (age 41.5 +/- 4.6) participated in a non-exercise control. DHEA (25 mg twice daily) or placebo was orally supplemented for 48 hours. Before exercise and 48 hours after the last exercise bout (14 hours after the last DHEA intake), an oral glucose tolerance test and an insulin concentration were determined. Levels of fasting serum cholesterol and triglyceride, tumor necrosis factor-alpha (TNF-alpha), creatine kinase (CK) were also measured. The DHEA administration significantly elevated the fasting dehydroepiandrosterone sulfate (DHEA-S) level by approximately 3-fold. Both acute resistance exercise and DHEA administration improved glucose tolerance, but no addictive effect was found. Furthermore, exercise and DHEA administration did not affect serum triglyceride and cholesterol levels, but both lipids were significantly lowered when DHEA was given following exercise. Resistance exercise induced elevations in serum CK and TNFalpha levels, but these increases were attenuated by the DHEA administration. The new finding of this study was that post-exercise DHEA administration decreased serum triglycerides and cholesterol. This effect appeared to be associated with its TNF-alpha lowering action.

Yen SS. Aging and the adrenal cortex. Exp Gerontol 1998 Nov-Dec; 33(7-8):897-910 Aging in humans is accompanied by an increase in adrenal glucocorticoid secretion and a decline in adrenal androgen synthesis and secretion. The intense interest in adrenal function in aging individuals in recent years is in large measure related to the potential impact of cortisol excess in the development of cognitive impairment and hippocampal neuronal loss, and to the desire to provide hormone replacement and healthy aging. Although the preliminary data is tantalizing, solid scientific evidence are not at hand. It is apparent that both issues are extremely complex. Dehydroepiandrosterone (DHEA) and its 3 beta-sulfate are fascinating molecules, including their synthesis and actions in the brain. Recent studies have shown that DHEA-sulfate (DHEA-S), but not DHEA, activates peroxisome proliferator-activated receptor alpha (PPAR alpha) in the liver, an intracellular receptor belonging to the steroid receptor superfamily. Thus, DHEA-S may serve as a physiological modulator of liver fatty acid metabolism and peroxisomal enzyme expression, and thereby may contribute to the anticarcinogenic and chemoprotective properties of this intriguing class of endogenous steroids. The life-sustaining role of adrenal cortisol secretion and its regulation of metabolism via catabolic actions may be modulated by its partner DHEA and DHEA-S. During the anabolic growth period (childhood and early adulthood) the body is exposed to relatively high levels of DHEA/DHEA-S but to relatively or absolutely high levels of cortisol during infancy and the aging phase. The cortisol/DHEA-S ratio during the life span follows a U-shape curve, which may be telling us to explore these two critical adrenal steroids in tandem

Zwain IH, Yen SS. Neurosteroidogenesis in astrocytes, oligodendrocytes, and neurons of cerebral cortex of rat brain. Endocrinology 1999 Aug; 140(8):3843-52 The brain is a steroidogenic organ that expresses steroidogenic enzymes and produces neurosteroids. Although considerable information is now available regarding the steroidogenic capacity of the brain, little is known regarding the steroidogenic pathway and relative contributions of astrocytes, oligodendrocytes, and neurons to neurosteroidogenesis. In the present study, we investigated differential gene expression of the key steroidogenic enzymes using RT-PCR and quantitatively evaluated the production of neurosteroids by highly purified astrocytes, oligodendrocytes, and neurons from the cerebral cortex of neonatal rat brains using specific and sensitive RIAs. Astrocytes appear to be the most active steroidogenic cells in the brain. These cells express cytochrome P450 side-chain cleavage (P450scc), 17alpha-hydroxylase/C17-20-lyase (P450c17), 3beta-hydroxysteroid dehydrogenase (3betaHSD), 17beta-hydroxysteroid dehydrogenase (17betaHSD), and cytochrome P450 aromatase (P450arom) and produce pregnenolone (P5), progesterone (P4), dehydroepiandrosterone (DHEA), androstenedione (A4), testosterone (T), estradiol, and estrone. Oligodendrocytes express only P450scc and 3betaHSD and produce P5, P4, and A4. These cells do not express P450c17, 17betaHSD, or P450arom or produce DHEA, T, or estrogen. Neurons express P450scc, P450c17, 3betaHSD, and P450arom and produce P5, DHEA, A4, and estrogen, but do not express 17betaHSD or produce T. By comparing the ability of each cell type in the production of neurosteroids, astrocytes are the major producer of P4, DHEA, and androgens, whereas oligodendrocytes are predominantly the producer of P5 and neurons of estrogens. These findings serve to define the neurosteroidogenic pathway, with special emphasis on the dominant role of astrocytes and their interaction with oligodendrocytes and neurons in the genesis of DHEA and active sex steroids. Thus, we propose that neurosteroidogenesis is accomplished by a tripartite contribution of the three cell types in the brain.

CHAPTER 7

Pregnenolone:

Pregnenolone is derived from cholesterol, as are all other steroidal hormones. The conversion of cholesterol to Pregnenolone occurs in the mitochondria via P450scc (CYP11A1). Pregnenolone is produced in the mitochondria in the brain and in the adrenal glands. As we age, our pregnenolone levels decline by as much as 60% by the time we are 75 years old. Pregnenolone is known as the "grandmother" hormone in the body because it is a precursor to progesterone and to DHEA (dehydroepiandrosterone), which, in turn, is a precursor to the sex hormones testosterone and estrogen.

Our steroidal hormones are the body's best source of defense against stress. Pregnenolone also plays an important role in neutralizing cellular toxins. Pregnenolone modulates calcium-protein bindings, gene activation, protein turnover and the intra-cellular distribution of compounds and enzyme reactions involved in the storage and retrieval of memory.

Large concentrations of pregnenolone are found in the brain and Pregnenolone supplementation has been shown to improve many of our mental functions, including mood and cognition. Some patients with bipolar disorders have very low levels of Pregnenolone, as do some patients with ADHD and schizophrenia. The symptoms of these disorders are, to varying degrees, improved by Pregnenolone supplementation. Since Pregnenolone is known to have a protective effect on the neurons in the brain, restoring adequate levels of Pregnenolone has been shown to improve memory and rapid eye movement (REM) sleep. There is accumulating evidence that pregnenolone and other neurosteroids (all derived from Pregnenolone) have strong influences on learning and memory by facilitating neurotransmission in the hippocampus, amygdala, and prefrontal cortex of the brain. Specifically, Pregnenolone sulfate has been found to improve the survival of hippocampal neurons and improve aspects of neuronal structuring (via increased microtubule assembly).

In the 1940's, Pregnenolone was used successfully to treat many of the symptoms of arthritis including muscle and joint pain, decreased energy levels, decreased strength and decreased mobility without any of the unwanted side effects associated with the current standard cortisone treatments prescribed so frequently today. Pregnenolone has a protective action against the unwanted effects of elevated cortisol levels. Pregnenolone has been shown to improve mood, decrease fatigue, enhance memory and improve a person's ability to cope with stress. Pregnenolone may also be an important component in repairing the myelin sheath. Patients with multiple sclerosis, where the myelin sheath is destroyed, experience many debilitating symptoms. These patients also exhibit low levels of Pregnenolone and DHEA (amongst other neurosteroids), which, when supplemented, may ameliorate some symptoms. Endogenous Pregnenolone has also been demonstrated to play a role in recovery from spinal cord injury— accordingly, its supplementation may improve recovery.

When clinically indicated, we prescribe Pregnenolone to our patients. Dosage usually ranges from 100 mg to 200 mg per day and should be taken in the morning. If DHEAS levels are suboptimal, Pregnenolone levels may also be suboptimal. No significant adverse side effects from Pregnenolone supplementation have been observed; though there is some indication that low doses may be more effective than higher doses for some symptoms.

Pregnenolone treatment has been found to provide benefit in a variety of complications including:

- Anxiety
- Fatigue
- Sleep disorders
- Depression
- Memory loss
- ADHD
- Arthritis
- Spinal injury
- Multiple sclerosis

Management:

Lab testing has not been shown to significantly help clinical treatment. If DHEAS levels are suboptimal, Pregnenolone levels will probably also be suboptimal.

It can be prescribed in a capsule compounded with DHEA or separately.

Men 25-200 mg
Women: 12-50 mg.

PREGNENELONE ABSTRACTS

Akwa Y Neurosteroids: behavioral aspects and physiological implications J Soc Biol 1999;193(3):293-8 The term "neurosteroids" applies to those steroids that are both formed in the nervous system from sterol precursors, and accumulate in the nervous system, at least in part, independently of peripheral steroidogenic glands secretion. Neurosteroids that are active on the central nervous system include, mainly, pregnenolone (PREG), dehydroepiandrosterone (DHEA) and their sulfate esters (PREG-S and DHEA-S), as well as the reduced metabolite of progesterone, 3 alpha,5 alpha-TH PROG also called allopregnanolone. These neuroactive neurosteroids alter neuronal excitability by modulating the activity of several neurotransmitter receptors and thus can influence behavior. PREG-S decreases the sleeping time in rats anesthetized with a barbiturate, which is consistent with its antagonist action on the GABAA receptor (GABAA-R). Allopregnanolone is anxiolytic in rats tested in a conflict paradigm, through an interaction at a site specific for the benzodiazepine (BZ) receptor inverse agonist RO15-4513 and/or at the picrotoxinin site on GABAA-R. The contribution of the amygdala, a key region involved in the control of anxiety, is also demonstrated for the anxiolytic action of allopregnanolone. An anti-agressive effect of DHEA can be observed in castrated male mice who become agressive in the presence of lactating females. This inhibition of agressiveness by DHEA is associated to a selective decrease in the brain of PREG-S, which may, in turn, trigger an increase of endogenous GABAergic tone. Finally, cognitive performances of aged rats tested in the Morris water maze and the Y-maze can be correlated with individual concentrations of PREG-S in the hippocampus, i.e. poor performance in both tasks with low levels of PREG-S. Remarkably, the memory deficits are significantly improved, albeit transiently, by an intra-hippocampal injection of PREG-S in impaired aged rats. Promnesiant PREG-S may then reinforce some neurotransmitter systems that can decline with age. This brief review provides evidence of the pharmacology and physiological correlates of neurosteroids involved in behavioral phenomena. However, neurobiological mechanisms of behavioral effects of neurosteroids await further investigation.

Charalampopoulos I, Remboutsika E, Margioris AN, & Gravanis A. Neurosteroids as modulators of neurogenesis and neuronal survival. Trends Endocrinol Metab. 2008 Oct;19(8):300-7. Neurons and glia in the central nervous system express the necessary enzymes for the synthesis of neurosteroids that are produced in concentrations high enough to exert paracrine effects. Synthesis of brain neurosteroids declines with age, during stressful conditions (including major depression, chronic psychological stress), and in chronic inflammatory and neurodegenerative diseases. Recent reports associate the decrease of brain neurosteroids to neuronal dysfunction and degeneration. This review summarizes the recent findings on how the most studied neurosteroids (dehydroepiandrosterone, pregnenolone and their sulphate esters, progesterone and allopregnanolone) affect neuronal survival, neurite outgrowth and neurogenesis; furthermore, this review discusses potential applications of these neurosteroids in the therapeutic management of neurodegenerative conditions, including that of age-related brain atrophy.

Darnaudéry M, Koehl M, Pallarés M, Le Moal MJ, Mayo W. The neurosteroid preg- nenolone sulfate increases cortical acetyl- choline release: A microdialysis study of freely moving rats. J Neurochem. 1998 Nov;71(5):2018-22.The effects of pregnenolone sulfate (Preg-S) administrations (0, 12, 48, 96, and 192 nmol intracerebroventricularly) on acetylcholine (ACh) release in the frontal cortex and dorsal striatum were investigated by on-line microdialysis in freely moving rats. Following Preg-S administration, extracellular ACh levels in the frontal cortex increased in a dose-dependent manner, whereas no change was observed in the striatum. The highest doses (96 and 192 nmol) induced a threefold increase above control values of ACh release, the intermediate dose of 48 nmol led to a twofold increase, whereas after the dose of 12 nmol, the levels of ACh were not different from those observed after vehicle injection. The increase in cortical ACh reached a maximum 30 min after administration for all the active doses. Taken together, these results suggest that Preg-S interacts with the cortical cholinergic system, which may account, at least in part, for the promnesic and/or antiamnesic properties of this neurosteroid.

Darnaudery M, Pallares M, Piazza PV, Le Moal M, Mayo W. The neurosteroid preg- nenolone sulfate infused into the medial sep- tum nucleus increases hippocampal acetyl- choline and spatial memory in rats. Brain Res. 2002 Oct 4; 951(2):237-42. The effects of an infusion of the neurosteroid pregnenolone sulfate into the medial septum on acetylcholine release in the hippocampus and on spatial memory were evaluated in two experiments. Results show that pregnenolone sulfate enhanced acetylcholine release by more than 50% of baseline and improved recognition memory of a familiar environment. Therefore, our results suggest that the septo-hippocampal pathway could be involved in the promnesic properties of this neurosteroid.

George M, Guidotti A, Rubinow D, Pan B, Mikalauskas K, Post R. CSF neuroactive steroids in affective disorders: pregnenolone, progesterone and DBI. Biolog Psychiatry. 1994 May 15; 35(10):775-80.Recently several steroid compounds have been discovered to act as neuromodulators in diverse central nervous system (CNS) functions. We wondered if neuroactive steroids might be involved in affective illness or in the mode of action of mood-regulating medications such as carbamazepine. Levels of the neuroactive steroids pregnenolone and progesterone, as well as the neuropeptide diazepam binding inhibitor (DBI) (known to promote steroidogenesis), were analyzed from cerebrospinal fluid (CSF) obtained by lumbar puncture (LP) from 27 medication-free subjects with affective illness and 10 healthy volunteers. Mood-disordered subjects who were clinically depressed at the time of the LP had lower CSF pregnenolone (n = 9, 0.16 ng/ml) compared with euthymic volunteers (n = 10, 0.35 ng/ml; p < 0.01). In addition, pregnenolone was lower in all affectively ill subjects (n = 26, 0.21 ng/ml), regardless of mood state on the LP day, than healthy volunteers (p < 0.05). No differences were found for progesterone or DBI levels by mood state or diagnosis. Progesterone, pregnenolone, and DBI did not change significantly or consistently in affectively ill subjects after treatment with carbamazepine. CSF pregnenolone is decreased in subjects with affective illness, particularly during episodes of active depression. Further research into the role of neuroactive steroids in mood regulation is warranted.

Heydari B, Le Melledo JM. Low preg- nenolone sulfate plasma concentrations in patients with generalized social phobia. Psychol Med. 2002 Jul2; 32(5):929-33. BACKGROUND: Animal studies have shown that neuroactive steroids modulate the activity of the gamma-aminobutyric acid type A/benzodiazepine receptor complex and that these steroids display anxiolytic or anxiogenic activity depending on their positive (e.g. allopregnanolone) or negative allosteric modulation (e.g. dehydroepiandrosterone sulphate) of this receptor. This study compared plasma levels of allopregnanolone, dehydroepiandrosterone sulphate and pregnenolone sulphate in healthy controls and in patients with generalized social phobia, as assessed with the Mini-International Neuropsychiatric Interview. METHODS: Plasma concentrations of allopregnanolone, pregnenolone sulphate, and dehydroepiandrosterone sulphate were measured in 12 unmedicated male patients with generalized social phobia and 12 matched healthy male volunteers. RESULTS: Concentrations of pregnenolone sulphate were significantly lower in patients with generalized social phobia than in healthy controls. No statistically significant differences were found for the concentrations of allopregnanolone and dehydroepiandrosterone sulphate in plasma. CONCLUSIONS: These results are particularly interesting since we also observed lower pregnenolone sulphate concentrations in male patients suffering from generalized anxiety disorder. Their relevance to the pathophysiology of social anxiety disorder remains to be determined

Lanthier A, Patwardhan VV. Sex steroids and 5-en-3b-hydrosteroids in specific regions of the human brain and cranial nerves. J Steroid Biochem. 1986 Sep; 25(3):445-9. Sex steroids and 5-en-3 beta-hydroxysteroids were determined by radioimmunoassay in specific regions of the human brain, in the anterior and posterior pituitary, in one sensory organ, the retina and in the cranial nerves. Progesterone, androstenedione, testosterone and estrone were found in all areas of the brain and in all the cranial nerves but not in all cases. There was no sex difference except in the case of androstenedione where values were higher in women in some brain areas. Estrone values were always higher than those of estradiol in both men and women. No 5 alpha-dihydrotestosterone was detected in any of the samples studied. The values for pregnenolone, dehydroepiandrosterone and their sulfates were much higher than those of the sex steroids in all areas of the brain and in all the cranial nerves. Values for pregnenolone were greater than those of its sulfate while those of dehydroepiandrosterone were in general equal to or higher than those of its sulfate. The values for pregnenolone were greater than those of dehydroepiandrosterone. There were no obvious regional differences in the concentrations of the 5-en-3 beta-hydroxysteroids either in specific areas of the brain or in the cranial nerves. But there was a definite trend for the free dehydroepiandrosterone values to be higher in women. The possible significance of these observations is discussed.

Marx CE et al. Proof of concept trial with the neurosteroid pregnenolone targeting cognitive and negative symptoms in schizophrenia. Neuropsychopharmacology. 2009 July; 34(8):1885-903. The neurosteroid pregnenolone and its sulfated derivative enhance learning and memory in rodents. Pregnenolone sulfate also positively modulates NMDA receptors and could thus ameliorate hypothesized NMDA receptor hypofunction in schizophrenia. Furthermore, clozapine increases pregnenolone in rodent hippocampus, possibly contributing to its superior efficacy. We therefore investigated adjunctive pregnenolone for cognitive and negative symptoms in patients with schizophrenia or schizoaffective disorder receiving stable doses of second-generation antipsychotics in a pilot randomized, placebo-controlled, double-blind trial. Following a 2-week single-blind placebo lead-in, patients were randomized to pregnenolone (fixed escalating doses to 500 mg/day) or placebo, for 8 weeks. Primary end points were changes in BACS and MCCB composite and total SANS scores. Of 21 patients randomized, 18 completed at least 4 weeks of treatment (n=9/group). Pregnenolone was well tolerated. Patients receiving pregnenolone demonstrated significantly greater improvements in SANS scores (mean change=10.38) compared with patients receiving placebo (mean change=2.33), $p=0.048$. Mean composite changes in BACS and MCCB scores were not significantly different in patients randomized to pregnenolone compared with placebo. However, serum pregnenolone increases predicted BACS composite scores at 8 weeks in the pregnenolone group ($r(s) =0.81$, $p=0.022$). Increases in allopregnanolone, a GABAnergic pregnenolone metabolite, also predicted BACS composite scores ($r(s) =0.74$, $p=0.046$). In addition, baseline pregnenolone ($r(s) =-0.76$, $p=0.037$), pregnenolone sulfate ($r(s) =-0.83$, $p=0.015$), and allopregnanolone levels ($r(s) =-0.83$, $p=0.015$) were inversely correlated with improvements in MCCB composite scores, further supporting a possible role for neurosteroids in cognition. Mean BACS

223

and MCCB composite scores were correlated (r(s) =0.74, p<0.0001). Pregnenolone may be a promising therapeutic agent for negative symptoms and merits further investigation for cognitive symptoms in schizophrenia.

Mayo M et al. Pregnenolone Sulfate and Aging of Cognitive Functions: Behavioral, Neurochemical and Morphological Investigations. Hormones and Behavior 40, 215-217 (2001)
Neurosteroids are a subclass of steroids that can be synthesized in the central nervous system independently of peripheral sources. Several neurosteroids influence cognitive functions. Indeed, in senescent animals we have previously demonstrated a significant correlation between the cerebral concentration of pregnenolone sulfate (PREG-S) and cognitive performance. Indeed, rats with memory impairments exhibited low PREG-S concentrations compared to animals with correct memory performance. Furthermore, these memory deficits can be reversed by intracerebral infusions of PREG-S. Neurotransmitter systems modulated by this neurosteroid were unknown until our recent report of an enhancement of acetylcholine (ACh) release in basolateral amygdala, cortex, and hippocampus induced by central administrations of PREG-S. Central ACh neurotransmission is involved in the regulation of memory processes and is affected in normal aging and in human neurodegenerative pathologies like Alzheimer's disease. ACh neurotransmission is also involved in the modulation of sleep-wakefulness cycle and relationships between paradoxical sleep and memory are well documented in the literature. PREG-S infused at the level of ACh cell bodies induces a dramatic increase of paradoxical sleep in young animals. Cognitive dysfunctions, particularly those observed in Alzheimer's disease, have also been related to alterations of cerebral plasticity. Among these mechanisms, neurogenesis has been recently studied. Preliminary data suggest that PREG-S central infusions dramatically increase neurogenesis. Taken together these data suggest that PREG-S can influence cognitive processes, particularly in senescent subjects, through a modulation of ACh neurotransmission associated with paradoxical sleep modifications; furthermore our recent data suggest a role for neurosteroids in the modulation of hippocampal neurogenesis.

Mayo W, George O, Darbra S, et al. Individual differences in cognitive aging: implication of pregnenolone sulfate. Prog Neurobio. 2003 Sep; 71(1):43-8.
In humans and animals, individual differences in aging of cognitive functions are classically reported. Some old individuals exhibit performances similar to those of young subjects while others are severely impaired. In senescent animals, we have previously demonstrated a significant correlation between the cognitive performance and the cerebral concentration of a neurosteroid, the pregnenolone sulfate (PREG-S).Neurotransmitter systems modulated by this neurosteroid were unknown until our recent report of an enhancement of acetylcholine (ACh) release in basolateral amygdala, cortex and hippocampus induced by intracerebroventricular (i.c.v.) or intracerebral administrations of PREG-S. Central ACh neurotransmission is known to be involved in the

regulation of memory processes and is affected in normal aging and severely altered in human neurodegenerative pathologies like Alzheimer's disease.In the central nervous system, ACh neurotransmission is also involved in the modulation of sleep-wakefulness cycle, and particularly the paradoxical sleep (PS). Relationships between paradoxical sleep and memory are documented in the literature in old animals in which the spatial memory performance positively correlates with the basal amounts of paradoxical sleep. PREG-S infused at the level of ACh cell bodies (nucleus basalis magnocellularis, NBM, or pedunculopontine nucleus, PPT) increases paradoxical sleep in young animals.Finally, aging related cognitive dysfunctions, particularly those observed in Alzheimer's disease, have also been related to alterations of mechanisms underlying cerebral plasticity. Amongst these mechanisms, neurogenesis has been extensively studied recently. Our data demonstrate that PREG-S central infusions dramatically increase neurogenesis, this effect could be related to the negative modulator properties of this steroid at the GABA(A) receptor level.Taken together these data suggest that neurosteroids can influence cognitive processes, particularly in senescent subjects, through a modulation of ACh neurotransmission associated with paradoxical sleep modifications; furthermore, our recent data suggest a critical role for neurosteroids in the modulation of cerebral plasticity, mainly on hippocampal neurogenesis.

Myers GN et al . Further observations in the use of pregnenolone in rheumatoid arthritis. Ann Rheum Dis. 1951 Dec;10(4):432-40. No abstract available

Roberts E, Sherman MA. GABA—the quintessential neurotransmitter: electroneutrality, fidelity, specificity, and a model for the ligand binding site of GABAa receptors. Neurochem Res. 1993 Apr; 18(4):365-76. Alone of the known neurotransmitters, GABA is an electroneutral zwitterion (pI = 7.3) at physiological pH. This confers the highest probability of successfully traversing densely packed synaptic gaps without interacting electrostatically with charged entities enroute, making GABA a high fidelity neurotransmitter. Inhibitory tone in the nervous system is coordinately coupled with physiological activity by means of the GABA system, acidification increasing GABA formation and its Cl-channel-opening efficacy, while decreasing its removal by transport and metabolic degradation. The above, together with diminution upon acidification of the postsynaptic efficacy of glutamate on excitatory NMDA receptors constitutes a sensitively responsive mechanism by which protons control levels of neural activity, locally and globally. A model made of the GABA binding site of GABAA receptors based on H-bond and hydrophobic interactions makes it seem unlikely that any other substance known to occur in nerve tissue would give rise to a high noise level at GABAA receptors.

Schumacher M Neurosteroids in the Hippocampus: Neuronal Plasticity and Memory Stress 1997 Oct;2(1):65-78 The hippocampus, which is critically involved in learning and memory processes, is known to be a target for the neuromodulatory actions of steroid hormones produced by the adrenal glands and gonads. Much of the work of B.S. McEwen and collaborators has focused on the role of glucocorticosteroids and estrogen in modulating hippocampal plasticity and functions. In addition to hormones derived from the endocrine glands, cells in the hippocampus may be exposed to locally synthesized neurosteroids, including pregnenolone, dehydroepiandrosterone and their sulfated esters as well as progesterone and its reduced metabolites. In contrast to hormones derived from the circulation, neurosteroids have paracrine and/or autocrine activities. In the hippocampus, they have been shown to have trophic effects on neurons and glial cells and to modulate the activity of a variety of neurotransmitter receptors and ion channels, including type A gamma-aminobutyric acid, N-methyl-D-aspartate and sigma receptors and N- and L-type $Ca2+$ channels. There is accumulating evidence that some neurosteroids, in particular pregnenolone sulfate, have strong influences on learning and memory processes, most likely by regulating neurotransmission in the hippocampus. However, the hippocampus is not the only target for the amnesic effects of neurosteroids. Associated brain regions, the basal nuclei of the forebrain and the amygdaloid complex, are also involved. Some neurosteroids may thus be beneficial for treating age- or disease-related cognitive impairments.

Semeniuk, T et al. Neuroactive steroid levels in patients with generalized anxiety disorder.The Journal of Neuropsychiatry and Clinical Neurosciences 2001; 13:396-398 Serum levels of allopregnanolone, pregnenolone sulfate, and dehydroepiandrosterone sulfate were measured in 8 male patients with generalized anxiety disorder (GAD) and 8 healthy control subjects. Results suggest that patients with GAD have significantly lower levels of pregnenolone sulfate than control subjects.

Strous RD et al. Analysis of neurosteroid levels in attention deficit hyperactivity disorder. Int JNeuropsychopharmacol 2001 Sep; 4(3):259-64 Neurosteroids are important neuroactive substrates with demonstrated involvement in several neurophysiological and disease processes. Attention deficit hyperactivity disorder (ADHD) has been associated with dysregulation of the catecholaminergic and serotonergic systems; however its relationship to irregularities or changes in neurosteroid levels remains unknown. We examined the relationship between blood levels of dehydroepiandrosterone (DHEA), its principal precursor pregnenolone and its principal metabolite dehydroepiandrosterone sulphate (DHEAS) in 29 young male subjects aged 7-15 years with DSM-IV criteria of ADHD. Subjects were evaluated by a specially designed scale, following which patients were divided into two groups according to severity of symptomatology. Results indicated significant inverse correlations between clinical symptomatology and levels of

DHEA and pregnenolone in the total group. These inverse correlations were particularly evident in the less severe group of subjects. Levels of DHEA and DHEAS were inversely correlated with the hyperactivity subscale. Furthermore, using median blood levels as a cut-off indicator, higher blood levels of DHEA and DHEAS were associated with fewer ADHD symptoms, in particular hyperactivity symptomatology. Our findings suggest a possible protective effect of various neurosteroids on the expression of ADHD symptomatology.

Vallee M Neurosteroids: deficient cognitive performance in aged rats depends on low pregnenolone sulfate levels in the hippocampus Proc Natl Acad Sci U S A 1997 Dec 23;94(26):14865-70 Pregnenolone sulfate (PREG S) is synthesized in the nervous system and is a major neurosteroid in the rat brain. Its concentrations were measured in the hippocampus and other brain areas of single adult and aged (22-24 month-old) male Sprague-Dawley rats. Significantly lower levels were found in aged rats, although the values were widely scattered and reached, in about half the animals, the same range as those of young ones. The spatial memory performances of aged rats were investigated in two different spatial memory tasks, the Morris water maze and Y-maze. Performances in both tests were significantly correlated and, accompanied by appropriate controls, likely evaluated genuine memory function. Importantly, individual hippocampal PREG S and distance to reach the platform in the water maze were linked by a significant correlation, i.e., those rats with lower memory deficit had the highest PREG S levels, whereas no relationship was found with the PREG S content in other brain areas (amygdala, prefrontal cortex, parietal cortex, striatum). Moreover, the memory deficit of cognitively impaired aged rats was transiently corrected after either intraperitoneal or bilateral intrahippocampal injection of PREG S. PREG S is both a gamma-aminobutyric acid antagonist and a positive allosteric modulator at the N-methyl-D-aspartate receptor, and may reinforce neurotransmitter system(s) that decline with age. Indeed, intracerebroventricular injection of PREG S was shown to stimulate acetylcholine release in the adult rat hippocampus. In conclusion, it is proposed that the hippocampal content of PREG S plays a physiological role in preserving and/or enhancing cognitive abilities in old animals, possibly via an interaction with central cholinergic systems. Thus, neurosteroids should be further studied in the context of prevention and/or treatment of age-related memory disorders.

Vallée M, Mayo W, Le Moal M. Role of pregnenolone, dehydroepiandrosterone and their sulfate esters on learning and memory in cognitive aging. Brain Res Rev. 2001 Nov; 37(1-3):301-12. Aging is a general process of functional decline which involves in particular a decline of cognitive abilities. However, the severity of this decline differs from one subject to another and inter-individual differences have been reported in humans and animals. These differences are of great interest especially as concerns investigation of the neurobiological factors involved in cognitive aging. Intensive pharmacological studies suggest that neurosteroids, which are steroids synthesized in the brain in an independent manner from peripheral steroid sources, could be involved in learning and memory processes. This review summarizes data in animals and humans in favor of a role of neurosteroids in cognitive aging. Studies in animals demonstrated that the neurosteroids pregnenolone (PREG) and dehydroepiandrosterone (DHEA), as sulfate derivatives (PREGS and DHEAS, respectively), display memory-enhancing properties in aged rodents. Moreover, it was recently shown that memory performance was correlated with PREGS levels in the hippocampus of 24-month-old rats. Human studies, however, have reported contradictory results. First, improvement of learning and memory dysfunction was found after DHEA administration to individuals with low DHEAS levels, but other studies failed to detect significant cognitive effects after DHEA administration. Second, cognitive dysfunctions have been associated with low DHEAS levels, high DHEAS levels, or high DHEA levels; while in other studies, no relationship was found. As future research perspectives, we propose the use of new methods of quantification of neurosteroids as a useful tool for understanding their respective role in improving learning and memory impairments associated with normal aging and/or with pathological aging, such as Alzheimer's disease.

CHAPTER 8

Melatonin:

Melatonin is a hormone and powerful antioxidant synthesized principally in the pineal gland, a brain structure that Rene Descartes (1596-1650) called "the seat of the soul". Melatonin is evolutionarily conserved and almost every living species produces melatonin, from bacteria and fungi to plants and primates. It conveys information about day length and circadian rhythm to the organism and connects the organism to days, seasons and years.

Melatonin is synthesized from tryptophan, which is converted via 5-HTP into serotonin, which is bio transformed into melatonin. Melatonin is a natural sleep inducer, as it is the body's primary signal of nightfall: melatonin production is suppressed by light and stimulated by darkness, with levels peaking during the night and falling off toward the morning. Melatonin reduces body temperature and blood pressure, contributing to the induction of sleep. Even a brief exposure to light at night can inhibit melatonin production. Melatonin supplementation promotes deep sleep (both latency and duration) as well as growth hormone release during sleep.

Melatonin's anti-oxidant and anti-inflammatory actions are perhaps even more salient than its role in sleep. Melatonin triggers a powerful cascade of anti-oxidant activity, with its metabolites continuing to act as further anti-oxidants. Melatonin's anti-inflammatory effects include a reduction of many pro-inflammatory enzymes and cytokines. It is the most effective known scavenger of the hydroxyl radical, more so than Glutathione or Vitamin E, and endogenously protects the mitochondria and nuclear DNA from injury and oxidation—effects that become more pronounced at pharmacological concentrations. Melatonin is quickly distributed throughout all the body's tissues, protecting many lipids and proteins as well. Melatonin additionally stimulates other endogenous anti-oxidant enzymes, including superoxide dismutase and glutathione peroxidase, and increases the free radical scavenging and antioxidant efficacy of glutathione, vitamin E, and vitamin C. Melatonin protects against cellular and DNA damage from ionizing radiation and ischemia/reperfusion injury. Melatonin controls inflammatory cytokines and enhances immune function.

Melatonin exhibits potent and pleiotropic anti-inflammatory effects. It inhibits Cycloxigenase 2 (COX-2), & Nuclear Factor Kappa Beta, (NFκB) signaling and activation, reduces the expression of pro-inflammatory enzymes such as induced nitric oxide synthase, iNOS, and reduces the expression of inflammatory cytokines, including TNF-α, IL-1, IL-2, IL-6, interferon-γ, and GM-CSF. Melatonin up regulates IκBα, contributing to the inhibition of NFκB. These effects are heightened in response to inflammatory stressors.

Literature Review

Lifespan, health span and immune function are improved by melatonin supplementation in a wide range of animal studies. Stress and seasonally-induced immunosuppression is counteracted, (Nelson, 2000), and tumor growth is inhibited in humans (Edward et al 2005), while CD4, or 'natural killer' cells are increased (Kriegsfeld, 2001). Improved outcome in several human cancers, as well as amelioration of treatment side effects, is seen when melatonin is added to conventional therapy (Edward et al 2005). Melatonin's role in cancer risk is powerfully demonstrated in a study of 1,392 women by Flynn-Evans et al. (2009), in which total visual blindness (blocking the inhibitory effect of light perception on melatonin production and release) was associated with a 50% reduction in breast cancer prevalence, as compared to blindness with light perception intact (and all other variables being equal). Outcome appears to be improved by melatonin in Acute MI and the ongoing MARIA study is a prospective study of infarct size and clinical outcome (Dominquez-Rodriguez 2007). Melatonin reduces blood pressure and overall cholesterol (while stimulating HDL). Melatonin is neuroprotective in TBI (Samantaray 2009) and perhaps in Parkinson's and Alzheimer's Dementia (Rosales-Corral 2003), in addition to conferring resistance to aging-associated mitochondrial impairment in the brain and lungs (Carratero 2009). A variety of cognitive impairments are improved by melatonin supplementation, as well as some mood disorders, including depression, anxiety, and sleep disorders. Lowered melatonin levels, likewise, often accompany these issues.

Melatonin also has positive effects on aspects of obesity and metabolic syndrome, including a reduction of body weight, visceral adiposity, triglyceride levels, circulating glucose, insulin, and leptin, and the amelioration of insulin resistance (Walden-Hanson 2000). In addition to melatonin's defense against oxidative stress from diabetes, melatonin also directly affects physiological components underlying metabolic syndromes (Veneroso 2009).

Melatonin has been found to produce potent dose-dependent analgesic effects (Pang et al 2001, Ebad et al

1998), improving symptoms of fibromyalgia, irritable bowel syndrome, and migraine (Peres et al 2006).

As we age, mean melatonin levels decrease, as does peak melatonin amplitude at night. Melatonin levels decline by about 10-15% per decade after 20 years old. Decreases in melatonin levels are also associated with a number of conditions, including cardiovascular disease, Alzheimer's disease, breast cancer, obesity, type II diabetes, severe coronary artery disease, and depression. (Dominguez-Rodriquez 2009, Reiter et al 2003 and 2005, Simko 2009) Conversely, melatonin supplementation counteracts many aspects of these conditions. No melatonin toxicity has been seen even in doses of up to 300mg per day.

Management:

When using melatonin for sleep it is important to see what kind of sleep issue is occurring. If getting to sleep is an issue then we start with 2.5-3 mg of sublingual melatonin before bedtime. If staying asleep is important then we use timed release preparations that usually start at 3 mg and increase if needed. If you want to just take melatonin for the benefits it can generate and you have no sleep issues then you can use regular preparations of melatonin at 0.5-1mg of melatonin orally one hour before bedtime and increase the dose to 2-3 mg in about two to three weeks. Though no melatonin toxicity has been observed even in doses up to 300mg/day, some patients may feel a bit drowsy for one or two days after starting melatonin (this usually resolves) or have vivid dreams that can be perceived as interesting or frightening and unpleasant. If reactions are negative, melatonin should be discontinued. Rarely melatonin will produce alertness instead of sleep and then should not be used at night. Doses of melatonin vary for each patient. Doses may range from 500 mcg to 20 mg per night. Melatonin is helpful for preventing or treating jet lag. Use one 3 mg timed-release capsule on the airplane at the bedtime hour of the destination. Allow bring light to hit the face in the morning of arrival. Take 3 mg timed-release melatonin at bedtime for the next few nights.

While most could benefit from melatonin's sleep-promoting effects, there also exist individuals, particularly those of advanced age, with pathologically low melatonin levels, whose overall health and quality of life could be significantly improved by melatonin supplementation. Though melatonin supplementation regardless of endogenous levels appears to ameliorate many age-related issues, a melatonin serum level could be used to make a specific diagnosis of low melatonin. However, due to melatonin's pleiotropic benefits, coupled with its extremely low toxicity, lack of a formal diagnosis should not preclude therapeutic melatonin supplementation.

Health issues that may be improved by melatonin supplementation:
- Depression, anxiety, SAD
- Sleep disturbances
- Alzheimer's disease and dementia
- Type II diabetes
- Obesity
- Cancer and radio chemotherapy side-effects
- Hypertension
- Myocardial infarction
- Coronary heart disease
- Stroke
- Osteoporosis
- Migraine and headache disorders

MELATONIN ABSTRACTS

Brzezinski A. Mechanisms of Disease: Melatonin in Humans The New England Journal of Medicine -- January 16, 1997 -- Vol. 336, No. 3 – No abstract

Bubenik GA Prospects of the clinical utilization of melatonin. Biol Signals Recept 1998 Jul-Aug; 7(4):195-219 This review summarizes the present knowledge on melatonin in several areas on physiology and discusses various prospects of its clinical utilization. Ever increasing evidence indicates that melatonin has an immuno-hematopoietic role. In animal studies, melatonin provided protection against gram-negative septic shock, prevented stress-induced immunodepression, and restored immune function after a hemorrhagic shock. In human studies, melatonin amplified the antitumoral activity of interleukin-2. Melatonin has been proven as a powerful cytostatic drug in vitro as well as in vivo. In the human clinical field, melatonin appears to be a promising agent either as a diagnostic or prognostic marker of neoplastic diseases or as a compound used either alone or in combination with the standard cancer treatment. Utilization of melatonin for treatment of rhythm disorders, such as those manifested in jet lag, shift work or blindness, is one of the oldest and the most successful clinical application of this chemical. Low doses of melatonin applied in controlled-release preparation were very effective in improving the sleep latency, increasing the sleep efficiency and rising sleep quality scores in elderly, melatonin-deficient insomniacs. In the cardiovascular system, melatonin seems to regulate the tone of cerebral arteries; melatonin receptors in vascular beds appear to participate in the regulation of body temperature. Heat loss may be the principal mechanism in the initiation of sleepiness caused by melatonin. The role of melatonin in the development of migraine headaches is at present uncertain but more research could result in new ways of treatment. Melatonin is the major messenger of light-dependent periodicity, implicated in the seasonal reproduction of animals and pubertal development in humans. Multiple receptor sites detected in brain and gonadal tissues of birds and mammals of both sexes indicate that melatonin exerts a direct effect on the vertebrate reproductive organs. In a clinical study, melatonin has been used successfully as an effective female contraceptive with little side effects. Melatonin is one of the most powerful scavengers of free radicals. Because it easily penetrates the blood-brain barrier, this antioxidant may, in the future, be used for the treatment of Alzheimer's and Parkinson's diseases, stroke, nitric oxide, neurotoxicity and hyperbaric oxygen exposure. In the digestive tract, melatonin reduced the incidence and severity of gastric ulcers and prevented severe symptoms of colitis, such as mucosal lesions and diarrhea.

Carretero, M et al. Long-term melatonin administration protects brain mitochondria from aging. Journal of Pineal Research. 47(2):192-200, September 2009. We tested whether chronic melatonin administration in the drinking water would reduce the brain mitochondrial impairment that accompanies aging. Brain mitochondria from male and female senescent prone (SAMP8) mice at 5 and 10 months of age were studied. Mitochondrial oxidative stress was determined by measuring the levels of lipid peroxidation and nitrite, glutathione/glutathione disulfide ratio, and glutathione peroxidase and glutathione reductase activities. Electron transport chain activity and oxidative phosphorylation capability of mitochondria were also determined by measuring the activity of the respiratory chain complexes and the ATP content. The results support a significant age-dependent mitochondrial dysfunction with a diminished efficiency of the electron transport chain and reduced ATP production, accompanied by an increased oxidative/nitrosative stress. Melatonin administration between 1 and 10 months of age completely prevented the mitochondrial impairment, maintaining or even increasing ATP production. There were no major age-dependent differences between males in females, although female mice seemed to be somewhat more sensitive to melatonin treatment than males. Thus, melatonin administration as a single therapy maintained fully functioning brain mitochondria during aging, a finding with important consequences in the pathophysiology of brain aging.

Castagnino HE, Lago N, Centrella JM, Calligaris SD, Farina S, Sarchi MI, Cardinali DP. Cytoprotection by melatonin and growth hormone in early rat myocardial infarction as revealed by Feulgen DNA staining. Neuroendocrinol Lett 2002 Oct-Dec;23(5/6):391-395 OBJECTIVE: To examine the cytoprotective effect of melatonin or recombinant human growth hormone (hGH) on the early phase of a running myocardial infarction in rats by using the Feulgen staining. METHODS: Rats were subjected to surgical ligature of the left coronary artery or its sham-operation and were studied 1.5 3 h later. Melatonin was administered in the drinking water (100 microg/ml water) for 7 days before surgery. Recombinant hGH (2 IU/kg) was given ip at the time of surgery. Feulgen-stained histological cardiac sections were examined by light microscopy and image analysis. RESULTS: Infarcted rats receiving vehicle exhibited large, diffuse cardiac lesions with a marked positivity for Feulgen reaction. About 18 20% of the total area recorded became injured 1.5 or 3 h after infarction, respectively. Infarcted rats treated with melatonin or hGH, or the combination of both, and killed 3 h after surgery, showed cardiac sections with scattered lesions and only a few isolated injured muscle fibers. A similar effectiveness of melatonin and hGH, alone or in combination, to decrease injured area by 86 87% and the number of cardiac lesions by 75 80% was observed. CONCLUSION: A significant cytoprotective effect of melatonin or hGH is demonstrable in an early phase of myocardial infarction in rats.

Cervantes, M et al. Melatonin and ischemia-reperfusion injury of the brain. J Pineal Res. 2008 Aug; 45(1):1-7. This review summarizes the reports that have documented the neuroprotective effects of melatonin against ischemia/reperfusion brain injury. The studies were carried out on several species, using models of acute focal or global cerebral ischemia under different treatment schedules. The neuroprotective actions of melatonin were observed during critical evolving periods for cell processes of immediate or delayed neuronal death and brain injury, early after the ischemia/reperfusion episode. Late neural phenomena accounting either for brain damage or neuronal repair, plasticity and functional recovery taking place after ischemia/reperfusion have been rarely examined for the protective actions of melatonin. Special attention has been paid to the advantageous characteristics of melatonin as a neuroprotective drug: bioavailability into brain cells and cellular organelles targeted by morpho-functional derangement; effectiveness in exerting several neuroprotective actions, which can be amplified and prolonged by its metabolites, through direct and indirect antioxidant activity; prevention and reversal of mitochondrial malfunction, reducing inflammation, derangement of cytoskeleton organization, and pro-apoptotic cell signaling; lack of interference with thrombolytic and neuroprotective actions of other drugs; and an adequate safety profile. Thus, the immediate results of melatonin actions in reducing infarct volume, necrotic and apoptotic neuronal death, neurologic deficits, and in increasing the number of surviving neurons, may improve brain tissue preservation. The potential use of melatonin as a neuroprotective drug in clinical trials aimed to improve the outcome of patients suffering acute focal or global cerebral ischemia should be seriously considered.

Dominguez-Rodriguez A et al. Prognostic value of nocturnal melatonin levels as a novel marker in patients with ST-segment elevation myocardial infarction. Am J Cardiol. 2006 Apr 15; 97(8):1162-4. We evaluated the possible relation between circulating levels of nocturnal melatonin, C-reactive protein, and the development of adverse cardiovascular events in patients with ST-segment elevation myocardial infarction. Patients who had developed adverse events during follow-up had significantly lower nocturnal melatonin levels than patients without events.

Dominguez-Rodriguez et al. A unicenter, randomized, double-blind, parallel-group, placebo-controlled study of Melatonin as an Adjunct in patients with acute myocaRdial Infarction undergoing primary Angioplasty The Melatonin Adjunct in the acute myocaRdial Infarction treated with Angioplasty (MARIA) trial: study design and rationale.Contemp Clin Trials 2007 Jul;28(4):532-9. BACKGROUND: Experimental studies have documented the beneficial effects of the endogenously produced antioxidant, melatonin, in reducing tissue damage and limiting cardiac pathophysiology in models of experimental ischemia-reperfusion. Melatonin confers cardioprotection against ischemia-reperfusion injury most likely through its direct free radical scavenging activities and its indirect actions in stimulating antioxidant enzymes. These actions of melatonin permit it to reduce molecular damage and limit infarct size in experimental models of transient ischemia and subsequent reperfusion.STUDY DESIGN: The

Melatonin Adjunct in the acute myocaRdial Infarction treated with Angioplasty (MARIA) trial is an unicenter, prospective, randomized double-blind, placebo-controlled, phase 2 study of the intravenous administration of melatonin. The primary efficacy end point of this study is to determine whether melatonin treatment reduces infarct size determined by the cumulative release of alpha-hydroxybutyrate dehydrogenase (area under the curve: 0 to 72 h). Other secondary end points will be the clinical events occurring within the first 90 days: death, sustained ventricular arrhythmias, resuscitation from cardiac arrest, cardiogenic shock, heart failure, major bleedings, stroke, need for revascularization, recurrent ischemia, re-infarctions and rehospitalization.IMPLICATIONS: The MARIA trial tests a novel pharmacologic agent, melatonin, in patients with acute myocardial infarction and the hypothesis that it will confer cardioprotection against ischemia-reperfusion injury. If successful, the finding would support the use of melatonin in therapy of ischemic-reperfusion injury of the heart.

Dominguez-Rodriguez A et al. Clinical aspects of melatonin in the acute coronary syndrome. Curr Vasc Pharmacol. 2009 Jul; 7(3):367-73. This review considers the actions of an endogenously produced molecule, melatonin, on heart diseases. Recent research has shown that inflammation plays a key role in coronary heart disease (CHD) and other manifestations of atherosclerosis. Immune cells dominate early atherosclerotic lesions, their effector molecules accelerate progression of the lesions and activation of inflammation can elicit acute coronary syndromes (ACS). Scientific evidence from the last 15 years has suggested that melatonin has positive effects on the cardiovascular system. The presence of vascular melatoninergic receptor binding sites has been demonstrated; these receptors are functionally linked to vasoconstrictor or vasodilatory effects of melatonin. It has been shown that patients with CHD have a low melatonin production rate, especially those with higher risk of cardiac infarction and /or sudden death. Similarly to other organs and systems, the cardiovascular system exhibits diurnal and seasonal rhythms, including those in the heart rate, cardiac output and blood pressure. The suprachiasmatic nuclei of hypothalamus and, possibly, the melatoninergic system modulate the cardiovascular rhythms. The melatonin attenuates molecular and cellular damages resulting from cardiac ischemia/reperfusion in which destructive free radicals are involved. Anti-inflammatory and antioxidative properties of melatonin are also involved in the protection against vascular disease, i.e. atherosclerosis. The current brief summary of the literature provides an overview on the role of melatonin in the ACS.

Ebadi M et al. Pineal opioid receptors and analgesic action of melatonin. J Pineal Res. 1998 May; 24(4):193-200. Physicians have noted since antiquity that their patients complained of less pain and required fewer analgesics at night times. In most species, including the humans, the circulating levels of melatonin, a substance with analgesic and hypnotic properties, exhibit a pronounced circadian rhythm with serum levels being high at night and very low during day times. Moreover, melatonin exhibits maximal analgesic effects at night, pinealectomy abolishes the analgesic effects of melatonin, and mu opioid receptor antagonists disrupt the day-night rhythm of nociception. It is believed that melatonin, with its sedative and analgesic effects, is capable of providing a pain free sleep so that the body may recuperate and restore itself to function again at its peak capacity. Moreover, in conditions when pain is associated with extensive tissue injury, melatonin's ability to scavenge free radicals and abort oxidative stress is yet another beneficial effect to be realized. Since melatonin may behave as a mixed opioid receptor agonist-antagonist, it is doubtful that a physician simply could potentiate the analgesic efficacy of narcotics such as morphine by coadministering melatonin. Therefore, future research may synthesize highly efficacious melatonin analogues capable of providing maximum analgesia and hopefully being devoid of addiction liability now associated with currently available narcotics.

Flynn-Evans EEet al. Total visual blindness is protective against breast cancer. Cancer Causes Control. 2009 Aug 1. OBJECTIVE: Observational data, though sparse and based on small studies with limited ability to control for known breast cancer risk factors, support a lower risk of breast cancer in blind women compared to sighted women. Mechanisms influenced by ocular light perception, such as melatonin or circadian synchronization, are thought to account for this lower risk.METHODS: To evaluate whether blind women with no perception of light (NPL) have a lower prevalence of breast cancer compared to blind women with light perception (LP), we surveyed a cohort of 1,392 blind women living in North America (66 breast cancer cases).RESULTS: In multivariate-logistic regression models controlling for breast cancer risk factors, women with NPL had a significantly lower prevalence of breast cancer than women with LP (odds ratio, 0.43; 95% confidence interval, 0.21-0.85). We observed little difference in these associations when restricting to postmenopausal women, non-shift workers or when excluding women diagnosed with breast cancer within 2 or 4 years of onset of blindness. Blind women with NPL appear to have a lower risk of breast cancer, compared to blind women with LP. More research is needed to elucidate the impact of LP on circadian coordination and melatonin production in the blind and how these factors may relate to breast cancer risk.

Golombek DA et al. Chronopharmacology of melatonin: inhibition by benzodiazepine antagonism Chronobiol Int. 1992 Apr; 9(2):124-31. We endeavored to determine whether three behavioral effects of melatonin in rodents, i.e., depression of locomotor activity in hamsters, analgesia in mice, and impairment of 3-mercaptopropionic acid (3-MP) convulsions, exhibited the time dependency known to occur for several neuroendocrine effects of the hormone. Activity was monitored and registered by means of an optical actometer, and analgesia was assessed by the hot-plate procedure. Locomotor activity, analgesia, and seizure susceptibility were maximal at the beginning of the scotophase and minimal at noon. The effects of melatonin on the three parameters peaked at early night. The administration of the benzodiazepine antagonist flumazenil, although unable by itself to modify locomotor activity, pain, or seizure threshold, blunted the activity of melatonin. These results suggest that the time-dependent effects of melatonin on specific rodent behaviors may be mediated by central synapses employing gamma-aminobutyric acid (GABA) as an inhibitory transmitter.

Herrera J Melatonin prevents oxidative stress resulting from iron and erythropoietin administration Am J Kidney Dis 2001 Apr; 37(4):750-7 Intravenous iron (Fe) and recombinant human erythropoietin (rHuEPO) are routine treatments in the management of anemia in patients with chronic renal failure. We investigated the oxidative stress acutely induced by these therapies and whether pretreatment with oral melatonin (MEL) would have a beneficial effect. Nine patients (four women) were studied within 1 month of entering a chronic hemodialysis program in the interdialytic period. Plasma malondialdehyde (MDA), red blood cell glutathione (GSH), and catalase (CAT) activity were measured in blood samples obtained before (baseline) and 1, 3, and 24 hours after the administration of Fe (100 mg of Fe saccharate intravenously over 1 hour) or rHuEPO (4,000 U intravenously). One hour before these treatments, patients were administered a single oral dose of MEL (0.3 mg/kg) or placebo. Each patient was studied on four occasions, corresponding to studies performed using either placebo or MEL in association with intravenous Fe and rHuEPO administration. Baseline data showed increased oxidative stress in patients with end-stage renal failure. Increments in oxidative stress induced by Fe were more pronounced at the end of the administration: MDA, baseline, 0.74 +/- 0.09 nmol/mL; 1 hour, 1.50 +/- 0.28 nmol/mL (P: < 0.001); GSH, baseline, 2.51 +/- 0.34 nmol/mg of hemoglobin (Hb); 1 hour, 1.66 +/- 0.01 nmol/mg Hb (P: < 0.001); and CAT activity, baseline, 27.0 +/- 5.7 kappa/mg Hb; 1 hour, 23.3 +/- 4.2 kappa/mg Hb (P: < 0.001). rHuEPO-induced increments in oxidative stress were more pronounced (P: < 0.001) at 3 hours (MDA, 1.24 +/- 0.34 nmol/mL; GSH, 1.52 +/- 0.23 nmol/mg Hb; CAT activity, 18.0 +/- 3.1 kappa/mg Hb). MEL administration prevented the changes induced by Fe and rHuEPO and had no adverse side effects. These studies show that intravenous Fe and rHuEPO in doses commonly used to treat anemia in chronic hemodialysis patients acutely generate significant oxidative stress. Oral MEL prevents such oxidative stress and may be of clinical use.

Kriegsfeld LJ In vitro melatonin treatment enhances cell-mediated immune function in male prairie voles J Pineal Res 2001 May;30(4):193-8 The present study was designed (1) to determine the extent to which male prairie voles (Microtus ochrogaster) alter immune status in response to short-day lengths, (2) to evaluate the role of melatonin in coordinating these alterations in immune function, and (3) to assess the association between alterations in immune function and reproductive responsiveness to photoperiod. Male voles were housed in either long- or short-day lengths for 10 wk; voles in short days were subdivided into reproductive "responders" (R) or "non-responders" (NR) based on testicular mass at autopsy. After 10 wk of exposure to photoperiodic conditions, cell-mediated immune function was evaluated using an in vitro splenocyte proliferation assay. The direct effects of melatonin on immune cells were evaluated by adding melatonin to one-half of the cultures in each experimental condition. Melatonin treatment led to enhanced splenocyte proliferation for all experimental groups. Neither photoperiodic condition nor reproductive status was associated with alterations in immune function or the degree of immuno-enhancing effects of melatonin. Taken together, the results of the present study suggest that melatonin is capable of enhancing immune function in male voles potentially by acting directly on immune cells.

Lenoir V et al. Preventive and curative effect of melatonin on mammary carcinogenesis induced by dimethylbenz[a]anthracene in the female Sprague-Dawley rat. Breast Cancer Res. 2005; 7(4):R470-6. INTRODUCTION: It has been well documented that the pineal hormone, melatonin, which plays a major role in the control of reproduction in mammals, also plays a role in the incidence and growth of breast and mammary cancer. The curative effect of melatonin on the growth of dimethylbenz [a]anthracene-induced (DMBA-induced) mammary adenocarcinoma (ADK) has been previously well documented in the female Sprague-Dawley rat. However, the preventive effect of melatonin in limiting the frequency of cancer initiation has not been well documented.METHODS: The aim of this study was to compare the potency of melatonin to limit the frequency of mammary cancer initiation with its potency to inhibit tumor progression once initiation, at 55 days of age, was achieved. The present study compared the effect of preventive treatment with melatonin (10 mg/kg daily) administered for only 15 days before the administration of DMBA with the effect of long-term (6-month) curative treatment with the same dose of melatonin starting the day after DMBA administration. The rats were followed up for a year after the administration of the DMBA.RESULTS: The results clearly showed almost identical preventive and curative effects of melatonin on the growth of DMBA-induced mammary ADK. Many hypotheses have been proposed to explain the inhibitory effects of melatonin. However, the mechanisms responsible for its strong preventive effect are still a matter of debate. At least, it can be envisaged that the artificial amplification of the intensity of the circadian rhythm of melatonin could markedly reduce the DNA damage provoked by DMBA and therefore the frequency of cancer initiation.CONCLUSION: In view of the present results, obtained in the female Sprague-Dawley rat, it can be envisaged that the long-term inhibition of mammary ADK promotion by a brief, preventive treatment with melatonin could also reduce the risk of breast cancer induced in women by unidentified environmental factors.

Li JH et al. Melatonin reduces inflammatory injury through inhibiting NF-kappaB activation in rats with colitis.Mediators Inflamm. 2005 Aug 31; 2005(4): Proinflammatory mediators are important in the pathogenesis of IBD, which are regulated by activation of NF-kappaB. The aim of this study was to investigate whether melatonin reduces inflammatory injury and inhibits proinflammatory molecule and NF-kappaB in rats with colitis. Rat colitis model was established by TNBS enema. NF-kappaB p65, TNF-alpha, ICAM-1, and IkappaBalpha in colon tissue were examined by immunohistochemistry, EMSA, RT-PCR, and Western blot analysis. Expression of proinflammatory molecule and activation of NF-kappaB were upregulated and IkappaB level decreased in rats with colitis. Melatonin reduces colonic inflammatory injury through downregulating proinflammatory molecule mediated by NF-kappaB inhibition and blockade of IkappaBalpha degradation.

Mills Edward et al. Melatonin in the treatment of cancer: a systematic review of randomized controlled trials and meta-analysis Journal of Pineal Research. 39(4):360-366, November 2005. Most observational studies show an association between melatonin and cancer in humans. We conducted a systematic review of randomized controlled trials (RCTs) of melatonin in solid tumor cancer patients and its effect on survival at 1 yr. With the aid of an information specialist, we searched 10 electronic databases from inception to October 2004. We included trials using melatonin as either sole treatment or as adjunct treatment. Prespecified criteria guided our assessment of trial quality. We conducted a meta-analysis using a random effects model. We included 10 RCTs published between 1992 and 2003 and included 643 patients. All trials included solid tumor cancers. All trials were conducted at the same hospital network, and were unblinded. Melatonin reduced the risk of death at 1 yr (relative risk: 0.66, 95% confidence interval: 0.59-0.73, I2=0%, heterogeneity P<or=0.56). Effects were consistent across melatonin dose, and type of cancer. No severe adverse events were reported. The substantial reduction in risk of death, low adverse events reported and low costs related to this intervention suggest great potential for melatonin in treating cancer. Confirming the efficacy and safety of melatonin in cancer treatment will require completion of blinded, independently conducted RCTs.

Nelson RJ Melatonin mediates seasonal changes in immune function Ann N Y Acad Sci 2000; 917:404-15. Field studies indicate that immune function is compromised and the prevalence of many diseases are elevated during winter when energetic stressors are extensive. Presumably, individuals would enjoy a survival advantage if seasonally recurring stressors could be anticipated and countered by shunting energy reserves to bolster immune function. The primary environmental cue that permits physiological anticipation of season is daily photoperiod, a cue that is mediated by melatonin. However, other environmental factors, including low food availability and ambient temperatures, may interact with photoperiod to affect immune function and disease processes. This paper will review laboratory studies that consistently report enhanced immune function in short day lengths. Prolonged melatonin treatment mimics short days, and both in vitro and in vivo melatonin treatment enhances various aspects of immune function, especially cell-mediated immune function, in nontropical rodents. Reproductive responsiveness to melatonin appears to affect immune function. In sum, melatonin may be part of an integrative system to coordinate reproductive, immunologic, and other physiological processes to cope successfully with energetic stressors during winter.

Pang CS et al. Effects of melatonin, morphine and diazepam on formalin-induced nociception in mice. Life Sci. 2001 Jan 12; 68(8):943-51. The possible analgesic effect of melatonin was investigated in young male ICR mice. The formalin test which elicits typically 2 phases of pain response, the acute (first) phase and tonic (second) phase, was used. The test was performed in the late light period when the mice have been reported to be more sensitive to pain. Compared to control mice, no significant difference in nociceptive response was observed when melatonin was injected intraperitoneally at doses of 0.1, 5, and 20, mg/kg body weight. The combined effects of melatonin with diazepam and/or morphine were also investigated. Melatonin, injected at 20 mg/kg 15 min before formalin test, significantly increased the antinociceptive response of diazepam (1 mg/kg) or morphine (5 mg/kg) in the second phase. In addition, when melatonin was given at 20 mg/kg together with diazepam and morphine, antinociceptive responses in both the first and second phase were increased. These data indicate the synergistic analgesia effect of melatonin with morphine and diazepam and suggest the possible involvement of melatonin as an adjunct medicine for pain patients.

Peres MF et al. Potential therapeutic use of melatonin in migraine and other headache disorders. Expert Opin Investig Drugs. 2006 Apr; 15(4):367-75. There is increasing evidence that headache disorders are connected with melatonin secretion and pineal function. Some headaches have a clearcut seasonal and circadian pattern, such as cluster and hypnic headaches. Melatonin levels have been found to be decreased in both migraine and cluster headaches. Melatonin mechanisms are related to headache pathophysiology in many ways, including its anti-inflammatory effect, toxic free radical scavenging, reduction of pro-inflammatory cytokine upregulation, nitric oxide synthase activity and dopamine release inhibition, membrane stabilisation, GABA and opioid analgesia potentitation, glutamate neurotoxicity protection, neurovascular regulation, 5-HT modulation and the similarity in chemical structure to indometacin. The treatment of headache disorders with melatonin and other chronobiotic agents, such as melatonin agonists (ramelteon and agomelatin), is promising and there is a great potential for their use in headache treatment.

Pierpaoli W, Regelson W. Pineal control of aging: effect of melatonin and pineal grafting on aging mice. Proc Natl Acad Sci U S A 1994; 91:787-91. Dark-cycle, night administration of the pineal hormone melatonin in drinking water to aging mice (15 months of age) prolongs survival of BALB/c females from 23.8 to 28.1 months and preserves aspects of their youthful state. Similar results were seen in New Zealand Black females beginning at 5 months and C57BL/6 males beginning at 19 months. As melatonin is produced in circadian fashion from the pineal, we grafted pineals from young 3- to 4-month-old donors into the thymus of 20-month-old syngeneic C57BL/6 male recipients, and a 12% increase in survival was induced. Prolongation of survival was also seen on pineal transplant to the thymus in C57BL/6, BALB/cJ, and hybrid female mice at 16, 19, and 22 months. In all studies, the endogenous pineal of grafted mice was left in situ. Pineal grafted aged mice display a remarkable maintenance of thymic structure and cellularity. Preservation of T-cell-mediated function, despite age, as measured by response to oxazolone is seen. Other evidence suggests that melatonin and/or pineal-related factors could produce their effects through an influence on thyroid function. These data indicate that pineal influences have a place in the physiologic regulation of aging.

Reiter RJ et al. Melatonin: a novel protective agent against oxidative injury of the ischemic/reperfused heart. Cardiovasc Res. 2003 Apr 1; 58(1):10-9. This brief review summarizes the recently obtained evidence which illustrates the beneficial effects of the endogenously produced antioxidant, melatonin, in reducing tissue damage and reversing cardiac pathophysiology in models of experimental ischemia/reperfusion. The report also describes the actions of other antioxidants, especially vitamin E and antioxidative enzymes, in altering the degree of ischemia/reperfusion damage in the heart. Based on the data available, melatonin seems to have advantages over other antioxidants tested in terms of ameliorating the hypoxia and reoxygenation-induced damage. While the bulk of the studies that have used melatonin to overcome cardiac injury following transient arterial occlusion and subsequent reperfusion have used pharmacological doses to achieve protection, two recent reports have further shown that merely reducing endogenous circulating concentrations of melatonin (by surgical removal of a source of melatonin, i.e. the pineal gland) exaggerates the degree of injury and reduces survival of animals as a result of induced ischemia/reperfusion of the heart. These findings are consistent with observations in other organs where the loss of physiological concentrations of melatonin results in increased oxidative damage during hypoxia and reoxygenation. These findings have implications for the elderly since in the aged endogenous levels of melatonin are naturally reduced thereby possibly predisposing them to more severe cardiac damage during a heart attack. To date, the bulk of the studies relating to the protective actions of melatonin in reducing cardiac ischemia/reperfusion injury have used the rat as the experimental model. Considering the high efficacy of melatonin in limiting ischemia/reperfusion damage as well as melatonin's low toxicity, the studies should be expanded to include other species and models of cardiac ischemia/reperfusion. The results of these investigations would help to clarify the potential importance of the use of melatonin in situations of oxidative damage to the heart in humans.

Reiter RJ et al. When melatonin gets on your nerves: its beneficial actions in experimental models of stroke. Exp Biol Med (Maywood). 2005 Feb; 230(2):104-17. This article summarizes the evidence that endogenously produced and exogenously administered melatonin reduces the degree of tissue damage and limits the biobehavioral deficits associated with experimental models of ischemia/reperfusion injury in the brain (i.e., stroke). Melatonin's efficacy in curtailing neural damage under conditions of transitory interruption of the blood supply to the brain has been documented in models of both focal and global ischemia. In these studies many indices have been shown to be improved as a consequence of melatonin treatment. For example, when given at the time of ischemia or reperfusion onset, melatonin reduces neurophysiological deficits, infarct volume, and the degree of neural edema, lipid peroxidation, protein carbonyls, DNA damage, neuron and glial loss, and death of the animals. Melatonin's protective actions against these adverse changes are believed to stem from its direct free radical scavenging and indirect antioxidant activities, possibly from its ability to limit free radical generation at the mitochondrial level and because of yet-undefined functions. Considering its high efficacy in overcoming much of the damage associated with ischemia/reperfusion injury, not only in the brain but in other organs as well, its use in clinical trials for the purpose of improving stroke outcome should be seriously considered.

Reiter RJ et al. Alterations in Lipid Levels of Mitochondrial Membranes Induced by Amyloid-β: A Protective Role of Melatonin. Int J Alzheimers Dis. 2012; 2012: 459806.
Alzheimer pathogenesis involves mitochondrial dysfunction, which is closely related to amyloid-β (Aβ) generation, abnormal tau phosphorylation, oxidative stress, and apoptosis. Alterations in membranal components, including cholesterol and fatty acids, their characteristics, disposition, and distribution along the membranes, have been studied as evidence of cell membrane alterations in AD brain. The majority of these studies have been focused on the cytoplasmic membrane; meanwhile the mitochondrial membranes have been less explored. In this work, we studied lipids and mitochondrial membranes in vivo, following intracerebral injection of fibrillar amyloid-β (Aβ). The purpose was to determine how Aβ may be responsible for beginning of a vicious cycle where oxidative stress and alterations in cholesterol, lipids and fatty acids, feed back on each other to cause mitochondrial dysfunction. We observed changes in mitochondrial membrane lipids, and fatty acids, following intracerebral injection of fibrillar Aβ in aged Wistar rats. Melatonin, a well-known antioxidant and neuroimmunomodulator indoleamine, reversed some of these alterations and protected mitochondrial membranes from obvious damage. Additionally, melatonin increased the levels of linolenic and n-3 eicosapentaenoic acid, in the same site where amyloid β was injected, favoring an endogenous anti-inflammatory pathway.

Rosales-Corral S et al. Orally administered melatonin reduces oxidative stress and proinflammatory cytokines induced by amyloid-

beta peptide in rat brain: a comparative, in vivo study versus vitamin C and E.J Pineal Res. 2003 Sep;35(2):80-4 To determine the efficacy of antioxidants in reducing amyloid-beta-induced oxidative stress, and the neuroinflammatory response in the central nervous system (CNS) in vivo, three injections of fibrillar amyloid-beta (fAbeta) or artificial cerebrospinal fluid (aCSF) into the CA1 region of the hippocampus of the rat were made. Concomitantly, one of the three free radical scavengers, i.e. melatonin, vitamin C, or vitamin E was also administered. Besides being a free radical scavenger, melatonin also has immunomodulatory functions. Antioxidant treatment reduced significantly oxidative stress and pro-inflammatory cytokines. There were no marked differences between melatonin, vitamin C, and vitamin E regarding their capacity to reduce nitrites and lipoperoxides. However, melatonin exhibited a superior capacity to reduce the pro-inflammatory response induced by fAbeta.

Samantaray, S et al. Therapeutic potential of melatonin in traumatic central nervous system injury.Mini Reviews Journal of Pineal Research. 47(2):134-142, September 2009. A vast literature extolling the benefits of melatonin has accumulated during the past four decades. Melatonin was previously considered of importance to seasonal reproduction and circadian rhythmicity. Currently, it appears to be a versatile anti-oxidative and anti-nitrosative agent, a molecule with immunomodulatory actions and profound oncostatic activity, and also to play a role as a potent neuroprotectant. Nowadays, melatonin is sold as a dietary supplement with differential availability as an over-the-counter aid in different countries. There is a widespread agreement that melatonin is nontoxic and safe considering its frequent, long-term usage by humans at both physiological and pharmacological doses with no reported side effects. Endeavors toward a designated drug status for melatonin may be enormously rewarding in clinics for treatment of several forms of neurotrauma where effective pharmacological intervention has not yet been attained. This mini review consolidates the data regarding the efficacy of melatonin as an unique neuroprotective agent in traumatic central nervous system (CNS) injuries. Well-documented actions of melatonin in combating traumatic CNS damage are compiled from various clinical and experimental studies. Research on traumatic brain injury and ischemia/reperfusion are briefly outlined here as they have been recently reviewed elsewhere, whereas the studies on different animal models of the experimental spinal cord injury have been extensively covered in this mini review for the first time.

Simko, F et al. Potential roles of melatonin and chronotherapy among the new trends in hypertension treatment. Journal of Pineal Research. 47(2):127-133, September 2009. The number of well-controlled hypertensives is unacceptably low worldwide. Respecting the circadian variation of blood pressure, nontraditional antihypertensives, and treatment in early stages of hypertension are potential ways to improve hypertension therapy. First, prominent variations in circadian rhythm are characteristic for blood pressure. The revolutionary MAPEC (Ambulatory Blood Pressure Monitoring and Cardiovascular Events) study, in 3000 adult hypertensives investigates, whether chronotherapy influences the cardiovascular prognosis beyond blood pressure reduction per se. Second, melatonin, statins and aliskiren are hopeful drugs for hypertension treatment. Melatonin, through its scavenging and antioxidant effects, preservation of NO availability, sympatholytic effect or specific melatonin receptor activation exerts antihypertensive and anti-remodeling effects and may be useful especially in patients with nondipping nighttime blood pressure pattern or with nocturnal hypertension and in hypertensives with left ventricular hypertrophy (LVH). Owing to its multifunctional physiological actions, this indolamine may offer cardiovascular protection far beyond its hemodynamic benefit. Statins exert several pleiotropic effects through inhibition of small guanosine triphosphate-binding proteins such as Ras and Rho. Remarkably, statins reduce blood pressure in hypertensive patients and more importantly they attenuate LVH. Addition of statins should be considered for high-risk hypertensives, for hypertensives with LVH, and possibly for high-risk prehypertensive patients. The direct renin inhibitor, aliskiren, inhibits catalytic activity of renin molecules in circulation and in the kidney, thus lowering angiotensin II levels. Furthermore, aliskiren by modifying the prorenin conformation may prevent prorenin activation. At present, aliskiren should be considered in hypertensive patients not sufficiently controlled or intolerant to other inhibitors of renin-angiotensin system. Third, TROPHY (Trial of Preventing Hypertension) is the first pharmacological intervention for prehypertensive patients revealing that treatment with angiotensin II type 1 receptor blocker attenuates hypertension development and thus decreases the risk of cardiovascular events.

Szarszoi O, Asemu G, Vanecek J, Ost'adal B, Kolar F. Effects of melatonin on ischemia and reperfusion injury of the rat heart. Cardiovasc Drugs Ther 2001; 15(3):251-7. Effects of melatonin on various manifestations of ischemia/reperfusion injury of the isolated perfused rat heart were examined. Ischemia- and reperfusion-induced ventricular arrhythmias were studied under constant flow in hearts subjected to 10, 15 or 25 min of regional ischemia (induced by LAD coronary artery occlusion) and 10-min reperfusion. Melatonin was added to the perfusion medium 5 min before ischemia at concentrations of 10 micromol/l or 10 nmol/l and was present throughout the experiment. Recovery of the contractile function was evaluated under constant perfusion pressure after 20-min global ischemia followed by 40-min reperfusion. Hearts were treated with melatonin at a high concentration (10 micromol/l) either 5 min before ischemia only (M1) or 5 min before ischemia and during reperfusion (M2) or only during reperfusion (M3). At the high concentration, melatonin significantly reduced the incidence of reperfusion-induced ventricular fibrillation and decreased arrhythmia score (10% and 2.2+/-0.3, respectively) as compared with the corresponding untreated group (62% and 4.1+/-0.3, respectively); the low concentration had no effect. This substance did not affect the incidence and severity of ischemic arrhythmias. Melatonin (M2, M3) significantly improved the recovery of the contractile function as compared with the untreated group; this protection did not appear if melatonin was absent in the medium during reperfusion (MI). Our results show that melatonin, in accordance with its potent antioxidant properties, effectively protects the rat heart against injury associated with reperfusion. It appears unlikely that melatonin is cardioprotective at physiological concentrations.

Veneroso, C et al. Melatonin reduces cardiac inflammatory injury induced by acute exercise. Journal of Pineal Research. 47(2):184-191, September 2009 Cardiac muscle tissue, when stimulated by acute exercise, presents increased signs of cell damage. This study was designed to investigate whether overexpression of inflammatory mediators induced in the heart by acute exercise could be prevented by melatonin and whether the protective effect of melatonin was related with inhibition of nuclear factor kappa B (NF-kappaB) activation. Male Wistar rats received melatonin i.p. at a dose of 1.0 mg/kg body weight 3 min before being exercised for 60 min on a treadmill at a speed of 25 m/min and a 10% slope. Exercise was associated with a significant increase in myeloperoxidase activity and in TNF-alpha, IL-1 and IL-6 mRNA levels. Both mRNA level and protein concentrations of intercellular adhesion molecule-1, inducible nitric oxide synthase, and cyclooxygenase-2 were also significantly elevated. A significant activation of nuclear factor kappa B (NF-kappaB) was observed in exercised rats. These effects were totally or partially prevented by melatonin administration. Data obtained indicate that melatonin protects against heart damage caused by acute exercise. Impaired production of noxious mediators involved in the inflammatory process and down-regulation of the NF-kappaB signal transduction pathway appear to contribute to the beneficial effects of melatonin.

Wolden-Hanson T Daily melatonin administration to middle-aged male rats suppresses body weight, intraabdominal adiposity, and plasma leptin and insulin independent of food intake and total body fat Endocrinology 2000 Feb;141(2):487-97. Pineal melatonin secretion declines with aging, whereas visceral fat, plasma insulin, and plasma leptin tend to increase. We have previously demonstrated that daily melatonin administration at middle age suppressed male rat intraabdominal visceral fat, plasma leptin, and plasma insulin to youthful levels; the current study was designed to begin investigating mechanisms that mediate these responses. Melatonin (0.4 microg/ml) or vehicle was administered in the drinking water of 10-month-old male Sprague Dawley rats (18/treatment) for 12 weeks. Half (9/treatment) were then killed, and the other half were submitted to cross-over treatment for an additional 12 weeks. Twelve weeks of melatonin treatment decreased (P<0.05) body weight (BW; by 7% relative to controls), relative intraabdominal adiposity (by 16%), plasma leptin (by 33%), and plasma insulin (by 25%) while increasing (P<0.05) locomotor activity (by 19%), core body temperature (by 0.5 C), and morning plasma corticosterone (by 154%), restoring each of these parameters toward more youthful levels.

Food intake and total body fat were not changed by melatonin treatment. Melatonin-treated rats that were then crossed over to control treatment for a further 12 weeks gained BW, whereas control rats that were crossed to melatonin treatment lost BW, but food intake did not change in either group. Feed efficiency (grams of BW change per g cumulative food intake), a measure of metabolic function, was negative in melatonin-treated rats and positive in control rats before cross-over (P<0.001); this relationship was reversed after cross-over (P<0.001). Thus, melatonin treatment in middle age decreased BW, intraabdominal adiposity, plasma insulin, and plasma leptin, without altering food intake or total adiposity. These results suggest that the decrease in endogenous melatonin with aging may alter metabolism and physical activity, resulting in increased BW, visceral adiposity, and associated detrimental metabolic consequences.

Xu M et al. Melatonin Protection Against Lethal Myocyte Injury Induced by Doxorubicin as Reflected by Effects on Mitochondrial Membrane Potential.J Mol Cell Cardiol 2002 Jan; 34(1):75-79 Melatonin (MLT) is highly protective against cardiotoxicity caused by doxorubicin (DOX). DOX induces cardiac damage via production of reactive oxygen species. This study tests the hypothesis that oxygen radicals generated by DOX disrupt mitochondrial membrane potential (Delta (psi) (m)) prior to severe cell injury. Myocytes were incubated with 20 micromol/l DOX for 24 h. Myocyte damage was estimated by lactate dehydrogenase (LDH) release. Mitochondrial membrane potential was determined by staining myocytes with 5, 5', 6, 6'-tetrachloro-1, 1', 3, 3'-tetraethylbenzimidazolcarbocyanine iodide (JC-1) using confocal microscope. A significant amount of LDH was observed after 24 h of treatment with DOX. Mitochondria in DOX-treated myocytes exhibited a collapse of Delta (psi) (m). Pretreatment with melatonin (1 mmol/l) for one hour prevented the release of LDH and restored Delta (psi) (m). The data support the hypothesis that DOX induces damage to mitochondria through radicals, and this is reflected in depolarization of Delta (psi) (m), which was prevented by melatonin.

CHAPTER 9

Human Growth Hormone:

"Growth hormone is essential for normal adult life and without it life expectancy is shortened, energy and vitality reduced and the quality of this life impaired. The medical case for growth hormone replacement is now proved beyond any reasonable medical and scientific doubt." (Sonksen, 1998).

Of all the interventions that preventive/regenerative medicine has brought to medicine and the patients who wish to slow and reverse the aging process, human growth hormone (GH) is perhaps the the most controversial. Controversies include doping in sports, cancer risk and unique prescribing laws.

.

GH Physiology:

The hypothalamus produces Growth Hormone Releasing Hormone (GHRH) that signals the anterior pituitary gland to release human growth hormone. GH is a peptide hormone and consists of a chain of 191 amino acids. GH is a relatively large molecule with a complex three-dimensional structure. Somatostatin, or growth hormone inhibiting hormone (GHIH), produced by the hypothalamus, signals the anterior pituitary gland to inhibit the release of growth hormone. Most of the GH produced by the pituitary gland is secreted at night, during stage III and IV sleep. GHRH is released constantly during deep sleep and Somatostatin (GHIH) is inhibited during deep sleep. So the inhibitor is inhibited and the net result is more GH in the body. GH is the only pituitary hormone that "has an on switch and an off switch."

There are other endogenous ligands known as growth hormone releasing peptides that also signal the pituitary to release growth hormone. One of the major effects of GH is to stimulate hepatic production of insulin-like growth factor 1 (IGF-1). Growth hormone and IGF-1 cross the blood brain barrier and optimize cognitive function. IGF-1 has a cytoprotective effect against beta amyloid plaque formation, which is associated with Alzheimer's dementia. IGF-1 increases dendritic formation of the cortical neurons. Patients with traumatic brain injury (TBI), and the resultant growth hormone deficiency, treated with growth hormone showed significant improvement in concentration, memory, depression, anxiety and fatigue when treated. Growth hormone increases connexin-43 in the brain, which mediates neuronal communication.

GH stimulates the production of binding proteins, which transport IGF-1 and function as hormones. Growth Hormone Binding Protein 3 (IGFBP 3) transports IGF 1 and is associated with decreasing cancer risks. (Ingermann). The mechanism may be through stimulation of the P53 gene. The molar ratio of IGF1 to IGFBP3 is usually constant when patients are treated with growth hormone replacement therapy. (Scire) Growth hormone is released in brief spurts during stage 3 and 4 sleep and has a half-life of 14 minutes. Since random serum GH levels do not give us useful information, the next best lab test for evaluating human growth hormone levels is IGF-1. IGF-1 is not a perfect test for GH levels but we know that if the IGF-1 level is low, the patient is not producing enough GH.

24 hour urine testing is another useful method for assessing GH production.

GH and IGF-1 affect all organs and tissues of the body including:

- Brain: improves cognitive function and mood
- Heart: improves blood flow and cardiac output
- Carotid arteries: promotes less atherosclerosis and improves intimal medial thickness
- Lungs: improves pulmonary function
- Body composition: promotes less fat, especially abdominal fat, helps to maintain muscle, improves bone mineral density
- Exercise: increases exercise capacity
- Immune: increases immune system function T and B cell maturation
- Metabolism: GH improves dyslipidemia, improves wound healing and decreases insulin resistance in most instances
- Inflammation: Improves inflammation and reduces TNF alpha, IL-1 beta, IL-6

Human growth hormone obtained its name from the fact that GH is necessary to make children grow. Children with pituitary dwarfism can and have been treated with GH for years to reach normal adult heights. Children with other causes of short stature have been successfully treated with GH. In adults, "growth hormone" is a misleading name for this hormone since it is also necessary for a vigorous and healthy adult life. A better name for GH might be repair hormone.

Classical causes of adult growth hormone deficiency are surgery, radiation, trauma or prior childhood growth hormone deficiency. When we look at the mental and physical functioning of these patients it looks a lot like "aging." Mild adult growth hormone deficiency can also occur with the normal aging process. Growth hormone released by the pituitary gland decreases steadily after thirty or forty years of age and the GH levels of a normal fifty or sixty year old may be as low as an adult with classical growth hormone deficiency. This is where the paradigm shift of preventive/regenerative medicine diverges from traditional endocrinology.

Literature Review:

GH is one of the most studied compounds in medicine with almost 100,000 journal references currently in Pubmed. There is an exponential decline in GH release after 18-21 years of age and a 14% decline per decade after puberty. In an article published in Hormone Research in 2000, Savine et al concluded that life without growth hormone is poor both in quantity and quality. The emphasis here should be placed on quality as maintaining a good quality of life is the goal. Savine found that GH peaks at puberty and starts decreasing at 21. At the age of 60, most adults have the same 24-hour secretion rate indistinguishable from those hypopituitary patients with organic lesions in the pituitary gland. Thus, a normal 60-year-old is the same as a sick 25-year-old in terms of GH levels. Savine also concluded that if an IGF-1 level of 300 is mean normal for a 20 to 30-year-old, almost everybody over the age of 40 has an IGF-1 deficit.

Low GH is associated with decreased longevity in humans, with more that 20 years decreased lifespan with low GH. (Beeson) Older men with higher IGF-1 down not show the same decrease in lean body mass and increase in fat mass. "GH determines life's potential" (Ruiz-Torres) Childhood or adult GH deficiency is associated with 2-3 times increase in mortality. (Stochholm)

Chronic inflammation is associated with most age-related diseases. Doing whatever we can to decrease chronic inflammation is important in the quest to stay healthy. A number of things can be done to help combat chronic inflammation. Control of free radicals, homocysteine, advanced glycation end products, and optimizing hormones to youthful levels, such as testosterone, estrogens, GH, IGF-1 all decrease inflammatory cytokines. Inflammation induces GH insensitivity, however GHRT decreases inflammation. GH replacement therapy decreases C - reactive protein (CRP) levels. Cappola et al carried out a study to investigate what factors were associated with a better quality of life in women aged 70 and over. The results showed that women who had the best quality of life in terms of functional capability – that is: walking limitation, mobility, activities of daily living, cognition – had high IGF-1 levels and low IL-6 levels, indicating high GH levels and minimal inflammation. Decreased GH levels and decreased IGF-1 levels lead to frailty. GH deficiency is associated with neurocognitive decline, and GHRT improves memory, alertness, and concentration. Aleman et al correlated IGF-1 with cognitive function in men – with higher IGF-1 levels being linked to better cognitive function. GH deficiency was correlated with poor emotional and psychosocial functioning. GH increases the strength and formation of cortical bone. Logobardi linked GH deficiency with reduced bone density, and GHRT with reversal of osteoporosis. Patients who sustain hip fractures tend to have lower IGF-1 levels. GH is synergistic with exercise and to get the maximum effect from GHRT it has to be combined with regular exercise.

Van der Lely et al. treated patients over 75 with hip fractures with GH at the time of fracture for six weeks. The end point was return to pre-fracture living arrangements. Results of the double-blind placebo-controlled trial showed that 94% of patients treated with GH returned to pre-fracture living within just six weeks, compared with 75% of control patients. GH increases bone mineral density. Gillberg et al. treated men with idiopathic osteoporosis with GH. Participants were randomly assigned to treatment with GH, either as continuous treatment with daily injections of 0.4 mg GH or as intermittent treatment with 0.8 mg GH for 14 days every 3 months. All patients were treated with GH for 24 months, with a follow-up period of 12 months. No positive effects of treatment were noted at the 12-month follow-up. But after 12 months there was a continued increase in bone mineral density and no significant adverse effects were reported. After two years of GH treatment significant improvement in bone mineral density were observed in both groups.

GH deficiency is associated with increased cardiovascular mortality, while GHRT is associated with improved cardiovascular function. Research suggests that GHRT may help to reverse atherosclerosis, improve cardiomyopathy, and reduce carotid intima medial thickness. Pro-inflammatory cytokines contribute to chronic and acute heart failure. Adamopoulos et al. treated patients with idiopathic dilated cardiomyopathy (IDC) with GH. Results showed that GH treatment led to a significant decrease in both TNF-α and IL-6 levels and significant improvements in exercise capacity. GH also correct endothelial dysfunction. In our opinion, too much emphasis is placed upon the cholesterol model of atherosclerosis. Inflammation and endothelial dysfunction are more important contributors to the process of atherosclerosis.

GH improves endothelial dysfunction, which plays a significant role in both heart failure and arteriosclerosis. Homocysteine is a strong predictor of cardiovascular disease. Sesmilo et al randomly assigned 40 men with GH deficiency to treatment with GH or a placebo for a period of 18 months. Homocysteine levels fell significantly in those treated with GH. IGF-1 has profound cardiac actions. It improves cardiac contractility, stroke volume, and ejection fraction. After myocardial infarction, IGF-1 is critical in preventing pathological remodeling of the heart. It improves recovery and reduces the incidence of congestive heart failure. IGF-1 is correlated with fitness. (Nindl)

GH is a key component to the neuroendocrine immune system. IGF-1 is vital for lymphocyte maturation. GH will restore age-related thymic involution in rodents. IGF-1 is needed to develop T-cells and B-cells, and the age-related decline in these important cells can be reversed with GHRT.

GHRT can decrease visceral abdominal fat by as much as 50%. According to Christiansen, GH deficiency is linked to:

- Abnormal body composition
- An increase in adipose mass and decrease in muscle mass
- Insulin resistance
- Decreased muscle strength

Long-term GHRT can normalize these abnormalities. GH secretion is impaired in obesity. Johannsson et al. studied middle-aged men with low GH and abdominal obesity.

After nine months of treatment with GH, abdominal visceral fat decreased by 18%, insulin sensitivity improved, total cholesterol, LDL, and triglyceride levels dropped, and diastolic blood pressure decreased. The men did not make any lifestyle changes during the study. Blackman et al. studied the effect of treating healthy men and women with sex steroids and GH. Results showed that visceral abdominal fat decreased by 16% in those given GH and testosterone. Women who were treated with GH alone did not lose abdominal fat, but when GH was combined with the HRT they did. A second study by the same group was published a year later in 2002 and VO2 max increased in both men and women, and muscle strength increased by 6.8% in men treated with both GH and testosterone. These changes occurred within six months, and the participants made no life-style changes. Frequent side effects were found including arthralgias and insulin resistance. The high rate of side effects seen with this study might be related to the dosage schedule – the fixed dose per weight, and the three times a week, and not adjusting the dose and no attempt to optimize life style. In clinical practice approximately 10% of patients may suffer from these side effects; however these are manageable by life style optimization, decreasing the dose or if that is not effective, discontuation of treatment. A possible side effect of GHRT is increasing glucose and insulin and even inducing type 2 diabetes. As demonstrated above and by Nam, when combined with diet and exercise this does not occur. Even if diabetes were to be induced it would be a temporary phenomenon that would be reversed and disappear when GHRT was discontinued. Type 2 diabetes will actually be improved by GHRT treatment. See the quote below from Nam.

"Low-dose GH treatment combined with dietary restriction resulted not only in a decrease of visceral fat but also in an increase of muscle mass with a consequent improvement of the insulin resistance observed in obese type 2 diabetic patients."

Gibney et al. found a link between GH deficiency and chronic fatigue and depression. GHRT was found to improve sense of well-being and was associated with an improved quality of life. Gilchrist found that GHRT significantly improved energy levels, vitality, anxiety, depression, well-being, and self-control.

Low GH and its downstream hormone IGF-1 are associated with poor health and quality of life outcomes. When AGHD is treated with GH, there are usually increases in GH, IGF-1 and IGF Binding Protein 3 (IGFBP-3) which all have a role in clinical results. Although IGF-1 is pro-mitotic and taken out of context could promote cancer, IGFBP-3 is anti cancer (Ingermann). The mechanism is explained by stimulation of anti-cancer gene p53. Teenagers with the highest GH and IGF-1 have low rates of cancer. When treating with GH a balance is produced between IGF-1 and IGFBP-3. (Scire) A central question in GHRT is "Does GHRT increase the risk of cancer." Multiple studies and reviews have concluded that there is no increase in cancer risk compared to the general population. Jenkins review is aptly titled, "Does Growth Hormone cause cancer?" and provides the conculsion:

"Extensive studies of the outcome of GH replacement in childhood cancer survivors show no evidence of an excess of de novo cancers, and more recent surveillance of children and adults treated with GH has revealed **no increase in observed cancer risk."**

Moltich's review has similar conclusions:

"Although there has been some concern about an increased risk of cancer, reviews of existing, well-maintained databases of treated patients have shown this theoretical risk to be nonexistent"

In children with brain tumors treated with GH there was no increased risk of tumor progression, recurrence or new CNS or non-CNS tumor or leukemia. (Bogarin) The recurrence rate of the brain tumor was significantly less in the children treated with GH. No studies have proven an association between GH and malignancy. Van Bunderen concludes, "Mortality due to malignancies was not elevated in adults receiving GH treatment." Savendaal recently reported results of mortality in over 2500 patients treated with GH as children for various causes including short stature. There were more than 46,000 person years of observation. The 21 deaths were mostly caused by accidents or suicide. The author's state, "Importantly, none of the patients died from cancer or from a cardiovascular disease"

Bell studied safety of GH in Children and concludes:

"The current data now comprise 20 yr of GH therapy, 54,996 patients, and a cumulative 192,345 patient-years of treatment. With the longer time and expanded patient numbers, we continue to see no increase in new malignancies or recurrences of CNS tumors in rhGHtreated children without risk factors, consistent with other reports."

Endothelial Progenitor cells (EPC's) are the stem cells that maintain and repair the cardiovascular system. The quantity and quality of EPC's is perhaps the best biomarker of aging with higher counts correlating with improved health outcomes. Any intervention that improves EPC's should be considered a major intervention to improve health. IGF-1 through GH improves the number and function of EPC's. EPC senescence is improved, probably thorough increasing telomerase activity and lengthening the telomeres of these critical stem cells. (Thum, Devin)

GH Management:

Prior to initiating AGHD replacement therapy, a thorough work up should be done including history, physical and laboratory evaluation. If active malignancy is present, then referral to appropriate specialist for consultation is indicated. If you suspect AGHD based on the phenotype, which can include suboptimal body composition (excess visceral fat), dyslipidemia, poor quality of life, decreased exercise capacity and a generalized inflammatory state as well as laboratory data suggestive of AGHD, then treatment should be considered. GH is administered subcutaneously daily either in the morning within one hour of waking or at bedtime. Since GH can be locally lipolytic it can be given in the "love handle" region of the body or in the abdomen or the thighs, rotating injection sites to avoid a divot effect.

GH is not given on a mg/kg dosing schedule. Fewer side effects occur with gradual increases or ramping up. Start on 0.2 mg SQ daily for 2 weeks. If no side effects then we increase to 0.4 mg SQ daily.

Adult Growth Hormone Deficiency

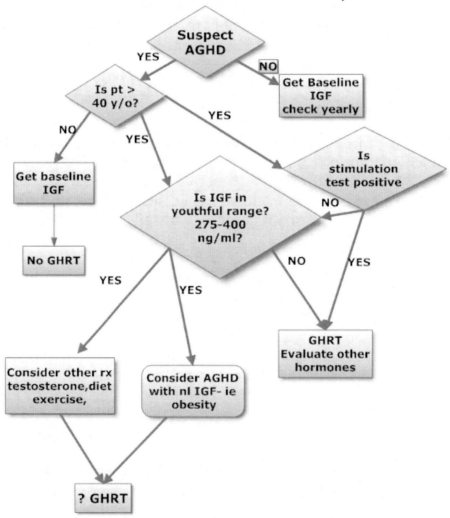

Adult Growth Hormone Deficiency -2-

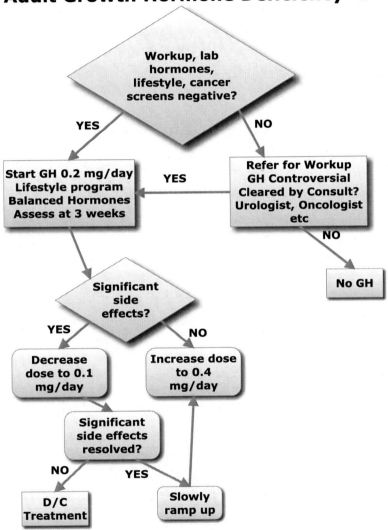

After 3 months a follow up laboratory testing and clinical assessment is done. The IGF 1 values are guidelines and we do not necessarily titrate dosing to hit specific values. For example, if IGF-1 was 80 ng/ml and follow up testing is 180, and significant clinical benefits are seen, no dosage increase may be necessary. An evaluation for side effects including, paresthesias, arthralgias, glucose elevation and edema is done, and dosage adjustments are made if indicated.

Adult Growth Hormone Deficiency -3-

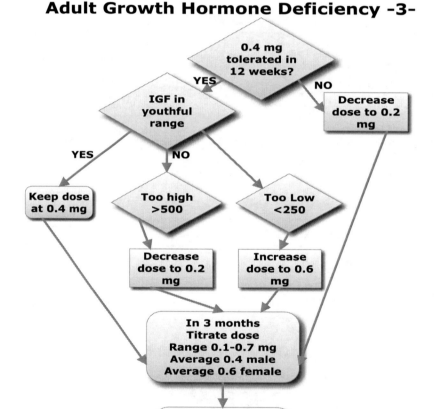

Side Effects of GH Replacement Therapy:

The side effects of GH replacement therapy, if any, are usually minor and are reversible by decreasing the dose or in a few cases discontinuing the treatment.

Possible side effects of GH administration may include paresthesias (numbness and tingling in hands most common), arthralgias, glucose intolerance and insulin resistance and edema, can be remembered with the acronym PAGE. The paresthesias are commonly referred to as carpal tunnel syndrome. However since this is not a median nerve syndrome, this description is inaccurate. There may be numbness in the hands or the arms after sleeping in one position during the night. Joint aching can be experienced in the wrists, knees or other joints. However these symptoms are common in life and a trial of 1-2 weeks off treatment to evaluate for symptom resolution will help to clarify etiology. Even though most studies on GH replacement therapy have shown decreased insulin resistance with GH, there can be an increase in insulin resistance in some patients. Following a low glycemic anti-inflammatory diet with moderate exercise can usually prevent this situation. If life style modification is not effective then decreasing the dose of GH may control insulin resistance. When TRT is used along with GH, the complication of increased insulin resistance is less likely to occur. Monitor patients closely for these possible side effects and adjust the GH dose accordingly. Edema and arthralgias can be symptomatically treated with diuretics and anti-inflammatory agents, but this is not usually necessary.

Adult Growth Hormone Deficiency -4-

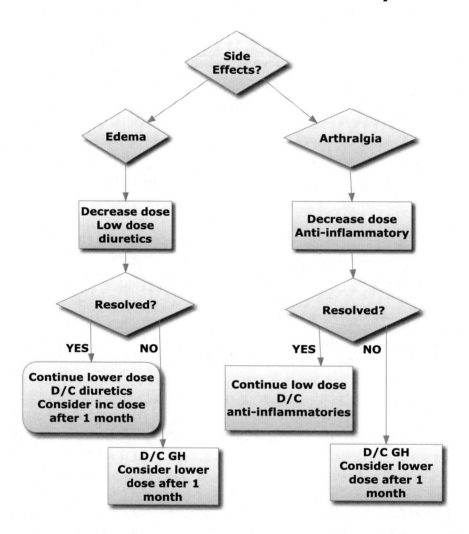

Adult Growth Hormone Deficiency -5-

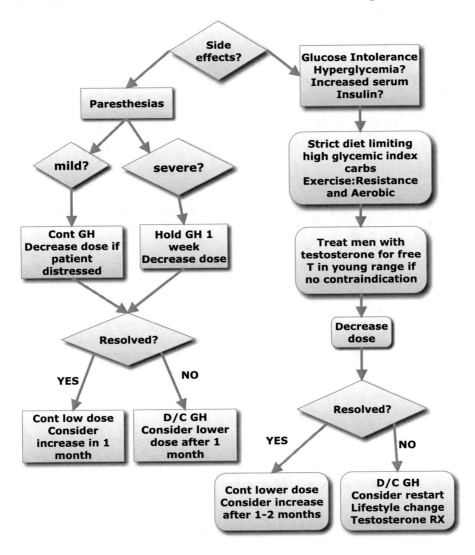

265

Conclusion:

Growth Hormone Replacement therapy for AGHD can help to restore a more youthful physiology and can have the benefits of better quality of life, body composition, cardiovascular function, immune function. A diagnosis of Adult Growth Hormone Deficiency should be made and documented in the patient's medical record.

Growth Hormone Abstracts

Aberg ND. Growth hormone increases connexin-43 expression in the cerebral cortex and hypothalamus. Endocrinology 2000 Oct; 141(10):3879-86 Several studies indicate that systemic GH influences various brain functions. Connexin-43 forms gap junctions that mediate intercellular communication and establish the astroglial syncytium. We investigated the effects of peripheral administration of bovine GH (bGH) and recombinant human insulin-like growth factor I (rhIGF-I) on the expression of connexin-43 in the rat brain. Hypophysectomized female Sprague Dawley rats were substituted with cortisol (400 microg/kg x day) and L-T4 (10 microg/kg x day) and treated with either bGH (1 mg/kg x day) or rhIGF-I (0.85 mg/kg x day) for 19 days. The abundance of connexin-43 messenger RNA (mRNA) and protein in the brainstem, cerebral cortex, hippocampus, and hypothalamus was quantified by means of ribonuclease protection assays and Western blots. Treatment with bGH increased the amounts of connexin-43 mRNA and protein in the cerebral cortex and hypothalamus. No changes were found in the brainstem or hippocampus. Infusion of rhIGF-I did not affect connexin-43 mRNA or protein levels in any of the brain regions studied. These results show that administration of bGH increases the abundance of cx43 in specific brain regions, suggesting that GH may influence gap junction formation and thereby intercellular communication in the brain.

Abs R. Update on the diagnosis of GH deficiency in adults. Eur J Endocrinol. 2003 Apr; 148 Suppl 2:S3-8. GH deficiency (GHD) in adults is associated with considerable morbidity and mortality. The diagnosis of GHD is generally straightforward in children as growth retardation is present; however, in adults, diagnosis of GHD is often challenging. Other markers are therefore needed to identify adults who have GHD and could potentially benefit from GH replacement therapy. Consensus guidelines for the diagnosis and treatment of adult GHD recommend provocative testing of GH secretion for patients who have evidence of hypothalamic-pituitary disease, patients with childhood-onset GHD, and patients who have undergone cranial irradiation or have a history of head trauma. Suspicion of GHD is also heightened in the presence of other pituitary hormone deficits. Tests for GHD include measurement of the hormone in urine or serum or measurement of stimulated GH levels after administration of various provocative agents. The results of several studies indicate that non-stimulated serum or urine measurements of GH levels cannot reliably predict deficiency in adults. Although glucagon and arginine tests produce a pronounced GH response with few false positives, the insulin tolerance test (ITT) is currently considered to be the gold standard of the GH stimulation tests available. Unfortunately, the ITT has some disadvantages and questionable reproducibility, which have prompted the development of several new tests for GHD that are based on pharmacological stimuli. Of these, GH-releasing hormone (GHRH) plus arginine and GHRH plus GH-releasing peptide (GHRP) appear to be reliable and practical. Thus, in cases where ITT is contraindicated or inconclusive, the combination of arginine and GHRH is an effective alternative. As experience with this test as well as with GHRH/GHRP-6 accumulates, they may supplant ITT as the diagnostic test of choice.

Adamopoulos S et al. Growth hormone administration reduces circulating proinflammatory cytokines and soluble Fas/soluble Fas ligand system in patients with chronic heart failure secondary to idiopathic dilated cardiomyopathy. Am Heart J 2002 Aug;144(2):359-64 BACKGROUND: Recent studies have shown that an abnormal proinflammatory cytokine expression and apoptotic process contribute to adverse left ventricular remodeling and progress of chronic heart failure. This study investigates the effects of growth hormone (GH) administration on serum levels of representative proinflammatory cytokines and soluble apoptosis mediators in patients with chronic heart failure secondary to idiopathic dilated cardiomyopathy (IDC). METHODS: Serum levels of tumor necrosis factor-alpha (TNF-alpha), its soluble receptors (sTNF-RI, sTNF-RII), interleukin-6 (IL-6), soluble IL-6 receptor (sIL-6R), soluble Fas (sFas) and soluble Fas Ligand (sFasL) were determined (enzyme-linked immunosorbent assay method) in 10 patients with IDC (New York Heart Association class III, ejection fraction 24% +/- 2%) before and after a 3-month subcutaneous administration of 4 IU GH every other day (randomized crossover design). Peak oxygen consumption (Vo (2) max) was also used to evaluate the functional status of patients with IDC. RESULTS: Treatment with GH produced a significant reduction in serum levels of TNF-alpha (8.2 +/- 1.2 vs 5.7 +/- 1.1 pg/mL, P <.05), sTNF-RI (3.9 +/- 0.4 vs 3.2 +/- 0.3 ng/mL, P <.05), sTNF-RII (2.6 +/- 0.3 vs 2.2 +/- 0.2 ng/mL, P <.05), IL-6 (5.5 +/- 0.6 vs 4.4 +/- 0.4 pg/mL, P =.05), sIL-6R (32.7 +/- 3.0 vs 28.2 +/- 3.0 ng/mL, P <.05), sFas (4.4 +/- 0.8 vs 3.1 +/- 0.6 ng/mL, P <.05), and sFasL (34.2 +/- 11.7 vs 18.8 +/- 7.3 pg/mL, P <.01). A significant improvement was also observed in VO2max after the completion of 3 months' treatment with GH (15.0 +/- 0.8 vs 17.2 +/- 1.0 mL/kg/min, P <.05). Good correlations were found between GH-induced reduction in TNF-alpha levels and increase in VO2max (r = -0.64, P <.05) as well as between GH-induced reduction in sFasL and increase in VO2max (r = -0.56, P =.08). CONCLUSIONS: GH administration reduces serum levels of proinflammatory cytokines and soluble Fas/FasL system in patients with IDC. These immunomodulatory effects may be associated with improvement in clinical performance and exercise capacity of patients with IDC.

Aimaretti G et al. Diagnostic reliability of a single IGF-I measurement in 237 adults with total anterior hypopituitarism and severe GH deficiency.Clin Endocrinol (Oxf). 2003 Jul; 59(1):56-61OBJECTIVE: Within an appropriate clinical context, GH deficiency (GHD) in adults must be demonstrated biochemically by a single provocative test. Insulin-induced hypoglycaemia (ITT) and GH-releasing hormone (GHRH) + arginine (ARG) are indicated as the tests of choice, provided that appropriate cut-off limits are defined. Although IGF-I is the best marker of GH secretory status, its measurement is not considered a reliable diagnostic tool. In fact, considerable overlap between GHD and normal subjects is present, at least when patients with suspected GHD are considered independently of the existence of other anterior pituitary defects. Considering the time and cost associated with provocative testing procedures, we aimed to re-evaluate the diagnostic power of IGF-I measurement. DESIGN: To this goal, in a large population [n = 237, 139 men, 98 women, age range 20-80 years, body mass index (BMI) range 26.4 +/- 4.3 kg/m2] of well-nourished adults with total anterior pituitary deficit including severe GHD (as shown by a GH peak below the 1st centile limit of normal response to GHRH + ARG tests and/or ITT) we evaluated the diagnostic value of a single total IGF-I measurement. IGF-I levels in hypopituitary patients were evaluated based on age-related normative values in a large population of normal subjects (423 ns, 144 men and 279 women, age range 20-80 years, BMI range 18.2-24.9 kg/m2). RESULTS: Mean IGF-I levels in GHD were lower than those in normal subjects in each decade, but not the oldest one (74.4 +/- 48.9 vs. 243.9 +/- 86.7 micro g/l for 20-30 years; 81.8 +/- 46.5 vs. 217.2 +/- 56.9 micro g/l for 31-40 years; 85.8 +/- 42.1 vs. 168.5 +/- 69.9 micro g/l for 41-50 years; 82.3 +/- 39.3 vs. 164.3 +/- 60.3 micro g/l for 51-60 years; 67.5 +/- 31.8 vs. 123.9 +/- 50.0 micro g/l for 61-70 years; P < 0.0001; 54.3 +/- 33.6 vs. 91.6 +/- 53.5 micro g/l for 71-80 years, P = ns). Individual IGF-I levels in GHD were below the age-related 3rd and 25th centile limits in 70.6% and 97.63% of patients below 40 years and in 34.9% and 77.8% of the remaining patients up to the 8th decade, respectively. CONCLUSIONS: Total IGF-I levels are often normal even in patients with total anterior hypopituitarism but this does not rule out severe GHD that therefore ought to be verified by provocative testing of GH secretion. However, despite the low diagnostic sensitivity of this parameter, very low levels of total IGF-I can be considered definitive evidence of severe GHD in a remarkable percentage of total anterior hypopituitary patients who could therefore skip provocative testing of GH secretion.

Albert SG et al. Low-dose recombinant human growth hormone as adjuvant therapy to lifestyle modifications in the management of obesity.Clin Endocrinol Metab. 2004 Feb; 89(2):695-701. Obese individuals are in a reduced GH/IGF-I state that may be maladaptive. Fifty-nine obese men and premenopausal menstruating women (body mass index, 36.9 +/- 5.0 kg/m (2)) were randomized to a double-blind, placebo-controlled trial of low dose recombinant human GH (rhGH). During the 6-month intervention, subjects self-administered daily rhGH or equivalent volume of placebo at 200 micro g (1.9 +/- 0.3 microg/kg for men, 2.0 +/- 0.3 microg/kg for women); after 1 month, the dose was increased to 400 microg (3.8 +/- 0.5 microg/kg) in men and 600 microg (6.0 +/- 0.8 microg/kg) in women. rhGH was then discontinued, and subjects were followed up after 3 months. Forty completed the intervention, and 39 completed the follow-up. Drop-out rates between rhGH vs. placebo groups were not different (chi (2) = 1.45; P = 0.228). One subject discontinued the drug due to an rhGH-related side effect. Body weight (BW) decreased with rhGH from 100.4 +/- 13.2 to 98.0 +/- 15.6 kg at 6 months (P = 0.04) and was sustained at 98.1 +/- 16.6 kg at 9 months (P = 0.02). BW loss was entirely due to loss of body fat (BF). Intention to treat analyses demonstrated changes from baseline between rhGH and placebo in BW (-2.16 +/- 4.48 vs. -0.04 +/- 2.67 kg; P = 0.03) and BF (-2.89 +/- 3.76 vs. -0.68 +/- 2.37 kg; P = 0.01). rhGH increased IGF-I from -0.72 to +0.10 SD (P = 0.0001). rhGH increased high-density lipoprotein cholesterol 19% from 1.11 +/- 0.34 to 1.32 +/- 0.28 mmol/liter (P < 0.001). Neither group had changes in fasting glucose, insulin sensitivity, or resting energy expenditure. In conclusion, in obesity, rhGH normalized IGF-I levels, induced loss of BW from BF, and improved lipid profile without untoward effects on insulin sensitivity.

Aleman et al. Insulin-Like Growth Factor-I and Cognitive Function in Healthy Older Men J Clin Endocrinol Metab 84:471–475, 1999 The GH/insulin-like growth factor-I (GH/IGF-I) axis is known to be involved in aging of physiological functions. Recent studies indicate that the GH/IGF-I axis may be associated with cognitive functioning. The aim of the present study was to determine whether the age-related decline in circulating levels of IGF-I, as an index of anabolic status, is associated with cognitive functions that are known to decline with aging, but not with cognitive functions not sensitive to aging. Twenty five healthy older men with well-preserved functional ability participated in the study. We also administered neuropsychological tests of general knowledge, vocabulary, basic visual perception, reading ability, visuoconstructive ability, perceptual-motor speed, mental tracking, and verbal long-term memory. Performance on the last four tests decline with aging, whereas the first four of these tests have been shown not to be sensitive to cognitive aging. Mean age of the subjects was 69.1 +/- 3.4 (SD) yr (range 65-76 yr), their mean body mass index was 27.0 +/- 2.4 kg/m2, and their mean IGF-I level was 122 ng/mL (range: 50-220). We found IGF-I levels to be significantly associated with the performances (controlled for education) on the Digit Symbol Substitution test (r = 0.52, P = 0.009) and the Concept Shifting Task (r = -0.55, P = 0.005), which measure perceptual-motor and mental processing speed. Subjects with higher IGF-I levels performed better on these tests, performance on which is known to decline with aging. In conclusion, the results of this study support the hypothesis that circulating IGF-I may play a role in the age-related reduction of certain cognitive functions, specifically speed of information processing.

Andreassen et al. Concentrations of the acute phase reactants high-sensitive C-reactive protein and YKL-40 and of interleukin-6 before and after treatment in patients with acromegaly and growth hormone deficiency. Clin Endocrinol (Oxf). 2007 Aug 28 BACKGROUND: Acromegaly is accompanied by increased cardiovascular mortality and a cluster of proatherogenic risk factors. In the general population, ischaemic heart disease (IHD) is associated with elevated levels of inflammatory markers. The acute phase reactant (APR) C-reactive protein (CRP) has been reported to be reduced in acromegaly and increase after treatment, suggesting that excess of GH/IGF-I could have anti-inflammatory effects. This is in accordance with results obtained in patients with growth hormone deficiency (GHD), where increased levels of CRP have been reported.OBJECTIVE: To investigate the hypothesis that the GH/IGF-I system is a suppressive regulator of inflammatory processes.SUBJECTS AND METHODS: Twenty-one acromegalic patients and 19 GH-deficient patients were studied. The two APRs CRP and YKL-40 and the proinflammatory cytokine interleukin-6 (IL-6) were measured before and after treatment and in healthy matched controls.RESULTS: In acromegalic patients, serum concentrations of high-sensitive CRP (hsCRP) and YKL-40 were reduced compared to controls (P < 0.001) and increased (P < 0.001) after treatment, together with IL-6 (P = 0.021), to levels comparable with controls. Pretreatment serum YKL-40 and IL-6 showed a significant inverse correlation with IGF-I and GH. In GH-deficient patients, hsCRP and YKL-40 were elevated compared to controls (P = 0.001 and P = 0.048). During treatment, levels of both APRs showed a trend towards a decrease (P = 0.087 and P = 0.060), and after treatment, levels of YKL-40 no longer differed from that of controls. Serum IL-6 was not different from controls and did not change during GH treatment.CONCLUSION: The results point to the possibility of a relationship between GH disturbances and inflammatory processes.

Baffa R et al. Low serum insulin-like growth factor 1 (IGF-1): a significant association with prostate cancer. Tech Urol 2000 Sep; 6(3):236-239 PURPOSE: Insulin-like growth factor 1 (IGF-1) is an important mitogenic and antiapoptotic peptide that affects the proliferation of normal and malignant cells. Contradictory reports on the association between serum IGF-1 level and prostate cancer have been highlighted in the recent literature. The purpose of this study was to investigate the relation between serum levels of IGF-1 and prostate cancer. MATERIALS AND METHODS: We analyzed a population of 57 patients who underwent radical prostatectomy (RP) for adenocarcinoma. Serum samples were collected before RP (T0), 6 months after RP (T6), and from 39 age-matched controls. IGF-1 levels were determined by the active IGF-1 Elisa kit (Diagnostic Systems Laboratories, Inc.). Parallel samples were evaluated for prostate-specific antigen (PSA) levels. Data between groups were analyzed using Welch's t-test and levels before RP and after 6 months were compared by paired t-test. RESULTS: The normal mean serum IGF-1 for case patients at T0 (124.6+/-58.2 ng/mL) was significantly lower than the control subjects (157.5+/-70.8 ng/mL; p = .0192). The normal mean serum IGF-1 for case patients at T0 (124.91+/-58.6 ng/mL) also was significantly lower when it was compared with the T6 group (148.49+/-57.2 ng/mL; p = .0056). No association was found between IGF-1 and PSA blood levels, or IGF-1 and patient weight (p = 0.2434). An inverse relation between IGF-1 levels and age in the normal controls (p = .0041) was observed. CONCLUSION: Findings of this study indicate a significant association between low serum levels of IGF-1 and prostate cancer.

Bartke A et al. Consequences of growth hormone (GH) overexpression and GH resistance. Neuropeptides 2002 Apr;36(2-3):201 Development of transgenic mice overexpressing GH and GHR-KO mice with GH resistance provided novel animal models for study of the somatotropic axis and for identifying GH actions that may be relevant to its current and contemplated use in medicine and agriculture. Studies of phenotypic characteristics of these animals revealed previously unsuspected actions of GH and IGF-I on neuroendocrine functions related to reproduction and to the release of "stress hormones" (glucocorticoids and prolactin). These studies also provided novel and still-disputed evidence for involvement of somatotropic axis in the control of aging and life span and in mediating the actions of longevity genes.

Baum HB et al. Effects of physiologic growth hormone therapy on bone density and body composition in patients with adult-onset growth hormone deficiency. A randomized, placebo-controlled trial. Ann Intern Med 1996 Dec 1; 125(11):883-90 BACKGROUND: Patients with adult-onset growth hormone deficiency have reduced bone density and increased fat mass. Growth hormone at high doses may decrease body fat in these patients, but the effects of growth hormone at more physiologic doses on bone density and body composition have not been convincingly shown. OBJECTIVE: To determine whether long-term growth hormone therapy at a dose adjusted to maintain normal insulin-like growth factor 1 (IGF-1) levels has clinical effects in patients with adult-onset growth hormone deficiency. DESIGN: Randomized, placebo-controlled study. SETTING: Tertiary referral center. PATIENTS: 32 men with adult-onset growth hormone deficiency. INTERVENTION: Growth hormone (initial daily dose, 10 micrograms/kg of body weight) or placebo for 18 months. The growth hormone dose was reduced by 25% if IGF-1 levels were elevated. MEASUREMENTS: Body composition and bone mineral density of the lumbar spine, femoral neck, and proximal radius were measured by dual energy x-ray absorptiometry at 6-month intervals. Markers of bone turnover were also measured during the first 12 months of the study. RESULTS: Growth hormone therapy increased bone mineral density in the lumbar spine by a mean (+/- SD) of 5.1% +/- 4.1%

and bone mineral density in the femoral neck by 2.4% +/- 3.5%. In the growth hormone group, significant increases were seen in the following markers of bone turnover: osteocalcin (4.4 +/- 3.6 mg/L to 7.2 +/- 4.6 mg/L) and urinary pyridinoline (39.0 +/- 19.8 nmol/mmol of creatinine to 55.7 +/- 25.5 nmol/mmol of creatinine) and deoxypyridinoline (8.4 +/- 7.1 nmol/mmol of creatinine to 14.9 +/- 9.4 nmol/mmol of creatinine). Percentage of body fat in the growth hormone group decreased (from 31.9% +/- 6.5% to 28.3% +/- 7.0%), and lean body mass increased (from 59.0 +/- 8.5 kg to 61.5 +/- 6.9 kg). These changes were significant compared with corresponding changes in the placebo group (P < 0.01 for all comparisons). CONCLUSIONS: Growth hormone administered to men with adult-onset growth hormone deficiency at a dose adjusted according to serum IGF-1 levels increases bone density and stimulates bone turnover, decreases body fat and increases lean mass, and is associated with a low incidence of side effects.

Bennett R Growth hormone in musculoskeletal pain states.Curr Rheumatol Rep. 2004 Aug; 6(4):266-73. Growth hormone is essential for normal linear growth and the attainment of an adult mature height. It also plays an important role in cartilage growth and the attainment of normal bone mass. There is only one rheumatic disorder, namely acromegaly, in which abnormalities of growth hormone production play a major etiologic role. However, there is increasing appreciation that suboptimal growth hormone secretion, leading to a state of adult growth hormone deficiency, may occur in the setting of chronic inflammatory disease, chronic corticosteroid use, and fibromyalgia. Therefore, the evaluation and effective management of growth hormone oversecretion and undersecretion is relevant to practicing rheumatologists.

Bennett RM et al. A randomized, double-blind, placebo-controlled study of growth hormone in the treatment of fibromyalgia Am J Med. 1998 Mar; 104(3):227-31. PURPOSE: The cause of fibromyalgia (FM) is not known. Low levels of insulin-like growth factor 1 (IGF-1), a surrogate marker for low growth hormone (GH) secretion, occur in about one third of patients who have many clinical features of growth hormone deficiency, such as diminished energy, dysphoria, impaired cognition, poor general health, reduced exercise capacity, muscle weakness, and cold intolerance. To determine whether suboptimal growth hormone production could be relevant to the symptomatology of fibromyalgia, we assessed the clinical effects of treatment with growth hormone. METHODS: Fifty women with fibromyalgia and low IGF-1 levels were enrolled in a randomized, placebo-controlled, double-blind study of 9 months' duration. They gave themselves daily subcutaneous injections of growth hormone or placebo. Two outcome measures--the Fibromyalgia Impact Questionnaire and the number of fibromyalgia tender points-were evaluated at 3-monthly intervals by a blinded investigator. An unblinded investigator reviewed the IGF-1 results monthly and adjusted the growth hormone dose to achieve an IGF-1 level of about 250 ng/mL. RESULTS: Daily growth hormone injections resulted in a prompt and sustained increase in IGF-1 levels. The treatment (n=22) group showed a significant improvement over the placebo group (n=23) at 9 months in both the Fibromyalgia Impact Questionnaire score (P <0.04) and the tender point score (P <0.03). Fifteen subjects in the growth hormone group and 6 subjects in the control group experienced a global improvement (P <0.02). There was a delayed response to therapy, with most patients experiencing improvement at the 6-month mark. After discontinuing growth hormone, patients experienced a worsening of symptoms. Carpal tunnel symptoms were more prevalent in the growth hormone group (7 versus 1); no other adverse events were more common in this group. CONCLUSIONS: Women with fibromyalgia and low IGF-1 levels experienced an improvement in their overall symptomatology and number of tender points after 9 months of daily growth hormone therapy. This suggests that a secondary growth hormone deficiency may be responsible for some of the symptoms of fibromyalgia.

Besson A et al. Reduced longevity in untreated patients with isolated growth hormone deficiency. J Clin Endocrinol Metab. 2003 Aug; 88(8):3664-7. Increased longevity of hypopituitary dwarf mice and GH-resistant knockout mice appears to be in contrast with observations made in clinical practice. In humans, on one hand hypopituitarism and GH deficiency (GHD) are believed to constitute risk factors for cardiovascular disease and, therefore, early death. But on the other hand, patients with a PROP-1 gene mutation, presenting with a combined pituitary-derived hormonal deficiency, can survive to a very advanced age, apparently longer than normal individuals in the same population. The aim of this study was to analyze the impact of untreated GHD on life span. Hereditary dwarfism was recognized in 11 subjects. Genetic analysis revealed an underlying 6.7-kb spanning deletion of genomic DNA encompassing the GH-1 gene causing isolated GHD. These patients (five males and six females) were never treated for their hormonal deficiency and thus provide a unique opportunity to compare their life span and cause of death directly with their unaffected brothers and sisters (11 males and 14 females) as well as with the normal population (100 males and females). Although the cause of death did not vary between the two groups, median life span in the GH-deficient group was significantly shorter than that of unaffected brothers and sisters [males, 56 vs. 75 yr (P < 0.0001); females, 46 vs. 80 yr (P < 0.0001)]. Therefore, with the wealth of information regarding the beneficial effects of GH replacement and the dramatic findings of this study, GH treatment in adult patients suffering from either childhood- or adult-onset GHD is crucially important.

Biller BM et al. Sensitivity and specificity of six tests for the diagnosis of adult GH deficiency. J Clin Endocrinol Metab. 2002 May; 87(5):2067-79. Although the use of the insulin tolerance test (ITT) for the diagnosis of adult GH deficiency is well established, diagnostic peak GH cut-points for other commonly used GH stimulation tests are less clearly established. Despite that fact, the majority of patients in the United States who are evaluated for GH deficiency do not undergo insulin tolerance testing. The aim of this study was to evaluate the relative utility of six different methods of testing for adult GH deficiency currently used in practice in the United States and to develop diagnostic cut-points for each of these tests. Thirty-nine patients (26 male, 13 female) with adult-onset hypothalamic-pituitary disease and multiple pituitary hormone deficiencies were studied in comparison with age-, sex-, estrogen status-, and body mass index-matched control subjects (n = 34; 20 male, 14 female). A third group of patients (n = 21) with adult-onset hypothalamic-pituitary disease and no more than one additional pituitary hormone deficiency was also studied. The primary end-point was peak serum GH response to five GH stimulation tests administered in random order at five separate visits: ITT, arginine (ARG), levodopa (L-DOPA), ARG plus L-DOPA, and ARG plus GHRH. Serum IGF-I concentrations were also measured on two occasions. For purposes of analysis, patients with multiple pituitary hormone deficiencies were assumed to be GH deficient. Three diagnostic cut-points were calculated for each test to provide optimal separation of multiple pituitary hormone deficient and control subjects according to three criteria: 1) to minimize misclassification of control subjects and deficient patients (balance between high sensitivity and high specificity); 2) to provide 95% sensitivity for GH deficiency; and 3) to provide 95% specificity for GH deficiency. The greatest diagnostic accuracy occurred with the ITT and the ARG plus GHRH test, although patients preferred the latter (P = 0.001). Using peak serum GH cut-points of 5.1 microg/liter for the ITT and 4.1 microg/liter for the ARG plus GHRH test, high sensitivity (96 and 95%, respectively) and specificity (92 and 91%, respectively) for GH deficiency were achieved. To obtain 95% specificity, the peak serum GH cut-points were lower at 3.3 microg/liter and 1.5 microg/liter for the ITT and ARG plus GHRH test, respectively. There was substantial overlap between patients and control subjects for the ARG plus L-DOPA, ARG, and L-DOPA tests, but test-specific cut-points could be defined for all three tests to provide 95% sensitivity for GH deficiency (peak GH cut-points: 1.5, 1.4 and 0.64 microg/liter, respectively). However, 95% specificity could be achieved with the ARG plus L-DOPA and ARG tests only with very low peak GH cut-points (0.25 and 0.21 microg/liter, respectively) and not at all with the L-DOPA test. Although serum IGF-I levels provided less diagnostic discrimination than all five GH stimulation tests, a value below 77.2 microg/liter was 95% specific for GH deficiency. In conclusion, the diagnosis of adult GH deficiency can be made without performing an ITT, provided that test-specific cut-points are used. The ARG plus GHRH test represents an excellent alternative to the ITT for the diagnosis of GH deficiency in adults

Blackman M et al. Growth Hormone and Sex Steroid Administration in Healthy Aged Women and Men. JAMA November 13, 2002. Vol 288 No 18. CONTEXT: Hormone administration to elderly individuals can increase lean body mass (LBM) and decrease fat, but interactive effects of growth hormone (GH) and sex steroids and their influence on strength and endurance are unknown. OBJECTIVE: To evaluate the effects of recombinant human GH and/or sex steroids on body composition, strength, endurance, and adverse outcomes in aged persons. DESIGN, SETTING, AND PARTICIPANTS: A 26-

week randomized, double-blind, placebo-controlled parallel-group trial in healthy, ambulatory, community-dwelling US women (n = 57) and men (n = 74) aged 65 to 88 years recruited between June 1992 and July 1998. INTERVENTIONS: Participants were randomized to receive GH (starting dose, 30 micro g/kg, reduced to 20 micro g/kg, subcutaneously 3 times/wk) + sex steroids (women: transdermal estradiol, 100 micro g/d, plus oral medroxyprogesterone acetate, 10 mg/d, during the last 10 days of each 28-day cycle [HRT]; men: testosterone enanthate, biweekly intramuscular injections of 100 mg) (n = 35); GH + placebo sex steroid (n = 30); sex steroid + placebo GH (n = 35); or placebo GH + placebo sex steroid (n = 31) in a 2 x 2 factorial design. MAIN OUTCOME MEASURES: Lean body mass, fat mass, muscle strength, maximum oxygen uptake (VO (2) max) during treadmill test, and adverse effects. RESULTS: In women, LBM increased by 0.4 kg with placebo, 1.2 kg with HRT (P =.09), 1.0 kg with GH (P =.001), and 2.1 kg with GH + HRT (P<.001). Fat mass decreased significantly in the GH and GH + HRT groups. In men, LBM increased by 0.1 kg with placebo, 1.4 kg with testosterone (P =.06), 3.1 kg with GH (P<.001), and 4.3 kg with GH + testosterone (P<.001). Fat mass decreased significantly with GH and GH + testosterone. Women's strength decreased in the placebo group and increased nonsignificantly with HRT (P =.09), GH (P =.29), and GH + HRT (P =.14). Men's strength also did not increase significantly except for a marginally significant increase of 13.5 kg with GH + testosterone (P =.05). Women's VO (2) max declined by 0.4 mL/min/kg in the placebo and HRT groups but increased with GH (P =.07) and GH + HRT (P =.06). Men's VO (2) max declined by 1.2 mL/min/kg with placebo and by 0.4 mL/min/kg with testosterone (P =.49) but increased with GH (P =.11) and with GH + testosterone (P<.001). Changes in strength (r = 0.355; P<.001) and in VO (2) max (r = 0.320; P =.002) were directly related to changes in LBM. Edema was significantly more common in women taking GH (39% vs 0%) and GH + HRT (38% vs 0%). Carpal tunnel symptoms were more common in men taking GH + testosterone (32% vs 0%) and arthralgias were more common in men taking GH (41% vs 0%). Diabetes or glucose intolerance occurred in 18 GH-treated men vs 7 not receiving GH (P =.006). CONCLUSIONS: In this study, GH with or without sex steroids in healthy, aged women and men increased LBM and decreased fat mass. Sex steroid + GH increased muscle strength marginally and VO (2) max in men, but women had no significant change in strength or cardiovascular endurance. Because adverse effects were frequent (importantly, diabetes and glucose intolerance), GH interventions in the elderly should be confined to controlled studies.

Bocchi EA et al. Growth hormone for optimization of refractory heart failure treatment. Arq Bras Cardiol 1999 Oct; 73(4):391-8 It has been reported that growth hormone may benefit selected patients with congestive heart failure. A 63-year-old man with refractory congestive heart failure waiting for heart transplantation, depending on intravenous drugs (dobutamine) and presenting with progressive worsening of the clinical status and cachexia, despite standard treatment, received growth hormone replacement (8 units per day) for optimization of congestive heart failure management. Increase in both serum growth hormone levels (from 0.3 to 0.8 microg/l) and serum IGF-1 levels (from 130 to 300ng/ml) was noted, in association with clinical status improvement, better optimization of heart failure treatment and discontinuation of dobutamine infusion. Left ventricular ejection fraction (by MUGA) increased from 13 % to 18 % and to 28 % later, in association with reduction of pulmonary pressures and increase in exercise capacity (rise in peak VO2 to 13.4 and to 16.2ml/kg/min later). The patient was "de-listed" for heart transplantation. Growth hormone may benefit selected patients with refractory heart failure.

Bohdanowicz-Pawlak A et al. Risk factors of cardiovascular disease in GH-deficient adults with hypopituitarism: a preliminary report. Med Sci Monit. 2006 Feb; 12(2):CR75-80. BACKGROUND: We estimated the influence of GH deficiency (GHD) in adults on chosen risk factors of cardiovascular disease and bone density. MATERIAL/METHODS: Fifty-four adults (mean age: 50.4 years) with hypopituitarism were studied. We measured blood pressure, body mass index, waist-to-hip ratio, total body fat, and bone mineral density and the serum levels of lipids, glucose, insulin, pituitary hormones, estradiol, testosterone, and thyroxine, and the excretion of free cortisol in 24-h urine. GHD was confirmed with the insulin intravenous test (IIT) with a GH response to IIT of <3 microg/ml. The control group consisted of 73 healthy adults. RESULTS: Increased levels of LDL-cholesterol and triglycerides and decreased levels of HDL-cholesterol in the GHD group were observed. Fasting serum glucose and insulin levels were significantly higher in the GHD group than in controls. Significant differences in the QUICKI and FIRI indexes were observed. Twenty-three percent of the hypopituitary patients were hypertensive and 65% were obese. The percentage of total body fat was significantly higher in the studied group than in controls. Thirty-seven percent of the GHD patients were osteoporotic and 23% were osteopenic. CONCLUSIONS: An atherogenic lipid profile, insulin resistance, obesity, and increased body and trunk fat in GHD adults may cause the higher risk of cardiovascular disease in these patients. GHD adults should receive human recombinant GH along with conventional replacement therapy. This may be a useful method in protecting against early onset of atherosclerosis, metabolic disturbances, and osteoporosis, especially in young patients.

Bogarin R et al. Growth hormone treatment and risk of recurrence or progression of brain tumors in children: a review. Childs Nerv Syst. 2009 Jan 14 INTRODUCTION: Brain tumors are one of the most common types of solid neoplasm in children. As life expectancy of these patients has increased with new and improved therapies, the morbidities associated with the treatments and the tumor itself have become more important.DISCUSSION: One of the most common morbidities is growth hormone deficiency, and since recombinant growth hormone (GH) became available, its use has increased exponentially. There is concern that in the population of children with brain tumors, GH treatment might increase the risk of tumor recurrence or progression or the appearance of a second neoplasm. In the light of this ongoing concern, the current literature has been reviewed to provide an update on the risk of tumor recurrence, tumor progression, or new intracranial tumor formation when GH is used to treat GH deficiency in children, who have had or have intracranial tumors.CONCLUSION: On the basis of this review, the authors conclude that the use of GH in patients with brain tumor is safe. GH therapy is not associated with an increased risk of central nervous system tumor progression or recurrence, leukemia (de novo or relapse), or extracranial non-leukemic neoplasms.

Borson-Chazot F. et al. Decrease in Carotid Intima-Media Thickness after One Year Growth Hormone (GH) Treatment in Adults with GH Deficiency J Clin Endocrinol Metab 84: 1329–1333, 1999 An increased carotid arterial intima-media thickness (IMT) has been reported in hypopituitary adults untreated for GH deficiency. In the present study, the effect of GH replacement on IMT and cardiovascular risk factors was prospectively investigated, in GH deficiency patients treated at a mean dose of 1 UI/day during 1 yr (n = 22) and 2 yr (n = 11). The IMT measurements were performed by the same experienced physician, and the coefficient of variation (calculated in two control groups) was below 6.5%. IMT at baseline was related to conventional risk factors. After 1 yr GH treatment, IMT decreased from 0.78 +/- 0.03 mm to 0.70 +/- 0.03 mm (P < 0.001). The decrement was observed in 21 of 22 patients. After 2 yr GH treatment, IMT had stabilized at 0.70 +/- 0.04 mm and remained significantly different from baseline values (P < 0.003). GH treatment resulted in a moderate decrease in waist circumference and body fat mass and an increase in VO2 max. Conventional cardiovascular risk factors were unmodified except for a transient 10% decrease in low-density lipoprotein cholesterol at 6 months. The contrast between the limited metabolic effect of treatment and the importance and precocity of the changes in IMT suggests that the decrease in IMT was not exclusively attributable to a reversal in the atherosclerotic process. A direct parietal effect of GH replacement on the arterial wall might also be involved. The consequences, in terms of cardiovascular risk, should be established by randomized prospective trials.

Branski LK et al. Randomized Controlled Trial to Determine the Efficacy of Long-Term Growth Hormone Treatment in Severely Burned Children., Ann Surg. 2009 Sep 2 BACKGROUND: Recovery from a massive burn is characterized by catabolic and hypermetabolic responses that persist up to 2 years and impair rehabilitation and reintegration. The objective of this study was to determine the effects of long-term treatment with recombinant human growth hormone (rhGH) on growth, hypermetabolism, body composition, bone metabolism, cardiac work, and scarring in a large prospective randomized single-center controlled clinical trial in pediatric patients with massive burns.PATIENTS AND METHODS: A total of 205 pediatric patients with massive burns over 40% total body surface area were prospectively enrolled between 1998 and 2007 (clinicaltrials.gov ID

NCT00675714). Patients were randomized to receive either placebo (n = 94) or long-term rhGH at 0.05, 0.1, or 0.2 mg/kg/d (n = 101). Changes in weight, body composition, bone metabolism, cardiac output, resting energy expenditure, hormones, and scar development were measured at patient discharge and at 6, 9, 12, 18, and 24 months postburn. Statistical analysis used Tukey t test or ANOVA followed by Bonferroni correction. Significance was accepted at P < 0.05.RESULTS: RhGH administration markedly improved growth and lean body mass, whereas hypermetabolism was significantly attenuated. Serum growth hormone, insulin-like growth factor-I, and IGFBP-3 was significantly increased, whereas percent body fat content significantly decreased when compared with placebo, P < 0.05. A subset analysis revealed most lean body mass gain in the 0.2 mg/kg group, P < 0.05. Bone mineral content showed an unexpected decrease in the 0.2 mg/kg group, along with a decrease in PTH and increase in osteocalcin levels, P < 0.05. Resting energy expenditure improved with rhGH administration, most markedly in the 0.1 mg/kg/d rhGH group, P < 0.05. Cardiac output was decreased at 12 and 18 months postburn in the rhGH group. Long-term administration of 0.1 and 0.2 mg/kg/d rhGH significantly improved scarring at 12 months postburn, P < 0.05.CONCLUSION: This large prospective clinical trial showed that long-term treatment with rhGH effectively enhances recovery of severely burned pediatric patients.

Burgess W et al. The immune-endocrine loop during aging: role of growth hormone and insulin-like growth factor-I. Neuroimmunomodulation 1999 Jan-Apr; 6(1-2):56-68 Why a primary lymphoid organ such as the thymus involutes during aging remains a fundamental question in immunology. Aging is associated with a decrease in plasma growth hormone (somatotropin) and IGF-I and this somatopause of aging suggests a connection between the neuroendocrine and immune systems. Several investigators have demonstrated that treatment with either growth hormone or IGF-I restores architecture of the involuted thymus gland by reversing the loss of immature cortical thymocytes and preventing the decline in thymulin synthesis that occurs in old or GH-deficient animals and humans. The proliferation, differentiation and functions of other components of the immune system, including T and B cells, macrophages and neutrophils, also demonstrate age-associated decrements that can be restored by IGF-I. Knowledge of the mechanism by which cytokines and hormones influence hematopoietic cells is critical to improving the health of aged individuals. Our laboratory has recently demonstrated that IGF-I prevents apoptosis in promyeloid cells, which subsequently permits these cells to differentiate into neutrophils. We also demonstrated that IL-4 acts much like IGF-I to promote survival of promyeloid cells and to activate the enzyme phosphatidylinositol 3'-kinase (PI 3-kinase). However, the receptors for IGF-I and IL-4 are completely different, with the intracellular beta chains of the IGF receptor possessing intrinsic tyrosine kinase activity and the alpha and gammac subunit of the heterodimeric IL-4 receptor utilizing the Janus kinase family of nonreceptor protein kinases to tyrosine phosphorylate downstream targets. Both receptors share many of the components of the PI 3-kinase signal transduction pathway, converging at the level of insulin receptor substrate-1 or insulin receptor subtrate-2 (formally known as 4PS, or IL-4 Phosphorylated Substrate). Our investigations with IGF-I and IL-4 suggest that PI 3-kinase inhibits apoptosis by maintaining high levels of the anti-apoptotic protein Bcl-2. The sharing of common activation molecules, despite vastly different protein structures of their receptors, forms a molecular explanation for the possibility of cross talk between IL-4 and IGF-I in regulating many of the events associated with hematopoietic differentiation, proliferation and survival.

Cappola AR et al. Association of IGF-I levels with muscle strength and mobility in older women. J Clin Endocrinol Metab 2001 Sep; 86(9):4139-46 The functional consequences of the age-associated decline in IGF-I are unknown. We hypothesized that low IGF-I levels in older women would be associated with poor muscle strength and mobility. We assessed this question in a population representative of the full spectrum of health in the community, obtaining serum IGF-I levels from women aged 70-79 yr, enrolled in the Women's Health and Aging Study I or II. Cross-sectional analyses were performed using 617 women with IGF-I levels drawn within 90 d of measurement of outcomes. After adjustment for age, there was an association between IGF-I and knee extensor strength ($P = 0.004$), but not anthropometry or other strength measures. We found a positive relationship between IGF-I levels and walking speed for IGF-I levels below 50 microg/liter ($P < 0.001$), but no relationship above this threshold. A decline in IGF-I level was associated with self-reported difficulty in mobility tasks. All findings were attenuated after multivariate adjustment. In summary, in a study population including frail and healthy older women, low IGF-I levels were associated with poor knee extensor muscle strength, slow walking speed, and self-reported difficulty with mobility tasks. These findings suggest a role for IGF-I in disability as well as a potential target population for interventions to raise IGF-I levels.

Cappola et al. Insulin-like growth factor I and interleukin-6 contribute synergistically to disability and mortality in older women JCEM, 2003 May; 88(5):2019-25. The physiology of age-related functional decline is poorly understood, but may involve hormones and inflammation. We hypothesized that older women with both low IGF-I and high IL-6 levels are at high risk for disability and death. We assessed walking speed and disability in 718 women enrolled in the Women's Health and Aging Study I, a 3-yr cohort study with 5-yr mortality follow-up. Women with IGF-I levels in the lowest quartile and IL-6 levels in the highest quartile had significantly greater limitation in walking and disability in mobility tasks and instrumental activities of daily living than those with neither risk factor (adjusted odds ratios, 10.77, 5.14, and 3.66). Women with both risk factors were at greater risk for death (adjusted relative risk, 2.10) as well as incident walking limitation, mobility disability, and disability in activities of daily living compared with those with high IGF-I and low IL-6 levels. The combination of low IGF-I and high IL-6 levels confers a high risk for progressive disability and death in older women, suggesting an aggregate effect of dysregulation in endocrine and immune systems. The joint effects of IGF-I and IL-6 may be important targets for treatments to prevent or minimize disability associated with aging.

Chan et al. Plasma insulin-like growth factor-I and prostate cancer risk: a prospective study. Science Vol 279 January 1998 Insulin-like growth factor-I (IGF-I) is a mitogen for prostate epithelial cells. To investigate associations between plasma IGF levels and prostate cancer risk, a nested case-control study within the Physicians' Health Study was conducted on prospectively collected plasma from 152 cases and 152 controls. A strong positive association was observed between IGF-I levels and prostate cancer risk. Men in the highest quartile of IGF-I levels had a relative risk of 4.3 (95 percent confidence interval 1.8 to 10.6) compared with men in the lowest quartile. This association was independent of baseline prostate-specific antigen levels. Identification of plasma IGF-I as a predictor of prostate cancer risk may have implications for risk reduction and treatment.

Cherbonnier C et al. Potentiation of tumour apoptosis by human growth hormone via glutathione production and decreased NF-kappaB activity. Br J Cancer. 2003 Sep 15;89(6):1108-15 In addition to its primary role as growth factor, human growth hormone (hGH) can also participate in cell survival, as already documented by its protective effect on human monocytes or human promyelocytic leukaemia U937 cells exposed to a Fas-mediated cell death signal. However, despite similarities in the molecular events following Fas and TNF-alpha receptor engagement, we report that U937 cells, genetically engineered to constitutively produce hGH, were made more sensitive to TNF-alpha-induced apoptosis than parental cells. This was due to overproduction of the antioxidant glutathione, which decreased the nuclear factor (NF)-kappaB activity known to control the expression of survival genes. These findings were confirmed in vivo, in nude mice bearing U937 tumours coinjected with recombinant hGH and the NF-kappaB -inducing anticancer drug daunorubicin, to avoid the in vivo toxicity of TNF-alpha. This study therefore highlights one of the various properties of hGH that may have potential clinical implications.

Christiansen, J. Influence of growth hormone and androgens on body composition in adults. Horm Res. 1996; 45(1-2):94-8. The secretion of both growth hormone (GH) and androgens declines with age which may play a role in the senescent changes in body composition and organ function. Among healthy adults abdominal adiposity is an important negative determinant of GH secretion. Surprisingly, abdominal or android obesity seems inversely correlated with testosterone levels in males but not in females. The ability of GH to promote lipolysis and preserve or increase lean body mass has been reappraised in substitution studies in GH-deficient adults. By comparison, adequately controlled studies of androgen replacement in hypogonadal and/or elderly males are few. In view of the physiological and clinical relevance of obtaining information about the aging process, there is a need for controlled experiments addressing similarities and differences between the action of GH and sex steroids in adults.

Colao A et al. Impaired cardiac performance in elderly patients with growth hormone deficiency J Clin Endocrinol Metab 1999 Nov; 84(11):3950-5 Several evidences indicate that GH and/or insulin-like growth factor I (IGF-I) are involved in the regulation of cardiovascular function. In patients with childhood and adulthood-onset GH deficiency (GHD), the impairment of cardiac performance is manifest primarily as a reduction in the left ventricular (LV) mass (LVM), inadequacy of LV ejection fraction both at rest and at peak exercise, and abnormalities of LV diastolic filling. No study has been reported to date in elderly GHD patients that investigated cardiac function. In particular, it is unknown whether cardiac function is modified in accordance with patients' age as a physiological response to aging, as in normal subjects the rate and extent of LV filling are reduced with age. This study was designed to evaluate heart morphology and function, by echocardiography and equilibrium radionuclide angiography, respectively, in rigorously selected elderly patients with GHD but without evidence of other complications able to affect cardiac performance. Eleven patients with hypopituitarism (6 men and 5 women, aged 60-72 yr) and 11 sex- age- and body mass index-matched healthy subjects entered this study. None of the patients and controls presented with or had previously suffered from other concomitant diseases, such as diabetes mellitus, coronary artery diseases, long-standing hypertension, and hyperthyroidism, which could affect cardiac function. All patients had been previously operated on via the transsphenoidal and/or transcranic route for nonfunctioning pituitary adenoma, meningioma, or craniopharyngioma, and 6 of them had been irradiated. Eight patients had FSH/LH insufficiency, 5 had TSH insufficiency and 6 had ACTH insufficiency, appropriately replaced. All subjects were tested with the combined arginine plus GHRH test showing a GH response below 9 microg/L. No significant difference was found in plasma IGF-I levels (49.2 +/- 8.5 vs. 71.8 +/- 7.5 microg/L) between patients and controls. However, IGF-I levels were lower than the normal range in 8 patients and 3 controls. Interventricular septum thickness (9.1 +/- 0.2 vs. 9.1 +/- 0.2 mm), LV posterior wall thickness (9.1 +/- 0.2 vs. 9.0 +/- 0.2 mm), and LVM after correction for body surface area (97.6 +/- 1.8 vs. 99.9 +/- 1.5 g/m2) were similar in patients and controls. Similarly, the LV ejection fraction at rest was similar in patients and controls (57.1 +/- 2% vs. 63.2 +/- 2.5%; P = NS), and it was normal (> or = 50%) in all controls and in 10 of 11 patients. By contrast, the LV ejection fraction at peak exercise was markedly depressed in elderly GHD patients compared to age-matched controls (51 +/- 2.5% vs. 73.3 +/- 3%; P < 0.001). A normal response (> or = 5% increase compared to basal value) of LV ejection fraction at peak exercise was found in 8 controls (72.7%) and in 2 of 11 patients (18.2%). No difference was found in the peak rate of LV filling, whether peak filling rate was normalized to end-diastolic volume (2.5 +/- 0.2 vs. 2.6 +/- 0.2 end-diastolic volume/s) or stroke volume (4.3 +/- 0.3 vs. 4.0 +/- 0.3 stroke volume/s), between patients and controls. Finally, exercise duration was significantly shorter in elderly GHD patients than in age-matched controls (7.2 +/- 2.1 vs. 9.1 +/- 0.2 min; P < 0.01). In the patient group, the GH peak after arginine plus GHRH test was significantly correlated with the LV ejection fraction at rest (r = 0.822; P < 0.01), whereas IGF-I was significantly correlated with the peak rate of LV filling whether the peak filling rate was normalized to end-diastolic volume (r = -0.863; P < 0.001) or stroke volume (r = -0.616; P < 0.05) or expressed as the ratio of peak filling rate to peak ejection fraction rate (r = -0.736; P < 0.01). Disease duration was significantly correlated with heart rate at peak exercise (r = 0.614; P < 0.05) and with systolic and diastolic blood pressures both at rest (r = 0.745; P < 0.01 and r = 0.650; P < 0.05) and at peak exercise (r = 0.684; P < 0.05

Colao A.Bone loss is correlated to the severity of growth hormone deficiency in adult patients with hypopituitarism. J Clin Endocrinol Metab 1999 Jun; 84(6):1919-24 Reduced bone mineral density (BMD) has been reported in patients with isolated GH deficiency (GHD) or with multiple pituitary hormone deficiencies (MPHD). To investigate whether the severity of GHD was correlated with the degree of bone mass and turnover impairment, we evaluated BMD at the lumbar spine and femoral neck; circulating insulin-like growth factor I (IGF-I), IGF-binding protein-3 (IGFBP-3), and osteocalcin levels, and urinary cross-linked N-telopeptides of type I collagen (Ntx) levels in 101 adult hypopituitary patients and 35 sex- and age-matched healthy subjects. On the basis of the GH response to arginine plus GHRH (ARG+/-GHRH), patients were subdivided into 4 groups: group 1 included 41 patients with a GH peak below 3 microg/L (0.9 +/- 0.08 microg/L), defined as very severe GHD; group 2 included 25 patients with a GH peak between 3.1-9 microg/L (4.7 +/- 0.4 microg/L), defined as severe GHD; group 3 included 18 patients with a GH peak between 9.1-16.5 microg/L (11.0 +/- 0.3 microg/L), defined as partial GHD; and group 4 included 17 patients with a GH peak above 16.5 microg/L (28.3 +/- 4.3 microg/L), defined as non-GHD. In all 35 controls (group 5), the GH response after ARG+/-GHRH was above 16.5 microg/L (40.7 +/- 2.2 microg/L). In patients in group 1, circulating IGF-I (P < 0.001), IGFBP-3 (P < 0.05), osteocalcin (P < 0.001), and urinary Ntx levels (P < 0.001) were lower than those in group 3-5, which were not different from each other; the t score at the lumbar spine (-1.99 +/- 0.2) and that at the femoral neck (-1.86 +/- 0.3) were lower than those in groups 3 (-0.5 +/- 0.7, P < 0.01 and -0.3 +/- 0.7, P < 0.01, respectively), 4 (-0.5 +/- 0.2, P < 0.01 and -0.3 +/- 0.7, P < 0.01, respectively), and 5 (-0.5 +/- 0.2, P < 0.001 and 0.0 +/- 0.02, P < 0.001, respectively). In patients in group 2, circulating IGF-I and IGFBP-3 levels were not different from those in group 1, whereas the t scores at the lumbar spine (-1.22 +/- 0.3) and femoral neck (-0.9 +/- 0.3) were significantly higher and lower, respectively, than those in groups 1 and 5 (P < 0.05) but not those in groups 3 and 4, and serum osteocalcin and urinary Ntx levels were significant higher than those in group 1 and lower than those in groups 3-5 (P < 0.001). To evaluate the effect of isolated GHD vs. MPHD, patients were subdivided according to the number of their hormonal deficits, such as panhypopituitarism with (10 patients) or without (31 patients) diabetes insipidus, GHD with 1 or more additional pituitary deficit(s) (36 patients), isolated GHD (7 patients), 1-2 pituitary hormone deficit(s) without GHD (10 patients), and normal anterior pituitary function (7 patients). The t score at the lumbar spine and femoral neck and the biochemical parameters of bone turnover were not significantly different among the different subgroups with similar GH secretions. A significant correlation was found between the GH peak after ARG+GHRH and IGF-I, osteocalcin, urinary Ntx levels, and the t score at the lumbar spine, but not that at the femoral neck level. A significant correlation was also found between plasma IGF-I levels and the t score at the lumbar spine and femoral neck, serum osteocalcin, and urinary Ntx. Multiple correlation analysis revealed that the t score at the lumbar spine, but not that at the femoral neck, was more strongly predicted by plasma IGF-I levels (t = 3.376; P < 0.005) than by the GH peak after ARG+GHRH (t = -0.968; P = 0.338). In conclusion, a significant reduction of BMD associated with abnormalities of bone turnover parameters was found only in patients with very severe or severe GHD, whereas normal BMD values were found in non-GHD hypopituitary patients. These abnormalities were consistently present in all patients with GHD regardless of the presence of additional hormone deficits, suggesting that GHD plays a central role in the development of osteopenia in hypopituitary patients.

Colao A et al. Beginning to end: Cardiovascular implications of growth hormone (GH) deficiency and GH therapy. Growth Horm IGF Res. 2006 May 9 BACKGROUND: Partial GH deficiency (GHD) in adults is poorly studied. OBJECTIVE: The objective of the study was to investigate the natural history and clinical implications of partial GHD. STUDY DESIGN: This was an analytical, observational, prospective, case-control study. PATIENTS: Twenty-seven hypopituitary patients (15 women, ages 20-60 yr) and 27 controls participated in the study. MAIN OUTCOME MEASURES: Measures included GH peak after GHRH plus arginine [(GHRH+ARG), measured by immunoradiometric assay]; IGF-I (measured after ethanol extraction) z-sd score (SDS); glucose, insulin, total cholesterol, high-density lipoprotein (HDL) cholesterol, and triglyceride levels; and common carotid arteries intima-media thickness (IMT) measured periodically. RESULTS: At study entry, partial GHD patients had significantly lower IGF-I and HDL-cholesterol levels and homeostasis model assessment index than controls. During the 60 months of median follow-up, 11 patients had severe GHD (40.7%); seven normalized their GH response (25.9%), and nine showed persistently partial GHD (33.3%). Patients with developed severe GHD at baseline had similar age and body mass index and lower GH peak (11.5 +/- 1.8 vs. 14.3 +/- 1.5 and 12.8 +/- 1.1 microg/liter, P = 0.008) and IGF-I SDS (-0.88 +/- 0.48 vs. 0.15 +/- 0.58 and -0.42 +/- 0.78; P = 0.01) than the patients with normal GH secretion or partial GHD. Severe GHD was accompanied by decreased IGF-I SDS and increased total to HDL cholesterol ratio, triglycerides, homeostasis model assessment index, and carotid intima-media thickness; normalization of GH secretion was accompanied by increased IGF-I SDS. By receiving-operator characteristic analysis, predictors of severe GHD were a baseline GH peak after GHRH+ARG of 11.5 microg/liter (sensitivity 64%, specificity 94%) and a baseline IGF-I SDS of -0.28 (sensitivity 91%, specificity 63%). CONCLUSIONS: Of 27 patients with partial GHD after pituitary surgery, 40.7% developed severe GHD and 25.9% normalized their GH response. With the assay used, changes in the GH peak response to GHRH+ARG were accompanied by changes in the IGF-I SDS, metabolic profile, and carotid IMT. A peak GH of 11.5 microg/liter or less and IGF-I SDS -0.28 or less were highly predictive of delayed deterioration of GH secretion.

Colao A et al. Effect of growth hormone (GH) and insulin-like growth factor I on prostate diseases: an ultrasonographic and endocrine study in acromegaly. J Clin Endocrinol Metab 1999 Jun; 84(6):1986-91 The role of insulin-like growth factor I (IGF-I) in prostate development is currently under thorough investigation because it has been claimed that IGF-I is a positive predictor of prostate cancer. To assess the effect of GH and IGF-I levels on prostate pathophysiology, 46 acromegalic (30 in active disease, 10 cured from acromegaly, and 6 affected from GH deficiency) and 30 age-matched male controls, free from previous or concomitant prostate disorders, underwent pituitary, androgen, and prostate hormonal assessments and transrectal ultrasonography. Compared to control values, GH (P < 0.0001), IGF-I (P < 0.0001), and IGFBP-3 (P < 0.001) levels were increased, whereas testosterone (P < 0.0001) and dihydrotestosterone levels (P < 0.0001) were reduced in active acromegalic patients. Hypogonadism was present in 28 of the 46 acromegalic patients (60.8%). The anteroposterior (P < 0.05), and transverse (P < 0.0001) prostate diameters and the transitional zone volume (P < 0.05) were increased in acromegalic patients compared to those in controls. Prostate volume (PV) was significantly higher in untreated acromegalic patients than in controls (41.7 +/- 3.2 vs. 21.9 +/- 1.4 mL; P < 0.0001), cured patients (23.6 +/- 1.6 mL; P < 0.0001), and GH-deficient patients (17.5 +/- 1.1 mL; P < 0.0001). In the patients, PV was correlated with disease duration (r = 0.606; P < 0.0001) and age (r = 0.496; P < 0.0001), whereas in controls it was correlated with age (r = 0.476; P < 0.01) and IGF-I levels (r = -0.448; P < 0.05). Benign prostate hyperplasia (PV > or = 30 mL) was found in 58% of the acromegalics and 26.6% of the controls. When grouped by age (<40, 40-60, and >60 yr), PV was increased in elderly patients compared to younger patients (P < 0.05) and to controls (P < 0.01). The prevalence of structural abnormalities, including calcifications, nodules, cysts, and vesicle inflammation, was significantly increased in patients compared to controls (78.2% vs. 23.3%; chi2 = 5.856; P < 0.05). No clinical, transrectal ultrasonography or cytological evidence of prostate cancer was detected in acromegalic or control subjects. In conclusion, chronic excess of GH and IGF-I cause prostate overgrowth and further phenomena of rearrangement, but not prostate cancer.

Collier SR et al. Growth hormone responses to varying doses of oral arginine.Growth Horm IGF Res. 2005 Apr; 15(2):136-9. Intravenous (IV) arginine invokes an increase in growth hormone (GH) concentrations, however, little is known about the impact of oral arginine ingestion on the GH response. OBJECTIVE: The purpose of this study was to determine the dose of oral arginine that elicits an optimal GH response and to determine the time course of the response. DESIGN: Eight healthy males (18-33 years - 24.8+/-1.2 years) were studied on 4 separate occasions. Following an overnight fast at 0700 h, a catheter was placed in a forearm vein. Blood samples were taken every 10 min for 5 h. Thirty minutes after sampling was initiated; the subject ingested a dose of arginine (5, 9 or 13 g) or placebo (randomly assigned). RESULTS: Mean resting GH values for the placebo, 5, 9 and 13 g day were 0.76, 0.67, 2.0 and 0.79 microg/L (n=6), respectively. Integrated area under the curve was not different with 13 g (197.8+/-65.7 min microg/L), yet it increased with 5 and 9 g compared with the placebo (301.5+/-74.6, 524.28+/-82.9 and 186.04+/-47.8 min microg/L, respectively, P<0.05). Mean peak GH levels were 2.9+/-0.69, 3.9+/-0.85, 6.4+/-1.3 and 4.73+/-1.27 microg/L on each day for the placebo, 5, 9 and 13 g days. CONCLUSION: In conclusion, 5 and 9 g of oral arginine caused a significant GH response. A 13 g dose of arginine resulted in considerable gastrointestinal distress in most subjects without augmentation in the GH response. The rise in GH concentration started approximately 30 min after ingestion and peaked approximately 60 min post ingestion.

Cook, D et al. Route of Estrogen Administration Helps to Determine Growth Hormone (GH) Replacement Dose in GH-Deficient Adults. J Clin Endocrinol Metab 1999Nov; 84: (11): 3956–3960, We prospectively studied two groups of GH-deficient patients during GH therapy based upon exposure of the liver to elevated (oral estrogen) or not elevated (endogenous or transdermal) sources of estrogen. We wondered whether higher concentrations of estrogen at the liver level (oral estrogen) might inhibit insulin-like growth factor I (IGF-I) secretion and alter exogenous GH requirements. In this study we compared GH replacement requirements in these two groups of women as well as with GH-treated adult hypopituitary males. The final GH dose was based upon maintenance IGF-I levels in the mid- to high normal range adjusted for age and sex or symptom tolerance. Each group [women taking oral estrogen (n = 12), women not taking oral estrogen (n = 13), and men (n = 12)] was similar in age and final IGF-I concentration. Women taking oral estrogen required 10.6 +/- 0.7 microg/kg x day or 867 +/- 45 microg/day GH, women not taking oral estrogen required 5.0 +/- 0.7 microg/kg x day or 424 +/- 57 microg/day, and men required 4.1 +/- 0.6 microg/kg x day or 376 +/- 49 microg/day to achieve similar IGF-I concentrations. GH requirements in men were not different from those in women not taking oral estrogen, but the GH requirements in both groups were significantly different from GH requirements in women taking oral estrogen. These observations may be useful in anticipating appropriate starting and final doses of GH in adult hypopituitary patients.

Cook DM.Shouldn't adults with growth hormone deficiency be offered growth hormone replacement therapy?Ann Intern Med 2002 Aug 6;137(3):197-201Growth hormone as therapy for adults with growth hormone deficiency has not been universally accepted by endocrinologists who treat adult patients. The following are addressed in this commentary: the evidence on safety and efficacy in the literature supporting the idea that growth hormone should be offered as replacement therapy to adults who are growth hormone deficient; common concerns of the average prescribing endocrinologist, including the purported association between insulin-like growth factor-I and malignant neoplasms and quality-of-life issues with long-term therapy; and controversial subjects, such as differences in dosing for adults versus children and diagnostic issues. This analysis should encourage reluctant practitioners to at least consider growth hormone replacement therapy for patients with definite growth hormone deficiency--that is, patients with symptomatic panhypopituitarism.

Corpas E et al. Oral arginine-lysine does not increase growth hormone or insulin-like growth factor-I in old men. J Gerontol 1993 Jul; 48(4):M128-33 BACKGROUND. Older adults tend to have reduced growth hormone (GH) secretion and insulin-like growth factor I (IGF-I) levels as well as changes in body composition which are partially reversed by GH injections. Arginine stimulates GH release, and lysine may amplify this response. We investigated whether oral arginine/lysine could be used to increase basal IGF-I and GH levels in non-obese old men (age 69 +/- 5 years; mean +/- SD) to values similar to those of untreated young men (age 26 +/- 4 years). METHODS. Two groups of 8 healthy old men were treated with 3 g of arginine plus 3 g of lysine or with placebo capsules twice daily for 14 days. Before and on day 14 of each treatment GH levels were determined in blood samples taken at 20-minute intervals from 2000-0800 h, IGF-I was measured at 0800 h, and a 1 microgram/kg GHRH stimulation test was done. RESULTS. At baseline, mean GH peak amplitude (p < .02) and serum IGF-I (p < .0001) were lower, whereas GHRH responses were similar, in old vs young men. Arginine/lysine did not significantly alter spontaneous or GHRH-stimulated GH levels, or serum IGF-I. Arginine absorption was age-independent. The correlation (p < .005) between measured increments in serum arginine and increases in serum GH after a single dose of arginine/lysine was similar in old and young groups. CONCLUSIONS. Our data suggest that oral arginine/lysine is not a practical means of chronically enhancing GH secretion in old men.

Cuatrecasas G et al. Growth hormone as concomitant treatment in severe fibromyalgia associated with low IGF-1 serum levels. BMC Musculoskelet Disord. 2007 Nov 30 BACKGROUND: There is evidence of functional growth hormone (GH) deficiency, expressed by means of low insulin-like growth factor 1 (IGF-1) serum levels, in a subset of fibromyalgia patients. The efficacy of GH versus placebo has been previously suggested in this population. We investigated the efficacy and safety of low dose GH as an adjunct to standard therapy in the treatment of severe, prolonged and well-treated fibromyalgia patients with low IGF-1 levels.METHODS: Twenty-four patients were enrolled in a randomized, open-label, best available care-controlled study. Patients were randomly assigned to receive either 0.0125 mg/kg/d of GH subcutaneously (titrated depending on IGF-1) added to standard therapy or standard therapy alone during one year. The number of tender points, the Fibromyalgia Impact Questionnaire (FIQ) and the EuroQol 5D (EQ-5D), including a Quality of Life visual analogic scale (EQ-VAS) were assessed at different time-points.RESULTS: At the end of the study, the GH group showed a 60% reduction in the mean number of tender points (pairs) compared to the control group (p < 0.05; 3.25 +/- 0.8 vs. 8.25 +/- 0.9). Similar improvements were observed in FIQ score (p < 0.05) and EQ-VAS scale (p < 0.001). There was a prompt response to GH administration, with most patients showing improvement within the first months in most of the outcomes. The concomitant administration of GH and standard therapy was well tolerated, and no patients discontinued the study due to adverse events.CONCLUSION: The present findings indicate the advantage of adding a daily GH dose to the standard therapy in a subset of severe fibromyalgia patients with low IGF-1 serum levels

Drake W et al Optimizing growth hormone replacement therapy by dose titration in hypopituitary adults. J Clin Endocrinol Metab 1998 Nov; 83(11):3913-9 Although growth hormone (GH) replacement therapy is increasingly utilized in the management of adult hypopituitary patients, optimum dosing schedules are poorly defined. The use of weight-based or surface area-based dosing may result in overtreatment, and individual variation in susceptibility on the basis of gender and other factors is now being recognized. To optimize GH replacement and to explore further gender differences in susceptibility, we used a dose titration regimen, starting at the initiation of GH replacement therapy, in 50 consecutive adult-onset hypopituitary patients, and compared the results with those in 21 patients previously treated using a weight-based regimen. Titrated patients commenced GH 0.8 IU/day subcutaneously (0.4 IU/day if hypertensive or glucose tolerance impaired). Serum insulin-like growth factor I (IGF-I) was measured at 0, 2, 4, 6, 8, 10, and 12 weeks in all patients. Serum IGF binding protein 3 and acid labile subunit were measured at the same time points in 17 patients (8 male, 9 female). Patients were reviewed every 4 weeks and the dose of GH increased, if necessary, to achieve a serum IGF-I level between the median and the upper end of the age-related reference range. There was no significant difference between mean serum IGF-I at 2 and 4 weeks, or between 6 and 8 weeks, indicating that the full effects of a change in dose are evident within 2 weeks of that change. Maintenance doses were significantly higher in females than males [1.2 (0.8-2.0) vs. 0.8 (0.4-1.6) IU/day; median (range); P < 0.0001], and the median time to achieve maintenance dose was significantly shorter in males [4 (2-12) vs. 9 (2-26) weeks; P < 0.0001]. Median maintenance dose was lower overall than in a group of 21 patients initially commenced on GH using a weight-based dosing schedule, with subsequent adjustment of dose during clinical follow-up [1.5 (0.4-3.2) IU/day; P = 0.02]. Reduction in waist measurement and waist to hip ratio at 6 and 12 months was similar in females (P < 0.001) and males (P < 0.01). Well-being improved significantly after 3 months of GH therapy (14.2 +/- 5.9 vs. 7.4 +/- 4.5 SD; P < 0.0001), and there were no gender differences. Adult Growth Hormone Deficiency Assessment (AGHDA) scores at 6 months were similar to maintenance scores in patients commenced on weight-based regimens. Measurements of ALS and IGFBP-3 added no useful extra information to IGF-I in managing the dose titration. The practical scheme outlined for dose titration of GH replacement resulted in rapid achievement of lower maintenance doses than those achieved using conventional weight-based regimens without loss of efficacy. It was particularly important in female patients who demonstrated decreased overall sensitivity to GH and required higher doses to achieve the same effects as males. This constitutes the first report of a uniform titration regimen based on a defined target range of serum IGF-I in a large patient cohort.

Fazio et al. A preliminary study of GH in the treatment of dilated cardiomyopathy. NEJM 1996:334:809-814 BACKGROUND. Cardiac hypertrophy is a physiologic response that allows the heart to adapt to an excess hemodynamic load. We hypothesized that inducing cardiac hypertrophy with recombinant human growth hormone might be an effective approach to the treatment of idiopathic dilated cardiomyopathy, a condition in which compensatory cardiac hypertrophy is believed to be deficient. METHODS. Seven patients with idiopathic dilated cardiomyopathy and moderate-to-severe heart failure were studied at base line, after three months of therapy with human growth hormone, and three months after the discontinuation of growth hormone. Standard therapy for heart failure was continued throughout the study. Cardiac function was evaluated with Doppler echocardiography, right-heart catheterization, and exercise testing. RESULTS. When administered at a dose of 14 IU per week, growth hormone doubled the serum concentrations of insulin-like growth factor I. Growth hormone increased left-ventricular-wall thickness and reduced chamber size significantly. Consequently, end-systolic wall stress (a function of both wall thickness and chamber size) fell markedly (from a mean [+/-SE] of 144+/-11 to 85+/-8 dyn per square centimeter, P<0.001). Growth hormone improved cardiac output, particularly during exercise (from 7.4+/-0.7 to 9.7+/-0.9 liters per minute, P=0.003), and enhanced ventricular work, despite reductions in myocardial oxygen consumption (from 56+/-6 to 39+/-5 ml per minute, P=0.005) and energy production (from 1014+/-100 to 701+/-80 J per minute, P=0.002). Thus, ventricular mechanical efficiency rose from 9+/-2 to 21+/-5 percent (P=0.006). Growth hormone also improved clinical symptoms, exercise capacity, and the patients' quality of life. The changes in cardiac size and shape, systolic function, and exercise tolerance were partially reversed three months after growth hormone was discontinued. CONCLUSIONS- Recombinant human growth hormone administered for three months to patients with idiopathic dilated cardiomyopathy increased myocardial mass and reduced the size of the left ventricular chamber, resulting in improvement in hemodynamics, myocardial energy metabolism, and clinical status.

Fiebig HH et al. No evidence of tumor growth stimulation in human tumors in vitro following treatment with recombinant human growth hormone Anticancer Drugs 2000 Sep;11(8):659-64 In a recent study we demonstrated that recombinant human growth hormone (r-hGH; Saizen) delayed tumor-induced cachexia in human tumor xenografts in vivo. Such a therapeutic effect could have a great impact in the supportive care of advanced cancer patients. Before large clinical studies are initiated possible growth stimulation should be excluded. This question was investigated in vitro in 20 human tumor models, which had been established in serial passage in nude mice. The effect of continuous exposure of r-hGH was investigated at dose levels ranging from 0.3 ng/ml up to 0.1 microg/ml in colorectal (n=2), gastric (n=1), non-small cell lung (n=4), small cell lung (n=1), mammary (n=3), ovarian (n=2), prostate (n=2) and renal cancers (n=2), and melanoma (n=3) using a modified Hamburger and Salmon clonogenic assay. The results show that there was neither tumor growth inhibition nor any evidence for tumor growth stimulation in any of the tumors studies. Therefore this preclinical study in 20 human tumor models indicated no direct risk for tumor growth enhancement.

Franco C et al. Growth hormone treatment reduces abdominal visceral fat in postmenopausal women with abdominal obesity: a 12-month placebo-controlled trial. J Clin Endocrinol Metab. 2005 Mar; 90(3):1466-74 Abdominal obesity is associated with blunted GH secretion and a cluster of cardiovascular risk factors that characterize the metabolic syndrome. GH treatment in abdominally obese men reduces visceral adipose tissue and has beneficial effects on the metabolic profile. There are no long-term data on the effects of GH treatment on postmenopausal women with abdominal obesity. Forty postmenopausal women with abdominal obesity participated in a randomized, double-blind, placebo-controlled, 12-month trial with GH (0.67 mg/d). The primary aim was to study the effect of GH treatment on insulin sensitivity. Measurements of glucose disposal rate (GDR) using a euglycemic, hyperinsulinemic glucose clamp; abdominal fat, hepatic fat content, and thigh muscle area using computed tomography; and total body fat and fat-free mass derived from (40)K measurements were performed at baseline and at 6 and 12 months. GH treatment reduced visceral fat mass, increased thigh muscle area, and reduced total and low-density lipoprotein cholesterol compared with placebo. Insulin sensitivity was increased at 12 months compared with baseline values in the GH-treated group. In the GH-treated group only, a low baseline GDR was correlated with a more marked improvement in insulin sensitivity ($r = -0.68$; $P < 0.001$). A positive correlation was found between changes in GDR and liver attenuation as a measure of hepatic fat content between baseline and 12 months ($r = 0.7$; $P < 0.001$) in the GH-treated group. In postmenopausal women with abdominal obesity, 1 yr of GH treatment improved insulin sensitivity and reduced abdominal visceral fat and total and low-density lipoprotein cholesterol concentrations. The improvement in insulin sensitivity was associated with reduced hepatic fat content.

French RA et al. Age-Associated Loss of Bone Marrow Hematopoietic Cells Is Reversed by GH and Accompanies Thymic Reconstitution Endocrinology Vol. 143, No. 2 690-699, Jan 2002 Deterioration of the thymus gland during aging is accompanied by a reduction in plasma GH. Here we report gross and microscopic results from 24-month-old Wistar-Furth rats treated with rat GH derived from syngeneic GH3 cells or with recombinant human GH. Histological evaluation of aged rats treated with either rat or human GH displayed clear morphologic evidence of thymic regeneration, reconstitution of hematopoietic cells in the bone marrow, and multiorgan extramedullary hematopoiesis. Quantitative evaluation of formalin-fixed, hematoxylin and eosin-stained sections of bone marrow from aged rats revealed at least a 50% reduction in the number hematopoietic bone marrow cells, compared with that of young 3-month-old rats. This age-associated decline in bone marrow leukocytes, as well as the increase in bone marrow adipocytes, was significantly reversed by in vivo treatment with GH. Restoration of bone marrow cellularity was caused primarily by erythrocytic and granulocytic cells, but all cell lineages were represented and their proportions were similar to those in aged control rats. On a per-cell basis, GH treatment in vivo significantly increased the number of in vitro myeloid colony forming units in both bone marrow and spleen. Morphological evidence of enhanced extramedullary hematopoiesis was observed in the spleen, liver, and adrenal glands from animals treated with GH. These results confirm that GH prevents thymic aging. Furthermore, these data significantly extend earlier findings by establishing that GH dramatically promotes reconstitution of another primary hematopoietic tissue by reversing the accumulation of bone marrow adipocytes and by restoring the number of bone marrow myeloid cells of both the erythrocytic and granulocytic lineages.

Genth-Zotz S et al. Recombinant growth hormone therapy in patients with ischemic cardiomyopathy: effects on hemodynamics, left ventricular function, and cardiopulmonary exercise capacity. Circulation. 1999 Jan 5-12; 99(1):18-21 BACKGROUND: We studied the effects of recombinant growth hormone (rhGH) on exercise capacity and cardiac function in patients with ischemic cardiomyopathy. METHODS AND RESULTS: Seven patients (aged 55+/-9 years) with mild to moderate congestive heart failure (ejection fraction 31+/-4%) who were on standard therapy were included. The patients were studied at baseline, after 3 months of rhGH treatment, and 3 months after rhGH discontinuation. Cardiac function was assessed by exercise capacity, right heart catheterization at rest and after submaximal exercise, MRI, echocardiography, and Holter monitoring. When administered at a dose of 2 IU/d, rhGH doubled the serum concentration of insulin-like growth factor-I. rhGH improved clinical symptoms and exercise capacity significantly (New York Heart Association class 2.4+/-0.5 initially versus 1.4+/-0.5 at 3 months [mean+/-SD], P<0.05; VO2max 13.6+/-3.8 versus 17.4+/-5.4 mL. kg-1. min-1, P<0.05). Additionally, pulmonary capillary wedge pressures at rest and after submaximal exercise were reduced significantly. Cardiac output increased, particularly at rest (5.0+/-1.1 versus 5.8+/-1.3 L/min; P<0.05). Posterior wall thickness was increased (1.08+/-0.1 versus 1. 24+/-0.3 cm; P<0.05), and the end-diastolic and end-systolic volume indexes decreased significantly after rhGH treatment. There was no significant increase in left ventricular ejection fraction. The improvements were partially reversed 3 months after rhGH discontinuation. CONCLUSIONS: The administration of rhGH for 3 months in patients with ischemic cardiomyopathy results in significant improvement in hemodynamics and clinical function. The attenuation of left ventricular remodeling persisted 3 months after discontinuation of treatment.

Ghigo E et al. Diagnosis of adult GH deficiency. Growth Horm IGF Res. 2008 Feb; 18(1):1-16. The current guidelines for the diagnosis of adult GHD are mainly based on the statements from the GH Research Society Consensus from Port Stevens in 1997. It is stated that diagnosis of adult GHD must be shown biochemically by provocative tests within the appropriate clinical context. The insulin tolerance test (ITT) was indicated as that of choice and severe GHD defined by a GH peak lower than 3 microg/L. The need to rely on provocative tests is based on evidence that that the measurement of IGF-I as well as of IGFBP-3 levels does not distinguish between normal and GHD subjects. Hypoglycemia may be contraindicated; thus, alternative provocative tests were considered, provided they are used with appropriate cut-off limits. Among classical provocative tests, arginine and glucagon alone were indicated as alternative tests, although less discriminatory than ITT. Testing with the combined administration of GHRH plus arginine was recommended as an alternative to ITT, mostly taking into account its marked specificity. Based on data in the literature in the last decade, the GRS Consensus Statements should be appropriately amended. Regarding the appropriate clinical context for the suspicion of adult GHD, one should evaluate patients with hypothalamic or pituitary disease or a history of cranial irradiation, as well as those with childhood-onset GHD are at obvious risk as adults for severe GHD. Brain injuries (trauma, subarachnoid hemorrage, tumours of the central nervous system) very often cause acquired hypopituitarism, including severe GHD. Given the epidemiology of brain injuries, the important role of the endocrinologist in providing major clinical benefit to brain injured patients who are still undiagnosed should be underscored. From the biochemical point of view, although normal IGF-I levels do not rule out severe GHD, very low IGF-I levels in patients highly suspected for GHD (i.e. patients with childhood-onset, severe GHD or with multiple hypopituitarism acquired in adulthood) can be considered as definitive evidence for severe GHD; thus, these patients would skip provocative tests. Patients suspected for adult GHD with normal IGF-I levels must be investigated by provocative tests. ITT remains a test of reference but it should be recognized that other tests are as reliable as ITT. Glucagon as classical test and, particularly, new maximal tests such as GHRH in combination with arginine or GH secretagogues (GHS) (i.e. GHRP-6) have well defined cut-off limits, are reproducible, able to distinguish between normal and GHD subjects. Overweight and obesity have confounding effect on the interpretation of the GH response to provocative tests. In adults cut-off levels of GH response below which severe GHD is demonstrated must be appropriate to lean, overweight and obese subjects to avoid false positive diagnosis in obese adults and false negative diagnosis in lean GHD patients. Finally, normative values of GH response to provocative tests may depend on age, particularly in the transitional age; the normative cut-off levels of GH response to ITT in this phase of life are now available.

Gibney et al. The effects of 10 years of GH in adult GH deficient patients J Endocrin Metab 1999 August The long term effects of GH replacement in adult GH-deficient (GHD) patients have not yet been clarified. We studied 21 GHD adults who originally took part in a randomized, double blind, placebo-controlled trial of GH treatment in 1987. After completion of that trial, 10 patients received continuous GH replacement for the subsequent 10 yr, whereas 11 did not. A group of 11 age- and sex-matched normal controls were also studied in 1987 and 1997. Lean body mass, as assessed by total body potassium measurement and computed tomography scanning of the dominant thigh, increased in the GH-treated group (P < 0.01 for both) only (P < 0.05 between groups for total body potassium). Low density lipoprotein cholesterol decreased in the GH-treated group (P < 0.05) only. Carotid intima media thickness was significantly greater (P < 0.05) in the untreated group than in the GH-treated group. Assessment of psychological well-being using the Nottingham Health Profile revealed improvement in overall score, energy levels, and emotional reaction in the GH-treated group compared with those in the untreated group (P < 0.02). In conclusion, GH treatment for 10 yr in GHD adults resulted in increased lean body and muscle mass, a less atherogenic lipid profile, reduced carotid intima media thickness, and improved psychological well-being.

Gilchrist FJ et al. The effect of long-term untreated growth hormone deficiency (GHD) and 9 years of GH replacement on the quality of life (QoL) of GH-deficient adults. Clin Endocrinol (Oxf) 2002 Sep; 57(3):363-70 BACKGROUND: Quality of life (QoL) is reduced in GH-deficient adults compared with the normal population. Further support for the role of GH in the maintenance of QoL is derived from short-term studies of GH replacement in severely GH-deficient adults; these have predominantly reported beneficial effects, although the degree of improvement has often been modest. To date, however, there are few data to demonstrate whether this beneficial effect on QoL is maintained in the long term. PATIENTS AND METHODS: This study consisted of the follow-up of 85 GH-deficient adults who completed the Nottingham Health Profile (NHP) and the Psychological General Well-Being Schedule (PGWB) self-rating questionnaires in 1992, as part of a

12-month double-blind randomized study of GH replacement. In 2001 we attempted to contact all 85 patients and asked them to complete the two questionnaires again. Follow-up data were obtained in 61 patients. The findings were analysed according to whether the individual had received GH continuously since completion of the initial study, received no further GH replacement, or received GH replacement for only part of the intervening time. Both the NHP and the PGWB give a total score and subsection scores for six specific areas of QoL. A high score correlates with increased morbidity in the NHP, and with reduced morbidity in the PGWB. RESULTS: Fifty-nine patients completed the NHP at both time points. The patients who continued GH (n = 17) had significantly greater morbidity at baseline than patients who opted to discontinue therapy (n = 27), as reflected by the higher scores overall (5.7 +/- 4.0 vs. 2.8 +/- 3.5; P = 0.01) and in the energy subsection (47.0 +/- 34.7 vs. 13.2 +/- 28.6; P < 0.001). Over the study period energy levels improved in the patients who remained on GH therapy (47.0 +/- 34.7 vs. 25.7 +/- 31.0; P = 0.04). By contrast, a deterioration in the physical mobility subsection (2.4 +/- 5.4 vs. 8.2 +/- 16.7; P = 0.04) occurred in the patients who did not continue GH therapy, and no change occurred in the energy subsection. In the 36 patients who completed the PGWB significant differences were observed at baseline between patients who received GH replacement continuously (n = 10) and those who discontinued therapy (n = 21) in the overall score (67.2 +/- 14.1 vs. 86.8 +/- 14.7; P = 0.001); and in the subsections for anxiety (P = 0.04), depression (P = 0.04), well-being (P = 0.001), self-control (P = 0.04) and vitality (P < 0.001); the greater morbidity at baseline being observed in the patients who continued GH replacement. In the patients receiving GH continuously for 9 years the vitality subsection score improved significantly (7.7 +/- 2.4 vs. 12.5 +/- 3.2; P = 0.003), whereas no change in vitality score occurred in patients who did not continue GH therapy. The change in the energy subsection of the NHP and vitality subsection of the PGWB over the 9 years of the study were significantly different between the patients who opted to continue GH replacement and those who discontinued therapy (P = 0.008 and P < 0.001, respectively). CONCLUSION: During this 9-year study, small but significant declines in health were observed in GH-deficient adults who remained untreated. By contrast, the patients who received GH continuously experienced improvements in energy levels while all other areas of QoL were maintained. The beneficial effects of GH on QoL are therefore maintained with long-term GH replacement and obviate the reduction in QoL seen over time in untreated GH-deficient adults.

Gillberg, P. et al. Two Years of Treatment with Recombinant Human Growth Hormone Increases Bone Mineral Density in Men with Idiopathic Osteoporosis J Clin Endocrinol Metab 2002 87: 4900-4906
We have investigated the effects of GH treatment on bone turnover, bone size, bone mineral density (BMD), and bone mineral content (BMC) in 29 men, 27-62 yr old, with idiopathic osteoporosis. The patients were randomly assigned to treatment with GH, either as continuous treatment with daily injections of 0.4 mg GH/d (group A, n = 14) or as intermittent treatment with 0.8 mg GH/d

for 14 d every 3 months (group B, n = 15). All patients were treated with GH for 24 months, with a follow-up period of 12 months, and also received 500 mg calcium and 400 U vitamin D3 daily during all 36 months. Fasting morning urine and serum samples were obtained for assay of IGF-I, bone markers, and routine laboratory tests at baseline, after 1, 12, 24, and 36 months. Body composition, BMD, and BMC were determined by dual-energy x-ray absorptiometry at baseline and every 6 months. After 2 yr, there was an increase in BMD in lumbar spine (by 4.1%) in group A, and in total body (by 2.6%) in group A and (by 2.7%) in group B. BMC of the total body and lean body mass increased, whereas fat mass decreased in both treatment groups. After 36 months, the BMD and BMC in lumbar spine and total body had increased further in both groups. We conclude that 2 yr of intermittent or continuous treatment with GH in men with idiopathic osteoporosis results in an increase in BMD and BMC that is sustained for at least 1 yr post treatment.

Gotherstrom G et al. A prospective study of 5 years of GH replacement therapy in GH-deficient adults: sustained effects on body composition, bone mass and metabolic indices. J Clin Endocrinol Metab 2001 Oct; 86(10):4657-65 GH replacement therapy has proved its efficacy and safety in short-term trials and in a few long-term trials with limited number of subjects. In this 1-center study, including 118 consecutive adults (70 men and 48 women; mean age, 49.3 yr; range, 22-74 yr) with adult-onset GH deficiency, the effects of 5 yr of GH replacement on body composition, bone mass, and metabolic indices were determined. The mean initial GH dose was 0.98 mg/d. The dose was gradually lowered, and after 5 yr the mean dose was 0.48 mg/d. The mean IGF-I SD score increased from -1.73 at baseline to 1.66 at study end. A sustained increase in lean body mass and a decrease in body fat were observed. The GH treatment increased total body bone mineral content as well as lumbar (L2-L4) and femur neck bone mineral contents. BMD in lumbar spine (L2-L4) and femur neck were increased and normalized at study end. Total cholesterol and low density lipoprotein cholesterol decreased, and high density lipoprotein cholesterol increased. At 5 yr, serum concentrations of triglycerides and hemoglobin A (1c) were reduced compared with baseline values. The treatment responses in IGF-I SD score, body fat as estimated by four- and five-compartment body composition models, total body protein and nitrogen, and lumbar bone mineral content and BMD were more marked in men than in women. One patient died during the period, four patients discontinued the study due to adverse events, and one dropped out due to lack of compliance. Four patients were lost to follow-up. However, all patients were retained in the statistical analysis according to the intention to treat approach used. In conclusion, 5 yr of GH substitution in GH-deficient adults is safe and well tolerated. The effects on body composition, bone mass and metabolic indices were sustained. The effects on body composition and low density lipoprotein cholesterol were seen after 1 yr, whereas the effects on bone mass, triglycerides, and hemoglobin A (1c) were first observed after years of treatment.

Harris, et al. Cytokines, insulin-like growth factor 1, sarcopenia, and mortality in very old community-dwelling men and women: the Framingham Heart Study. Am J Med. 2003 Oct 15; 115(6):429-35. BACKGROUND: Aging is associated with increased production of catabolic cytokines, reduced circulating levels of insulin-like growth factor 1 (IGF-1), and acceleration of sarcopenia (loss of muscle with age). We hypothesized that these factors are independently linked to mortality in community-dwelling older persons. METHODS: We examined the relation of all-cause mortality to peripheral blood mononuclear cell production of inflammatory cytokines (tumor necrosis factor alpha [TNF-alpha], interleukin 1 beta, interleukin 6), serum interleukin 6 and IGF-1, and fat-free mass and clinical status in 525 ambulatory, free-living participants in the Framingham Heart Study. RESULTS: Of the 525 subjects (aged 72 to 92 years at baseline), 122 (23%) died during 4 years of follow-up. After adjusting for age, sex, comorbid conditions, smoking, and body mass index, mortality was associated with greater cellular production of TNF-alpha (hazard ratio [HR] = 1.27 per log(10) difference in ng/mL; 95% confidence interval [CI]: 1.00 to 1.61; P = 0.05) and higher serum interleukin 6 levels (HR = 1.30 per log(10) difference in pg/mL; 95% CI: 1.04 to 1.63]; P = 0.02), but not with higher serum IGF-1 levels (HR = 0.70 per log(10) difference in pg/mL; 95% CI: 0.49 to 0.99; P = 0.04). In a subset of 398 subjects (55 deaths) in whom change in fat-free mass index during the first 2 years was measured, less loss of fat-free mass and greater IGF-1 levels were associated with reduced mortality during the next 2 years. CONCLUSION: Greater levels or production of the catabolic cytokines TNF-alpha and interleukin 6 are associated with increased mortality in community-dwelling elderly adults, whereas IGF-1 levels had the opposite effect.

Hedstrom M. Hip fracture patients, a group of frail elderly people with low bone mineral density, muscle mass and IGF-I levels. Acta Physiol Scand 1999 Dec; 167(4):347-50 Elderly women with hip fractures constitute an increasing group of patients in many western countries. The most significant of many factors contributing to the incidence of hip fractures are neuromuscular impairment and low bone mineral density (BMD). Both bone mass and muscle strength decrease during ageing as well as growth hormone (GH) and the anabolic, insulin-like growth factor I (IGF-I). We have found a lower IGF-I level and lower bone and lean body mass in hip fracture patients than in an age-matched group of patients. This sign of catabolism seems to continue postoperatively, with a significant decrease of both BMD and lean body mass possibly indicating GH/IGF-I therapy together with adequate nutrition to preserve bone and muscle losses in elderly patients with hip fractures.

Ho KK et al. Regulating of growth hormone sensitivity by sex steroids: implications for therapy. Front Horm Res. 2006;35:115-28 Growth hormone (GH) is an important regulator of body composition, reducing body fat by stimulating fat oxidation and enhancing lean body mass by stimulating protein accretion. The emergence of differences in body composition between the sexes during puberty suggests sex steroids modulate the action of GH. Work from our laboratory have investigated the influence of estrogens and androgens on the metabolic actions of GH in human adults. The liver is an important site of physiological interaction as it is a sex steroid responsive organ and a major target of GH action. Estrogen, when administered orally impairs the GH-regulated endocrine and metabolic function of the liver via a first-pass effect. It reduces circulating IGF-I, fat oxidation and protein synthesis, contributing to a loss of lean and a gain of fat mass. These effects occur in normal and in GH-deficient women and are avoided by transdermal administration of physiological doses of estrogen. In contrast, studies in hypopituitary men indicate that testosterone enhances the metabolic effects of GH. Testosterone alone stimulates fat oxidation and protein synthesis, both of which are enhanced by GH. Studies in GH deficiency adults have consistently reported women to be less sensitive to GH than men. In summary, estrogens and androgens exert divergent effects on the action of GH. The results provide an explanation for sexual dimorphism in body composition in adults and the gender-related response to GH replacement in hypopituitary subjects. In the management of hypopituitarism, estrogens should be administered by the parenteral route in women and testosterone be replaced in men to optimize the benefits of GH replacement.

Hong J et al.; IGFBP-3 mutants that do not bind IGF-I or IGF-II stimulate apoptosis in human prostate cancer cells. J Biol Chem 2002 Jan 9, 2002 Insulin-like growth factor (IGF)-binding protein-3 (IGFBP-3) can stimulate apoptosis and inhibit cell proliferation directly and independently of binding IGFs or indirectly by forming complexes with IGF-I and IGF-II that prevent them from activating the IGF-I receptor to stimulate cell survival and proliferation. To date, IGF-independent actions only have been demonstrated in a limited number of cells that do not synthesize or respond to IGFs. To assess the general importance of IGF-independent mechanisms, we have generated human IGFBP-3 mutants that cannot bind IGF-I or IGF-II by substituting alanine for six residues in the proposed IGF binding site, Ile(56)/Tyr(57)/Arg(75)/Leu(77)/Leu(80)/Leu(81), and expressing the 6m-hIGFBP-3 mutant construct in Chinese hamster ovary cells. Binding of both IGF-I and IGF-II to 6m-hIGFBP-3 was reduced >80-fold. The nonbinding 6m-hIGFBP-3 mutant still was able to inhibit DNA synthesis in a mink lung epithelial cell line in which inhibition by wild-type hIGFBP-3 previously had been shown to be exclusively IGF-independent. 6m-hIGFBP-3 only can act by IGF-independent mechanisms since it is unable to form complexes with the IGFs that inhibit their action. We next compared the ability of wild-type and 6m-hIGFBP-3 to stimulate apoptosis in serum-deprived PC-3 human prostate cancer cells. PC-3 cells are known to synthesize and respond to IGF-II, so that

IGFBP-3 could potentially act by either IGF-dependent or IGF-independent mechanisms. In fact, 6m-hIGFBP-3 stimulated PC-3 cell death and stimulated apoptosis-induced DNA fragmentation to the same extent and with the same concentration dependence as wild-type hIGFBP-3. These results indicate that IGF-independent mechanisms are major contributors to IGFBP-3-induced apoptosis in PC-3 cells and may play a wider role in the antiproliferative and antitumorigenic actions of IGFBP-3.

Isgaard J et al. GH improves cardiac function in rats with experimental MI. Eur J Clin Invest 1997;27:517-Accumulating evidence suggests from experimental and clinical studies beneficial effects of growth hormone (GH) on contractility, although concomitant cardiac hypertrophy, generally considered to be a cardiovascular risk factor, has also been reported. In the present study, we combine a rat model with impaired cardiac performance after myocardial infarction (MI) with echocardiographic evaluation of GH effects on cardiac structure and function. We have used a rat model with ligation of the left coronary artery in normal, growing male rats resulting in subsequent impaired cardiac performance. After 6 weeks' recovery, blind transthoracic echocardiography was performed to determine infarction size, cardiac geometry and performance. Rats with no signs of myocardial infarction were excluded from the study. After randomization, the rats were treated with daily s.c. injections of saline (n = 8) or recombinant human growth hormone (rhGH) (n = 6) at a dose of approximately 1 mg kg-1 body weight for 1 week. A new blind echocardiography examination was performed after treatment demonstrating a 13% increase in ejection fraction (EF) and a 50% increase in cardiac index in GH-treated rats compared with control rats (P < 0.01). Moreover, GH caused a significant decrease in end-systolic volume. There were no significant changes in left ventricular (LV) or interventricular wall thickness, LV dimensions, heart rate or diastolic function. No effects were seen on LV weight, cardiac insulin-like growth factor (IGF) I, IGF-I receptor and GH receptor mRNA content. GH in a physiological dose improves systolic function in an experimental model of heart failure without signs of hypertrophy, suggesting a potential role as a therapeutic agent in the treatment of heart failure and merits further investigation.

Isley WL. Growth hormone therapy for adults: not ready for prime time? Ann Intern Med 2002 Aug 6;137(3):190-6 Human growth hormone is now readily available and approved for treatment of the growth hormone deficiency syndrome in adults. However, physicians have been slow to adopt this therapeutic modality. Reasons for skepticism about the use of growth hormone for the growth hormone deficiency syndrome include doubts about whether growth hormone deficiency causes increased morbidity and mortality in patients with hypopituitarism; availability of highly efficacious, easier to use, and less expensive agents for certain aspects of the growth hormone deficiency syndrome, especially cardiovascular disease; and concerns about possible toxicity in adults. Long-term studies in patients receiving appropriate comprehensive management for other hormonal deficiencies and for concomitant abnormalities will be required to convince physicians of the utility and safety of growth hormone replacement therapy.

Janssen, Y et al. A Switch from Oral (2 mg/Day) to Transdermal (50 mg/Day) 17b-Estradiol Therapy Increases Serum Insulin-Like Growth Factor-I Levels in Recombinant Human Growth Hormone (GH)-Substituted Women with GH Deficiency. J. Clin Endo Metab. 85: January 2000 The response to GH therapy in adults with GH deficiency (GHD) is considerably variable. Generally, the response with regard to serum insulin-like growth factor (IGF)-I concentrations is significantly lower in females compared with males with GHD, which could at least partly be explained by the use of oral estrogen replacement therapy. In the present study, we investigated whether a switch from oral to transdermal estrogen therapy alters serum IGF-I concentrations in women with GHD on stable GH therapy. Six females with GHD and LH deficiency were investigated. During cycles 1 and 2, an oral dose of estradiol was given (2 mg/day), whereas during cycles 3, 4, and 5 estradiol was administered via the transdermal route at a dose of 50 microg/day. Serum estrone levels significantly decreased (2470+/-475 to 110+/-26 pmol/L, P = 0.005), serum sex hormone-binding globulin levels significantly decreased (102+/-13 to 63+/-7 nmol/L, P = 0.004), and serum estradiol levels also decreased albeit nonsignificantly with transdermal therapy (273+/-81 to 114+/-18, P = 0.083). Serum IGF-I levels significantly increased after the switch from oral to transdermal estrogen therapy (18.7+/-1.6 and 23.4+/-2.5 nmol/L, respectively, P = 0.008). Two of the six patients experienced fluid retention-related side effects, which disappeared after a reduction in dose at the end of the study. The results of the present study suggest that the potency of GH is altered in patients on transdermal compared to oral estradiol therapy. Further investigation should be undertaken to answer the question whether the increase in serum IGF-I levels is due to lower serum levels of estradiol or to differences in the mode of administration of estradiol.

Jenkins PJ et al. Does growth hormone cause cancer? Clin Endocrinol (Oxf). 2006 Feb; 64(2):115-21. The ability of GH, via its mediator peptide IGF-1, to influence regulation of cellular growth has been the focus of much interest in recent years. In this review, we will explore the association between GH and cancer. Available experimental data support the suggestion that GH/IGF-1 status may influence neoplastic tissue growth. Extensive epidemiological data exist that also support a link between GH/IGF-1 status and cancer risk. Epidemiological studies of patients with acromegaly indicate an increased risk of colorectal cancer, although risk of other cancers is unproven, and a long-term follow-up study of children deficient in GH treated with pituitary-derived GH has indicated an increased risk of colorectal cancer. Conversely, extensive studies of the outcome of GH replacement in childhood cancer survivors show no evidence of an excess of de novo cancers, and more recent surveillance of children and adults treated with GH has revealed no increase in observed cancer risk. However, given the experimental evidence that indicates GH/IGF-1 provides an anti-apoptotic environment that may favour survival of genetically damaged cells, longer-term surveillance is necessary; over many years, even a subtle alteration in the environmental milieu in this direction, although not inducing cancer, could result in acceleration of carcinogenesis. Finally, even if GH/IGF-1 therapy does result in a small increase in cancer risk compared to untreated patients with GH deficiency, it is likely that the eventual risk will be the same as the general population. Such a restoration to normality will need to be balanced against the known morbidity of untreated GH deficiency.

Johannsson G et al. GH treatment of abdominally obese men reduces abdominal fat mass, improves glusoce and lipoprotein metabolism and reduces diastolic BP. J Clin Endocinol Metab 1997;82:727-734 The most central findings in both GH deficiency in adults and the metabolic syndrome are abdominal/visceral obesity and insulin resistance. Abdominal obesity is associated with blunted GH secretion and low serum insulin-like growth factor-I concentrations. GH treatment in GH-deficient adults has demonstrated favorable effects on most of the features of GH deficiency in adults, but it is not known whether GH can improve some of the metabolic aberrations observed in abdominal/visceral obesity. Thirty men, 48-66 yr old, with abdominal/visceral obesity were treated with recombinant human GH (rhGH) in a 9-month randomized, double-blind, placebo-controlled trial. The daily dose of rhGH was 9.5 micrograms/kg. Body fat was assessed from total body potassium, and abdominal sc and visceral adipose tissue was measured using computed tomography. The glucose disposal rate (GDR) was measured during an euglycemic, hyperinsulinemic glucose clamp. In response to the rhGH treatment, total body fat and abdominal sc and visceral adipose tissue decreased by 9.2 +/- 2.4%, 6.1 +/- 3.2%, and 18.1 +/- 7.6%, respectively. After an initial decrease in the GDR at 6 weeks, the GDR increased in the rhGH-treated group as compared with the placebo-treated one (P < 0.05). The mean serum concentrations of total cholesterol (P < 0.01) and triglyceride (P < 0.05) decreased, whereas blood glucose and serum insulin concentrations were unaffected by the rhGH treatment. Furthermore, diastolic blood pressure decreased and systolic blood pressure was unchanged in response to rhGH treatment. This trial has demonstrated that GH can favorably affect some of the multiple perturbations associated with abdominal/visceral obesity. This includes a reduction in abdominal/visceral obesity, improved insulin sensitivity, and favorable effects on lipoprotein metabolism and diastolic blood pressure.

Johansen et al. Ipamorelin a new ghrp induces longitudinal bone growth in rats. GH and IGF Research 1999, 9 106-113 Ipamorelin is a new and potent synthetic pentapeptide which has distinct and specific growth hormone (GH)-releasing properties. With the objective of investigating the effects on longitudinal bone growth rate (LGR), body weight (BW), and GH release, ipamorelin in different doses (0, 18, 90 and 450 microg/day) was injected s.c. three times daily for 15 days to adult female rats. After intravital tetracycline labelling on days 0, 6, and 13, LGR was determined by measuring the distance between the respective fluorescent bands in the proximal tibia metaphysis. Ipamorelin dose-dependently increased LGR from 42 microm/day in the vehicle group to 44, 50, and 52 microm/day in the treatment groups (P<0.0001). There was also a pronounced and dose-dependent effect on BW gain. The treatment did not affect total IGF-I levels, IGFBPs, or serum markers of bone formation and resorption. The number of tartrate-resistant acid phosphatase-positive multinuclear cells in the metaphysis of the tibia did not change significantly with treatment. The responsiveness of the pituitary to a provocative i.v. dose of ipamorelin or GHRH showed that the plasma GH response was marginally reduced (P<0.03) after ipamorelin, but unchanged after GHRH. The pituitary GH content was unchanged by ipamorelin treatment. Whether ipamorelin or other GH secretagogues may have a place in the treatment of children with growth retardation requires demonstration in future clinical studies.

Johnsen P. et al. Insulin-Like Growth Factor (IGF) I, -II, and IGF Binding Protein-3 and Risk of Ischemic Stroke J Clin Endocrinol Metab 2005 90: 5937-5941; Background: Low IGF-I levels may be associated with the development of stroke; however, prospective data appear to be unavailable. Methods: This was a nested case-control study within a Danish follow-up study, including 57,053 men and women. Baseline data included circulating IGF-I, IGF-II, and IGF binding protein (IGFBP)-3 concentrations as well as lifestyle factors and medical history. We identified 254 cases with incident ischemic stroke and 254 gender- and age-matched controls. Results: Participants in the bottom quartiles of IGF-I and IGFBP-3 levels (median concentrations, 72 and 2937 ng/ml, respectively) were at increased risk of ischemic stroke, e.g. adjusted odds ratios (ORs) of 2.06 [95% confidence interval (CI), 1.05–4.03] and 2.29 (95% CI, 1.17–4.49), respectively, when compared with participants in the top quartiles (median concentrations, 125 and 4835 ng/ml, respectively). A negative, although weaker, association was also found for IGF-II (adjusted OR 1.44, 95% CI 0.79–2.64) when comparing the bottom quartile with the top quartile. No substantial associations were seen for IGF-I and IGF-II when also adjusting for IGFBP-3; adjusting IGFBP-3 for IGF-I and -II had only a minor impact on the risk estimates. Conclusion: These findings give some support to the hypothesis that the IGF axis is involved in the pathogenesis of ischemic stroke.

Khansari DN et al. Effects of long-term, low-dose growth hormone therapy on immune function and life expectancy of mice. Mech Ageing Dev 1991 Jan; 57(1):87-100 We have studied effects of long-term, low-dose growth hormone therapy on the immune function and life expectancy of Balb/c mice. Sixty male Balb/c mice were aged up to the time when they started showing signs of senescence and causal death (deaths started when they became 17 months old). The aged mice were divided into two groups of 26 mice each. One group received growth hormone (30 micrograms/mouse) subcutaneously twice a week for 13 weeks. The control group received an equal volume of saline for the same period. During this treatment period, 16

300

control mice died (61%) whereas only 2 of the hormone-treated mice died (7%). Four mice from each group were killed and immunological functions of splenocytes were evaluated. Hormone-treated mice had higher stimulation indices for pokeweed mitogen but not for Concanavalin-A. Total IgG production was decreased but IL-1, IL-2 and TNF production was increased. After a lag period of 4 weeks, growth hormone therapy was continued for another 6 weeks. One of the growth hormone treated mice died while the control group no longer existed. Splenocyte functions of the growth hormone treated mice were compared to those of young mice. The results showed no significant difference between cytokine production (IL-1, IL-2, TNF and IgG) in the young and the hormone treated groups. Stimulation induced by concanavalin-A and pokeweed mitogen however, was higher in the young group than the old group. The mortality curve obtained suggests that long-term low-dose growth hormone treatment prolongs life expectancy.

Kurek R et al. The significance of serum levels of insulin-like growth factor-1 in patients with prostate cancer BJU Int 2000 Jan; 85(1):125-9 OBJECTIVES: To compare the serum levels of insulin-like growth factor-1 (IGF-1) in patients with prostate cancer and in control patients with no malignancy, and to evaluate any possible influence of testicular androgen withdrawal on the level of IGF-1 in patients with prostate cancer. PATIENTS AND METHODS: IGF-1 was measured in serum samples from 238 patients using both a chemiluminescence method and a radio-immunoassay. From a subgroup of 19 patients presenting with newly diagnosed carcinoma of the prostate, IGF-1 and testosterone values were measured before and during the course of testicular androgen withdrawal, achieved by the administration of luteinizing hormone-releasing hormone (LHRH) analogues combined with anti-androgens. RESULTS: There were no significant differences in the mean serum levels of IGF-1 patients with and without prostate cancer (158.6 and 159.1 ng/mL, respectively). There were no significant differences in mean IGF-1 levels before and after antiandrogen therapy; the mean (median, SD, range) levels of testosterone (microg/L) and IGF-1 (ng/mL) before androgen withdrawal were 4.81 (4.84, 1.26, 3.11-6.93) and 157.1 (152.5, 26.7, 122.8-195. 1). After androgen withdrawal the corresponding values were 0.303 (0. 218, 0.24, 0.13-0.81) and 169.7 (31.7, 168.6, 124.9-227.6). A linear regression analysis (P = 0.76) and Spearman rank order correlation test (correlation coefficient -0.0613, P = 0.64) showed no association between levels of testosterone and IGF-1. Freeze and thaw cycles applied to the samples had no effect on the IGF-1 values measured. CONCLUSIONS: There was no significant association between IGF-1 serum levels and prostate cancer. Short-term androgen withdrawal using LHRH analogues combined with anti-androgens had no effect on the levels of IGF-1.

Lang CH et al. Cytokine inhibition of JAK-STAT signaling: a new mechanism of growth hormone resistance. Pediatr Nephrol. 2004 Nov 10 Growth hormone (GH) and insulin-like growth factor (IGF)-I are potent regulators of muscle mass in health and disease. This somatomedin axis is markedly deranged in various catabolic conditions in which circulating and tissue levels of inflammatory cytokines are elevated. The plasma concentration of IGF-I, which is primarily determined by hepatic synthesis and secretion of the peptide hormone, is dramatically decreased during catabolic and inflammatory conditions. Moreover, many of these conditions are also associated with an inability of GH to stimulate hepatic IGF-I synthesis. This defect results from an impaired phosphorylation and activation of the traditional JAK2/STAT5 signal transduction pathway. Numerous lines of evidence support the role of tumor necrosis factor (TNF)-alpha as a prominent but probably not the sole mediator of the sepsis-induced impairment in basal and GH-stimulated IGF-I synthesis in liver. Additionally, catabolic conditions produce comparable alterations in skeletal muscle. However, in contrast to liver, the GH resistance in muscle is not mediated by a defect in STAT5 phosphorylation. Muscle is now recognized to respond to infectious stimuli with the production of numerous inflammatory cytokines, including TNF-alpha. Furthermore, myocytes cultured with TNF-alpha are GH resistant and this defect appears mediated via a STAT5-independent but JNK-dependent mechanism. Collectively, these changes act to limit IGF-I availability in muscle, which disturbs protein balance and results in the loss of protein stores in catabolic and inflammatory conditions.

Laughlin GA et al. The prospective association of serum insulin-like growth factor I (IGF-I) and IGF-binding protein-1 levels with all cause and cardiovascular disease mortality in older adults: the Rancho Bernardo Study. J Clin Endocrinol Metab. 2004 Jan; 89(1):114-20 The IGF system has been implicated in cardiovascular disease (CVD) development. The prospective association of serum IGF-I and IGF-binding protein-1 (IGFBP-1) with all cause, ischemic heart disease (IHD), and non-IHD CVD mortality was examined in 633 men and 552 nonestrogen-using postmenopausal women, aged 51-98 yr (mean, 74 yr) in 1988-1992, who were followed through July 2001 (96% follow-up). During the 9- to 13-yr follow-up, there were 522 deaths; 224 were attributed to CVD, and 105 were caused by IHD. IGF-I and IGFBP-1 were independently and jointly related to risk of IHD mortality. In a proportional hazards model including both IGF-I and IGFBP-1 and adjusting for CVD risk factors, the relative risk of IHD mortality was 38% higher for every 40 ng/ml (1 SD) decrease in IGF-I (95% confidence interval, 1.09-1.76; P = 0.005) and 3.11 times greater for those in the lowest quintile of IGFBP-1 (95% confidence interval, 1.74-5.56; P < 0.001) compared with those with higher IGFBP-1 levels. IGF-I and IGFBP-1 (alone or in combination) were not related to risk of all cause or non-IHD CVD mortality. We conclude that low baseline levels of IGF-I and IGFBP-1 increase the risk of fatal IHD among elderly men and women independent of prevalent IHD and CVD risk factors.

Leal-Cerro A The growth hormone (GH)-releasing hormone-GH-insulin-like growth factor-1 axis in patients with fibromyalgia syndrome. J Clin Endocrinol Metab. 1999 Sep; 84(9):3378-81.

Fibromyalgia (FM) is a painful syndrome of nonarticular origin, characterized by fatigue and widespread musculoskeletal pain, tiredness, and sleep disturbances, without any other objective findings on examination. Interestingly, some of the clinical features of FM resemble the ones described in the adult GH-deficiency syndrome. Furthermore, insulin-like growth factor (IGF)-1 levels are frequently reduced in patients with FM. To gain further insight into the mechanisms leading to dysregulation of the GH-IGF-1 axis in these patients, we assessed 24-h spontaneous GH secretion, GH responses to GHRH, and IGF-1 and IGF binding protein (BP)-3 levels before and after 4 days treatment with human (h) GH. We found that, in comparison with controls, patients with FM exhibited a marked decrease in spontaneous GH secretion as assessed by mean GH secretion (2.5 +/- 0.4 microg/L in controls vs. 1.2 +/- 0.1 microg/L in FM, $P < 0.05$), pulse height (4.7 +/- 0.8 microg/L in controls vs. 2.5 +/- 0.3 microg/L in FM, $P < 0.05$), and pulse area (4.7 +/- 1 min/mg x L in controls vs. 2.3 +/- 0.3 min/mg x L in FM, $P < 0.05$). In contrast, GH responses to GHRH (100 microg, i.v.) were similar in controls (mean peak, 13.5 +/- 2.5 microg/L) and in patients with FM (12.2 +/- 3 microg/L). Finally, treatment with hGH (2 IU, s.c. daily), over 4 days, led to a clear-cut increase in plasma IGF-1 and IGFBP-3 levels in patients with FM. In conclusion, our data show that patients with FM exhibited a marked decrease in spontaneous GH secretion, but normal pituitary responsiveness to exogenously administered GHRH, thus suggesting the existence of an alteration at the hypothalamic level in the neuroendocrine control of GH in these patients. Furthermore, our finding of increased IGF-1 and IGFBP-3 levels after GH treatment, over 4 days, opens up the possibility of testing the therapeutic potential of hGH in patients with FM.

Longobardi, S et al Effects of two years of growth hormone (GH) replacement therapy on bone metabolism and mineral density in childhood and adulthood onset GH deficient patients. J Endocinol Invest, May 1999 The aim of the current study was to evaluate bone metabolism and mass before and after 2 years of GH replacement therapy in adults with childhood or adulthood onset GH deficiency. Thirty-six adults with GH deficiency, 18 with childhood onset, 18 with adulthood onset GH deficiency and 28 sex-, age-, height- and weight-matched healthy subjects entered the study. Biochemical indexes of bone turnover such as serum osteocalcin, serum carboxyterminal telopeptide of type-I procollagen, urinary hydroxyproline/creatinine and deoxypyridinoline/creatinine, of soft tissue formation such as aminoterminal propeptide of type-III and bone mineral density were evaluated. Childhood onset GH deficient patients had significantly decreased bone (osteocalcin: 2.5+/-1.3 vs 6.6+/-4.8 mcg/l, p<0.001) and soft tissue formation (aminoterminal propeptide of type III: 273+/-49 vs 454+/-23 U/I, p<0.001) indexes and normal bone resorption indexes (serum carboxyterminal telopeptide of type-I procollagen: 105+/-48 vs 128+/-28 mcg/l p=NS; urinary hydroxyproline/creatinine: 0.19+/-0.16 vs 0.28+/-0.16 mmol/mol, p=NS; urinary deoxypyridinoline/creatinine: 21 +/-10 vs 25+/-8 mcmol/mol, p=NS) compared to healthy subjects. On the contrary, no

303

significant difference in bone turnover indexes between adulthood onset GH deficient patients and healthy subjects was found. Moreover, significantly decreased bone mineral density at any skeletal site and at whole skeleton was found in GH deficient patients compared to healthy subjects (e.g. femoral neck: 0.74+/-0.13 vs 0.97+/-0.11 g/cm2, p<0.001). In addition, a significant reduction of bone mineral density was found in childhood compared to adulthood onset GH deficient patients at any skeletal site, except at femoral neck. After 3-6 months of treatment, both groups of patients had a significant increase in bone turnover and in soft tissue formation. In particular, in childhood onset GH deficient patients after 3 months osteocalcin increased from 2.5+/-1.3 to 7.9+/-2.1 mcg/l, p<0.001 aminoterminal propeptide of type-III from 273+/-49 to 359+/-15 U/I p<0.001; serum carboxyterminal telopeptide of type-I procollagen from 105+/-48 to 201+/-45 mcg/l, p<0.001; urinary hydroxyproline/creatinine from 0.19+/-0.16 to 0.81+/-0.17 mmol/mol, p<0.001; urinary deoxypyridinoline/creatinine from 21 +/-10 to 54+/-20 mcmol/mol, p<0.001; while in adulthood onset GH deficient patients after 6 months osteocalcin increased from 4.2+/-3.6 to 6.5+/-1.9 mcg/l, p<0.05; aminoterminal propeptide of type- III from 440+/-41 to 484+/-37 U/I, p<0.05; serum carboxyterminal telopeptide of type-I procollagen from 125+/-40 to 152+/-22 mcg/l, p<0.05; urinary hydroxyproline/creatinine from 0.24+/-0.12 to 0.54+/-0.06 mmol/mol, p<0.001; urinary deoxypyridinoline/creatinine from 23+/-8 to 42+/-5 mcmol/mol, p<0.001. No significant difference in bone turnover between pre- and post-treatment period was found after 18-24 months of GH therapy. Conversely, bone mineral density was slightly reduced after 3-6 months of GH therapy, while it was significantly increased after 18-24 months. In fact, femoral neck bone mineral density values significantly rose from 0.74+/-0.13 g/cm2 to 0.87+/-0.11 g/cm2 (pre-treatment vs 2 years of GH treatment values). In conclusion, patients with childhood or adulthood onset GH deficiency have osteopenia that can be improved by long-term treatment with GH.

Major J et al. Insulin-Like Growth Factor-I and Cancer Mortality in Older Men The Journal of Clinical Endocrinology & Metabolism Vol. 95, No. 3 1054-1059 March 2010 Context: Although numerous studies have explored the relation of IGF-I with cancer incidence, few have investigated the association between IGF-I and cancer mortality. Objective: This study examined the association of serum IGF-I levels with cancer mortality in older community-dwelling men. Design, Setting, and Participants: We conducted a prospective, population-based study of 633 men aged 50 yr and older (mean = 73) who attended a 1988-1991 research clinic visit when blood was obtained for measurement of IGF-I. Participants were followed for vital status through July 2006. Main Outcome Measure: All-cancer mortality was assessed. Results: Median IGF-I was 96 ng/ml. During the 18-yr follow-up, 368 deaths occurred; 74 (20%) were due to cancer. Cox regression analyses showed a significant quadratic association between IGF-I and all-cancer mortality (P = 0.039). Higher levels of IGF-I were associated with progressively higher risk of cancer death after adjusting for age, IGF-binding protein-1, adiposity, exercise, current smoking, and previous cancer. The adjusted risk of cancer death was statistically significant for IGF-I levels above 120 ng/ml, with magnitudes of effect ranging from 1.61 [95% confidence interval (CI) = 1.28-2.02] to 2.61 (95% CI = 1.46-4.64). For the 46% of men with IGF-I above 100 ng/ml, the risk of fatal cancer was 1.82 (95% CI = 1.11-2.96) compared to the risk with lower levels. Conclusions: Higher serum IGF-I in older men is associated with increased risk of cancer death, independent of age, adiposity, lifestyle, and cancer history. These results suggest caution in the use of IGF-I-enhancing therapies to slow the adverse effects of aging.

Marcell TJ et al. Oral arginine does not stimulate basal or augment exercise-induced GH secretion in either young or old adults. Gerontol A Biol Sci Med Sci 1999 Aug; 54(8):M395-9 BACKGROUND: Growth hormone (GH) helps maintain body composition and metabolism in adults. However, basal and peak GH decline with age. Exercise produces a physiologic GH response that is subnormal in elderly people. Arginine (Arg) infusion can augment GH secretion, but the efficacy of oral Arg to improve GH response to exercise has not been explored. We investigated whether oral Arg increases GH secretion in young and old people at rest and during exercise. METHODS: Twenty young (Y: 22.1 +/- 0.9 y; SEM) and 8 old (O: 68.5 +/- 2.1 y) male and female subjects underwent three different trials following determination of their one-repetition maximum strength (1-RM); exercise only (EO; 3 sets, 8-10 reps at 85% of 1-RM; on 12 separate resistive lifts), Arg only (5.0 g), or Arg + exercise. Blood samples were collected between successive lifts, and GH (ng x ml (-1)) was determined via RIA. RESULTS: In Y vs O: Basal GH secreted (area under the curve) was 543.6 +/- 84.0 vs 211.5 +/- 63.0. During EO, values were 986.6 +/- 156.6 and 517.8 +/- 85.5. Both were significantly lower in the older individuals (p < .05). Oral Arg alone did not result in any increase in GH secretion at rest (310.8 +/- 73.2 vs 262.9 +/- 141.2). When Arg was coadministered during exercise, GH release was not affected in either the young or old and appeared to be blunted in the young compared to the exercise only trial in the young. CONCLUSION: Based upon these findings, we concluded that oral Arg does not stimulate GH secretion and may impair GH release during resistive exercise.

Mitsi AC et al. Early, intracoronary growth hormone administration attenuates ventricular remodeling in a porcine model of myocardial infarction. Growth Horm IGF Res. 2006 Apr; 16(2):93-100. OBJECTIVE: Ventricular remodeling is a common corollary of myocardial infarction. We hypothesized that this process may be attenuated by growth hormone, administered as a single high-dose, selectively in the infarct zone, early postmyocardial infarction. DESIGN: In 35 pigs (29+/-4 kg), myocardial infarction was generated by inflation of an over-the-wire angioplasty balloon in the circumflex artery for 60 min and 5 further pigs were sham-operated. Ten minutes after reperfusion, the pigs were randomized (2:1) to either growth hormone (1 IU/kg) (n=23) or normal saline (n=12), delivered via the balloon catheter. All survivors were treated with captopril and were sacrificed 4 weeks after myocardial infarction. RESULTS: Compared to controls, growth hormone-treated animals displayed lower heart weight (4.1+/-0.5 g/kg body weight, versus 3.4+/-0.4 g/kg, respectively, p=0.003) and dimensions (left ventricular short axis diameter 46+/-7 mm versus 37+/-6 mm, p=0.01; right ventricular short axis diameter 38+/-7 mm versus 30+/-5 mm p=0.001). Growth hormone increased wall thickness in the infarct (6.0+/-1.8 in controls versus 9.9+/-3.7 in treated animals, p=0.004) and non-infarct zones (10.6+/-1.8 in controls versus 15.5+/-3.8 in treated animals, p=0.0006) and produced higher (p<0.05) microvascular density in both zones. CONCLUSION: Intracoronary administration of growth hormone attenuates left and right ventricular remodeling by inducing hypertrophy and by enhancing angiogenesis.

Mitsi AC et al. Early, selective growth hormone administration may ameliorate left ventricular remodeling after myocardial infarction. Med Hypotheses. 2005; 64(3):582-5. Left ventricular (LV) remodeling after myocardial infarction (MI) may lead to congestive heart failure, disability and death. It consists of expansion of the infarct zone and dilatation of the non-infarcted myocardium, causing shape distortion and ventricular enlargement. Experimental studies have shown that treatment with growth hormone (GH) stimulates cardiac repair, resulting in increased infarct zone collagen scar formation and possibly enhanced proteinosynthesis. These actions may ameliorate the process of LV remodeling. We hypothesize that these beneficial effects may be more prominent, if GH is delivered selectively in the infarct area, during the early phase of acute MI. Experimental and clinical studies are necessary to validate this hypothesis.

Muniyappa R et al. Long-Term Testosterone Supplementation Augments Overnight Growth Hormone Secretion in Healthy Older Men. Am J Physiol Endocrinol Metab. 2007. Circulating testosterone (T) and GH/IGF-I are diminished in healthy aging men. Short-term administration of high doses of T augments GH secretion in older men. However, effects of long-term, low-dose T supplementation on GH secretion are unknown. Our objective was to evaluate effects of long-term, low-dose T administration on nocturnal GH secretory dynamics and AM concentrations of IGF-I and IGFBP-3 in healthy older men (65-88 yr, n = 34) with low-normal T and IGF-I. In a double-masked, placebo-controlled, randomized study we assessed effects of low-dose T supplementation (100 mg im every 2 wk) for 26 wk on nocturnal GH secretory dynamics [8 PM to 8 AM, Q(20) min sampling, analyzed by multiparameter deconvolution and approximate entropy (ApEn) algorithms]. The results were that T administration increased serum total T by 33% (P = 0.004) and E (2) by 31% (P = 0.009) and decreased SHBG by 17% (P = 0.002) vs. placebo. T supplementation increased nocturnal integrated GH concentrations by 60% (P = 0.02) and pulsatile GH secretion by 79% (P = 0.05), primarily due to a twofold increase in GH secretory burst mass (P = 0.02) and a 1.9-fold increase in basal GH secretion rate (P = 0.05) vs. placebo. There were no significant changes in GH burst frequency or orderliness of GH release (ApEn). IGF-I levels increased by 22% (P = 0.02),

306

with no significant change in IGFBP-3 levels after T vs. placebo. We conclude that low-dose T supplementation for 26 wk increases spontaneous nocturnal GH secretion and morning serum IGF-I concentrations in healthy older men.

Munzer T et al., Effects of GH and/or sex steroid administration on abdominal subcutaneous and visceral fat in healthy aged women and men. J Clin Endocrinol Metab 2001 Aug; 86(8):3604-10 Aging is associated with reduced GH, IGF-I, and sex steroid axis activity and with increased abdominal fat. We employed a randomized, double-masked, placebo-controlled, noncross-over design to study the effects of 6 months of administration of GH alone (20 microg/kg BW), sex hormone alone (hormone replacement therapy in women, testosterone enanthate in men), or GH + sex hormone on total abdominal area, abdominal sc fat, and visceral fat in 110 healthy women (n = 46) and men (n = 64), 65-88 yr old (mean, 72 yr). GH administration increased IGF-I levels in women (P = 0.05) and men (P = 0.0001), with the increment in IGF-I levels being higher in men (P = 0.05). Sex steroid administration increased levels of estrogen and testosterone in women and men, respectively (P = 0.05). In women, neither GH, hormone replacement therapy, nor GH + hormone replacement therapy altered total abdominal area, sc fat, or visceral fat significantly. In contrast, in men, administration of GH and GH + testosterone enanthate decreased total abdominal area by 3.9% and 3.8%, respectively, within group and vs. placebo (P = 0.05). Within-group comparisons revealed that sc fat decreased by 10% (P = 0.01) after GH, and by 14% (P = 0.0005) after GH + testosterone enanthate. Compared with placebo, sc fat decreased by 14% (P = 0.05) after GH, by 7% (P = 0.05) after testosterone enanthate, and by 16% (P = 0.0005) after GH + testosterone enanthate. Compared with placebo, visceral fat did not decrease significantly after administration of GH, testosterone enanthate, or GH + testosterone enanthate. These data suggest that in healthy older individuals, GH and/or sex hormone administration elicits a sexually dimorphic response on sc abdominal fat. The generally proportionate reductions we observed in sc and visceral fat, after 6 months of GH administration in healthy aged men, contrast with the disproportionate reduction of visceral fat reported after a similar period of GH treatment of nonelderly GH deficient men and women. Whether longer term administration of GH or testosterone enanthate, alone or in combination, will reduce abdominal fat distribution-related cardiovascular risk in healthy older men remains to be elucidated.

Nam SY et al. Growth Hormone and Adipocyte Function in Obesity.Horm Res 2000 Jul; 53 Suppl S1:87-97 In obesity, growth hormone (GH) secretion is impaired which is considered a consequence rather than a cause of obesity. GH regulates the expression of GH receptor and the synthesis of insulin-like growth factor I (IGF-I) in adipocytes. Although GH hyposecretion in obesity may decrease the generation of IGF-I in each adipocyte, increased amounts of IGF-I and GH-binding protein could be secreted from the excessively enlarged amounts of adipose tissue. This may contribute to the normal/high serum-IGF-I and high GH-binding protein levels

307

in obesity. Hyperinsulinemia and increased GH receptor activity may also affect the GH-IGF-I axis. Favorable effects of GH treatment have been observed in obese children and adults. GH treatment decreases adiposity, reduces triglyceride accumulation by inhibiting lipoprotein lipase and enhances lipolysis both via increased hormone-sensitive lipase activity and via induction of beta adrenoreceptors. GH treatment also has a favorable effect on obesity-associated dyslipidemia, but the effects on insulin sensitivity have been conflicting.

Nam SY et al. Low-dose growth hormone treatment combined with diet restriction decreases insulin resistance by reducing visceral fat and increasing muscle mass in obese type 2 diabetic patients. Int J Obes Relat Metab Disord 2001 Aug;25(8):1101-7 OBJECTIVE: To evaluate the effects of low-dose growth hormone (GH) therapy combined with diet restriction on changes in body composition and the consequent change in insulin resistance in newly-diagnosed obese type 2 diabetic patients. DESIGN: Double-blind and placebo-controlled trial of 25-kcal/kg IBW diet daily with GH (n=9; rhGH, 0.15 IU/kg body weight/week) or placebo (n=9) for 12 weeks. SUBJECTS: Eighteen newly-diagnosed obese type 2 diabetic patients (age 42--56 y, body mass index 28.1+/-2.7 kg/m (2)). MEASUREMENTS: Body composition and fat distribution parameters (by bioelectrical impedance analyzer and CT scans), serum IGF-1; serum glucose, insulin and free fatty acid (FFA) during oral glucose tolerance test (OGTT); HbA (1c); serum lipid profiles; and glucose disposal rate (GDR) by euglycemic hyperinsulinemic clamp at baseline and after treatment. RESULTS: The fraction of body weight lost as fat lost was significantly greater (0.98+/-0.39 vs 0.52+/-0.32 kg/kg, P<0.05) and visceral fat area was decreased more in the GH-treated group compared to the placebo-treated group (27.9 vs 21.6%, P<0.05). Lean body mass and muscle area were reduced in the placebo-treated group, whereas an increase in both was observed in the GH-treated group. GDR the was significantly increased in only the GH-treated group (4.67+/-1.05 vs 6.95+/-0.91 mg/kg/min, P<0.05). The GH-induced increase in GDR was positively correlated with the decrease in the ratio of visceral fat area/muscle area (r=0.588, P=0.001). Serum glucose levels and insulin- and FFA-area under the curve during OGTT and HbA (1c) were significantly decreased after GH treatment. LDL-cholesterol level was decreased in only the GH-treated group. CONCLUSION: Low-dose GH treatment combined with dietary restriction resulted not only in a decrease of visceral fat but also in an increase of muscle mass with a consequent improvement of the insulin resistance observed in obese type 2 diabetic patients.

Niikura, T et al. Insulin-Like Growth Factor I (IGF-I) Protects Cells from Apoptosis by Alzheimer's V642I Mutant Amyloid Precursor Protein through IGF-I Receptor in an IGF-Binding Protein-Sensitive Manner The Journal of Neuroscience, March 15, 2001, 21(6):1902-1910 It has been found that insulin-like growth factor I (IGF-I) exerts cytoprotection against Abeta amyloid-induced neuronal cell death. Deposits of

Abeta amyloid are one of the pathological hallmarks of Alzheimer's disease (AD). Here, we examined whether IGF-I exerts protective activity against cell death induced by a familial AD (FAD)-linked mutant of amyloid precursor protein (APP), and we found that IGF-I protected cells from toxicity of FAD-associated V642I mutant of APP in multiple cell systems. IGFBP-3 blocked this action of IGF-I, but not of des (1-3) IGF-I, which was as active as IGF-I in the presence of IGFBP-3. The data also demonstrated that the IGF-I receptor (IGF-IR) mediates the protective activity of IGF-I. The antagonizing function of the IGF-I/IGF-IR system against V642I-APP, which is further antagonized by IGFBP-3, provides a molecular clue to the understanding of AD pathophysiology and to the establishment of potential therapy for AD.

Nyberg F. Growth Hormone in the Brain: Characteristics of Specific Brain Targets for the Hormone and Their Functional Significance. Front Neuroendocrinol 2000 Oct; 21(4):330-348 During the past decade studies have shown that growth hormone (GH) may exert profound effects on the central nervous system (CNS). For instance, GH replacement therapy was found to improve the psychological capabilities in adult GH deficient (GHD) patients. Furthermore, beneficial effects of the hormone on certain functions, including memory, mental alertness, motivation, and working capacity, have been reported. Likewise, GH treatment of GHD children has been observed to produce significant improvement in many behavioral problems seen in these individuals. Studies also indicated that GH therapy affects the cerebrospinal fluid levels of various hormones and neurotransmitters. Further support that the CNS is a target for GH emerges from observations indicating that the hormone may cross the blood-brain barrier (BBB) and from studies confirming the presence of GH receptors in the brain. It was previously shown that specific binding sites for GH are present in discrete areas in the CNS of both humans and rats. Among these regions are the choroid plexus, hippocampus, hypothalamus, and spinal cord. The density of GH binding in the various brain regions was found to decline with increasing age. More recently, we were able to clone and determine the structure of several GH receptors in the rat and human brain. Although the brain receptor proteins for the hormone were shown to differ in molecular size compared to those present in peripheral tissues the corresponding transcripts did not seem to differ from their peripheral congeners. GH receptors in the hypothalamus are likely to be involved in the regulatory mechanism for hormone secretion and those located in the choroid plexus have been suggested to have a role in the receptor-mediated transport of GH across the BBB. The functions mediated by the GH receptors identified in the hippocampus are not yet known but recently it was speculated that they may be involved in the hormone's action on memory and cognitive functions.

Perrot, A. et al. Growth Hormone Treatment in Dilated Cardiomyopathy J Card. Surg 2001; 16:127-131 Treatment with human recombinant growth hormone (GH) has yielded conflicting results in patients with congestive heart failure. We analyzed the baseline somatotrophic axis in

50 patients with dilated cardiomyopathy. Then, a double-blind, randomized, placebo-controlled study of GH was performed. We randomly allocated these patients to treatment with subcutaneous GH (2 IU daily) or placebo for a minimum of 12 weeks. The primary end-points were the effect on left ventricular (LV) mass and systolic wall stress. The secondary endpoint was LV ejection fraction. Severity of heart failure as determined by cardiac index, LV end-diastolic diameter, and plasma noradrenaline concentrations correlated markedly with baseline serum insulin-like growth factor-1 (IGF-1) levels. Patients in the GH group had an increase in LV mass compared with the placebo group (p = 0.0001). There was no significant difference in LV systolic wall stress, mean blood pressure, or systemic vascular resistance between the two groups. New York Heart Association (NYHA) functional classification and distance in 6-minute walk test remained unchanged. The change in IGF-1 concentrations between GH and placebo group was notably related (p = 0.0001) to the change in LV mass (p = 0.0001). The GH-induced increase of IGF-1 predicted the changes of ejection fraction (p < 0.05). A marked increase of ejection fraction of 7% was observed in patients whose IGF-1 increased by more than the median increase, in comparison to the patients with an increase below the median (p = 0.03). Serum levels of IGF-1 reflecting GH secretion are diminished in relation to severity of heart failure in patients with dilated cardiomyopathy. GH-induced increases of IGF-1 of more than 80 pg/mL caused notable improvement of ejection fraction. There is a marked increase in LV mass in patients with dilated cardiomyopathy given GH. Changes in LV mass are related to changes in serum IGF-1 concentrations.

Pfeifer M et al. Growth Hormone (GH) Treatment Reverses Early atherosclerotic Changes in GH-Deficient Adults J Clin Endocrinol Metab 84: 453–457, 1999 Hypopituitary patients have increased mortality from vascular disease, and in these patients, early markers of atherosclerosis [increased carotid artery intima-media thickness (IMT) and reduced distensibility] are more prevalent. As GH replacement can reverse some risk factors of atherosclerosis, the present study examined the effect of GH treatment on morphological and functional changes in the carotid and brachial arteries of GH-deficient (GHD) adults. Eleven GHD hypopituitary men (24-49 yr old) were treated with recombinant human GH (0.018 U/kg BW x day) for 18 months. IMT of the common carotid artery (CCA) and the carotid bifurcation (CB), and flow-mediated endothelium-dependent dilation (EDD) of the brachial artery were measured by B mode ultrasound before and at 3, 6, 12, and 18 months of treatment, and values were compared with those in 12 age-matched control men. Serum concentrations of lipids, lipoprotein (a), insulin-like growth factor I (IGF-I), and IGF-binding protein-3 (IGFBP-3) were also measured. In GHD men before treatment the IMTs of the CCA [mean (SD), 0.67(0.05) mm] and CB [0.75(0.04) mm] were significantly greater (P < 0.001) than those in control men [0.52(0.07) and 0.65(0.07) mm, respectively]. GH treatment normalized the IMT of the CCA by 6 months [0.53(0.04) mm] and that of the CB by 3 months [0.68(0.05) mm]. The IMT of the carotid artery (CCA and CB) was negatively correlated with serum IGF-I (r = -0.53; P < 0.0001). There was a significant improvement in flow-mediated EDD of the brachial artery at 3 months, which was sustained at 6 and 18 months of GH treatment (P < 0.05). GH treatment increased high density lipoprotein cholesterol at 3 and 6 months, but did not reduce total or low density lipoprotein cholesterol and was without effect on lipoprotein (a). There was no correlation between plasma lipids and changes in IMT or EDD of the arteries examined. In conclusion, GH treatment of hypopituitary GHD men reverses early morphological and functional atherosclerotic changes in major arteries and, if maintained, may reduce vascular morbidity and mortality. GH seems to act via IGF-I, which is known to have important effects on endothelial cell function.

Popovic V, et al Growth Horm IGF Res. 2005 Jun; 15(3):177-84. 2005 Mar 21. Hypopituitarism following traumatic brain injury. Hypopituitary patients have increased mortality from vascular disease, and in these patients, early markers of atherosclerosis [increased carotid artery intima-media thickness (IMT) and reduced distensibility] are more prevalent. As GH replacement can reverse some risk factors of atherosclerosis, the present study examined the effect of GH treatment on morphological and functional changes in the carotid and brachial arteries of GH-deficient (GHD) adults. Eleven GHD hypopituitary men (24-49 yr old) were treated with recombinant human GH (0.018 U/kg BW x day) for 18 months. IMT of the common carotid artery (CCA) and the carotid bifurcation (CB), and flow-mediated endothelium-dependent dilation (EDD) of the brachial artery were measured by B mode ultrasound before and at 3, 6, 12, and 18 months of treatment, and values were compared with those in 12 age-matched control men. Serum concentrations of lipids, lipoprotein (a), insulin-like growth factor I (IGF-I), and IGF-binding protein-3 (IGFBP-3) were also measured. In GHD men before treatment the IMTs of the CCA [mean (SD), 0.67(0.05) mm] and CB [0.75(0.04) mm] were significantly greater (P < 0.001) than those in control men [0.52(0.07) and 0.65(0.07) mm, respectively]. GH treatment normalized the IMT of the CCA by 6 months [0.53(0.04) mm] and that of the CB by 3 months [0.68(0.05) mm]. The IMT of the carotid artery (CCA and CB) was negatively correlated with serum IGF-I (r = -0.53; P < 0.0001). There was a significant improvement in flow-mediated EDD of the brachial artery at 3 months, which was sustained at 6 and 18 months of GH treatment (P < 0.05). GH treatment increased high density lipoprotein cholesterol at 3 and 6 months, but did not reduce total or low density lipoprotein cholesterol and was without effect on lipoprotein (a). There was no correlation between plasma lipids and changes in IMT or EDD of the arteries examined. In conclusion, GH treatment of hypopituitary GHD men reverses early morphological and functional atherosclerotic changes in major arteries and, if maintained, may reduce vascular morbidity and mortality. GH seems to act via IGF-I, which is known to have important effects on endothelial cell function.

Popovic, V et al. The effectiveness of arginine + GHRH test compared with GHRH + GHRP-6 test in diagnosing growth hormone deficiency in

adults. Clin Endocrinol (Oxf). 2003 Aug; 59(2):251-7. OBJECTIVE: The objective of this study is to investigate the performance of two novel tests in diagnosing growth hormone deficiency in adults. PATIENTS: Fifty patients presenting with long-standing hypopituitarism and two control groups consisting of 50 healthy subjects in each group [age-, sex- and body mass index (BMI)-matched] participated in a multicentre study. All underwent two provocative tests on different days within 3 months apart: (i) a combined GHRH + GHRP-6 test and (ii) arginine + GHRH test. Main outcome measures were sensitivity, specificity and areas under receiver operating characteristic curves (ROC) for GHRH + GHRP-6 and arginine + GHRH tests in the diagnosis of GH deficiency in adults. RESULTS: A peak GH level after GHRH + GHRP-6, under 15.0 microg/l had a sensitivity of 94.4% and specificity of 98.8% for diagnosing GHD and area under the ROC curve was 0.99 (95% confidence interval 0.95-0.99). For peak GH levels after arginine + GHRH, a level under 9.6 microg/l had a sensitivity of 88.4% and specificity of 95% and area under the ROC curve of 0.96 (95% confidence interval 0.91-0.98). The relationship between the increment in serum GH following GHRH + GHRP-6 and arginine + GHRH test was positive, i.e. r = 0.749, P = 0.001.Thus, there was high concordance between both tests. CONCLUSION: Both GHRH + GHRP-6 and/or arginine + GHRH test may serve as an alternative to the ITT in diagnosing GHD in adults.

Ren J et al. Insulin-like growth factor I as a cardiac hormone: physiological and pathophysiological implications in heart disease. J Mol Cell Cardiol 1999 Nov;31(11):2049-61 Accumulating evidence has indicated that insulin-like growth factor-1 (IGF-1) plays a specific role in the intricate cascade of events of cardiovascular function, in addition to its well established growth-promoting and metabolic effects. IGF-1 is believed to mediate many effects of growth hormone (GH), IGF-1 promotes cardiac growth, improves cardiac contractility, cardiac output, stroke volume, and ejection fraction. In humans, IGF-1 improves cardiac function after myocardial infarction by stimulating contractility and promoting tissue remodeling. Furthermore, IGF-1 facilitates glucose metabolism, lowers insulin levels, increases insulin sensitivity, and improves the lipid profile. These data suggest an attractive therapeutic potential of IGF-1. Both clinically observed and experimentally induced impairments of cardiac function are also found to be associated with abnormal IGF-1 levels. IGF-1 and its binding proteins have been considered as markers for the presence of certain cardiac abnormalities, indicating that IGF-1 may be a risk factor for certain cardiac disorders. The present review will emphasize the role of IGF-1 in the regulation of cardiac growth and function, and the potential pathophysiological role of IGF-1 in cardiac function.

Rousseau N et al. Effect of aging on growth hormone-induced insulin-like growth factor-I secretion from cultured rat chondrocytes   Growth Regulation 7 (1) 1997. The physiological roles of growth hormone (GH) and insulin-like growth factor-I (IGF-I) in adult other than their effects on tissue growth is to maintain the integrity of the organism. It has been proposed that reduced availability of both hormones in late adulthood may contribute to the initiation of the major alterations and senescent changes in body composition that characterize normal human aging. Since accumulated evidence points to a direct interplay of GH with chondrocytes in cartilage, we determined in the present study the effect of aging on both basal and GH-stimulated IGF-I production from rat cultured chondrocytes. Namely, we investigated the effect of 0, 10 and 100 ng/ml of growth hormone on IGF-I levels during 1, 2, 4 and 8 days in monolayer cultured costal chondrocytes from 2-, 6-, 14- and 18-month-old rats. Measurement of IGF-I levels was done by a radioimmunoassay following a validated formic acid-heating-acetone extraction procedure. In 6- and 14-month-old rat chondrocytes, basal IGF-I secretion was higher than that of the 2-month-old control rats. In 18-month-old rat chondrocytes, basal IGF-I secretion was lower than in any other age group. Whereas in 2-, 6- and 14-month-old rat chondrocytes, GH induced a dose-related IGF-I response which was highly significant on day 8, the 18-month-old rat chondrocytes no longer responded to GH treatments. Our results suggest that the decrease in IGF-I production from cultured rat chondrocytes could be related to the blunted GH secretion in the course of aging. Therefore, GH availability in the course of aging appears to be a determinant factor in tissue responsiveness and underscores the hypothesis that GH replacement could present a therapeutic potential against the aging senescent changes.

Ruiz-Torres A et al. Ageing and longevity are related to growth hormone/insulin-like growth factor-1 secretion. Gerontology. 2002 Nov-Dec; 48(6):401-7. BACKGROUND: It is known that the growth process is related to an individual's life-span, but the role of growth hormone (GH) secretion in human ageing remains unknown. OBJECTIVE: This study has focussed on the influence of GH on ageing parameters and on its relationship with human longevity. METHODS: To deal with the first issue, we compared ageing parameters of young (up to 39) and old (over 70) individuals having similar insulin-like growth factor-1 (IGF-1) blood levels. For the second one, the decline in IGF-1 levels was studied comparing its behaviour in the first half with that in the second half of adult life. The latter represents the period of life in which mortality progressively increases. Two hundred and five healthy individuals were chosen as subjects, well distributed by gender and age (between 19 and 93 years). RESULTS: old males with IGF-1 levels similar to young ones do not show the age-dependent decrease in serum testosterone and lean body mass, or the increase in fat body mass. Other hormone-metabolic and nutritional parameters do not reveal any change compared with the results of all individuals. In females, the results do not allow to assume any IGF-1 influence. The behaviour of the linear regression in the second half of adult life of males, which becomes flat because old men having low IGF-1 blood levels die earlier, is consistent with these results. This effect, which is supported by predictive analysis, is not observed in females, i.e. the IGF-1 level declines in the second half of the women's adult life are only a little flatter than in the first half. Finally, extrapolating the regressions obtained in the first half of adulthood, the age at which the curve crosses the x-axis is 110 years for males and 132 for females. CONCLUSIONS: The presented study of IGF-1 levels suggests that the GH secretion in adulthood plays a determinant role not only for some regressive manifestations, but also for life potential.

Sattler F et al. Testosterone Threshold Levels and Lean Tissue Mass Targets Needed to Enhance Skeletal Muscle Strength and Function: The HORMA Trial. J Gerontol A Biol Sci Med Sci. 2010 Nov 8. BACKGROUND: In the HORMA (Hormonal Regulators of Muscle and Metabolism in Aging) Trial, supplemental testosterone and recombinant human growth hormone (rhGH) enhanced lean body mass, appendicular skeletal muscle mass, muscle performance, and physical function, but there was substantial interindividual variability in outcomes.METHODS: One hundred and twelve men aged 65-90 years received testosterone gel (5 g/d vs 10 g/d via Leydig cell clamp) and rhGH (0 vs 3 vs 5 µg/kg/d) in a double-masked 2 × 3 factorial design for 16 weeks. Outcomes included lean tissue mass by dual energy x-ray absorptiometry, one-repetition maximum strength, Margaria stair power, and activity questionnaires. We used pathway analysis to determine the relationship between changes in hormone levels, muscle mass, strength, and function.RESULTS: Increases in total testosterone of 1046 ng/dL (95% confidence interval = 1040-1051) and 898 ng/dL (95% confidence interval = 892-904) were necessary to achieve median increases in lean body mass of 1.5 kg and appendicular skeletal muscle mass of 0.8 kg, respectively, which were required to significantly enhance one-repetition maximum strength (≥30%). Co-treatment with rhGH lowered the testosterone levels (quantified using liquid chromatography-tandem mass spectrometry) necessary to reach these lean mass thresholds. Changes in one-repetition maximum strength were associated with increases in stair climbing power (r = .26, p = .01). Pathway analysis supported the model that changes in testosterone and insulin-like growth factor 1 levels are related to changes in lean body mass needed to enhance muscle performance and physical function. Testosterone's effects on physical activity were mediated through a different pathway because testosterone directly affected Physical Activity Score of the Elderly.CONCLUSIONS: To enhance muscle strength and physical function, threshold improvements in lean body mass and appendicular skeletal muscle mass are necessary and these can be achieved by targeting changes in testosterone levels. rhGH augments the effects of testosterone. To maximize functional improvements, the doses of anabolic hormones should be titrated to achieve target blood levels

Sattler F et al. Testosterone and Growth Hormone Improve Body Composition and Muscle Performance in Older Men. JCEM 2009 94:1991-2001 March 17 CONTEXT: Impairments in the pituitary-gonadal axis with aging are associated with loss of muscle mass and function and accumulation of upper body fat.OBJECTIVES: We tested the hypothesis that physiological supplementation with testosterone and GH together improves body composition and muscle performance in older men.DESIGN, SETTING,

AND PARTICIPANTS: One hundred twenty-two community-dwelling men 70.8 +/- 4.2 yr of age with body mass index of 27.4 +/- 3.4 kg/m2, testosterone of 550 ng/dl or less, and IGF-I in lower adult tertile (< or =167 ng/dl) were randomized to receive transdermal testosterone (5 or 10 g/d) during a Leydig cell clamp plus GH (0, 3, or 5 microg/kg . d) for 16 wk.MAIN OUTCOME MEASURES: Body composition by dual-energy x-ray absorptiometry, muscle performance, and safety tests were conducted.RESULTS: Total lean body mass increased (1.0 +/- 1.7 to 3.0 +/- 2.2 kg) as did appendicular lean tissue (0.4 +/- 1.4 to 1.5 +/- 1.3 kg), whereas total fat mass decreased by 0.4 +/- 0.9 to 2.3 +/- 1.7 kg as did trunk fat (0.5 +/- 0.9 to 1.5 +/- 1.0 kg) across the six treatment groups and by dose levels for each parameter (P < or = 0.0004 for linear trend). Composite maximum voluntary strength of upper and lower body muscles increased by 14 +/- 34 to 35 +/- 31% (P < 0.003 in the three highest dose groups) that correlated with changes in appendicular lean mass. Aerobic endurance increased in all six groups (average 96 +/- 137 sec longer). Systolic and diastolic blood pressure increased similarly in each group with mean increases of 12 +/- 14 and 8 +/- 8 mm Hg, respectively. Other predictable adverse events were modest and reversible.CONCLUSIONS: Supplemental testosterone produced significant gains in total and appendicular lean mass, muscle strength, and aerobic endurance with significant reductions in whole-body and trunk fat. Outcomes appeared to be further enhanced with GH supplementation.

Savine R. et al Growth hormone replacement for the somatopause. Horm Res 2000; 53 Suppl 3:37-41 Twenty-four-hour growth hormone (GH) secretion reaches a peak at around puberty and by the age of 21 has begun to decrease. Thereafter the fall in GH secretion is progressive such that by the age of 60 most adults have total 24-hour secretion rates indistinguishable from those of hypopituitary patients with organic lesions in the pituitary gland. Patterns of GH secretion are similar to those in younger people but GH pulses are markedly reduced in amplitude. Sleep and exercise remain the major stimuli for GH secretion. The fall in GH secretion seen with ageing coincides with changes in body composition and lipid metabolism that are similar to those seen in adults with GH deficiency. In elderly subjects, although GH secretion is markedly reduced, remaining GH secretion correlates closely with body composition (particularly with lean body mass and inversely with central abdominal fat). Pioneering studies carried out by Rudman showed that GH administration to elderly subjects with low insulin-like growth factor-I levels resulted in reversal of many of the changes associated with GH deficiency, namely an increase in lean body mass and bone mineral density and a reduction in body fat and plasma cholesterol. These changes were remarkably similar to those shown a year earlier in adults with GH deficiency given GH replacement. Subsequent studies of GH replacement in elderly adults have confirmed Rudman's initial observations but have been dominated by side effects which have led to a high number of dropouts. It is now clear that the elderly are very sensitive to GH and the doses used need to be very low, increased very slowly and tailored to the individual needs of each patient.

Using this more cautious approach, recent studies have been very positive. A series of papers from Blackman's group, presented at the US endocrine meeting in San Diego in 1999, investigated the effects of GH with or without testosterone supplements (in men) and oestrogen supplements (in women). Their results showed positive effects of GH on lean body mass, central fat, low-density lipoprotein cholesterol and aerobic capacity. In many instances there was a positive interaction between GH and hormone replacement with testosterone and oestrogen, but it appeared that GH showed the most potent anabolic effects. Clearly more studies are needed before GH replacement for the elderly becomes established. Safety issues will require close scrutiny, but the data available so far are sufficiently positive to undertake large multicentre, placebo-controlled trials, particularly looking at endpoints associated with prevention of frailty and loss of independence.

Schernhammer ES et al. Insulin-like growth factor-I, its binding proteins (IGFBP-1 and IGFBP-3), and growth hormone and breast cancer risk in The Nurses Health Study II. Endocr Relat Cancer. 2006 Jun; 13(2):583-592 Earlier data suggest that the relationship between circulating insulin-like growth factor I (IGF-I) levels and breast cancer risk differs according to menopausal status. We evaluated the association between IGF levels as well as the primary regulator of IGF-I production, growth hormone (GH), and breast cancer risk in the Nurses' Health Study II (NHS II) cohort, a large cohort of primarily premenopausal women. We conducted a case-control study nested within the prospective NHS II cohort. Plasma concentrations of IGF-I, IGF binding protein (IGFBP)-3, IGFBP-1, and GH were measured in blood samples collected between 1996 and 1999. Totally 317 women were identified who had a diagnosis of invasive or in situ breast cancer between the date of blood collection and June 1 2003; 75% of these women were premenopausal at blood collection. To each of the 317 women, two controls were age-matched for a total of 634 controls. We used conditional logistic regression models to estimate the relative risk of breast cancer. Overall, plasma IGF-I, IGFBP-1, IGFBP-3, and GH levels were not associated with breast cancer risk (relative risks, top vs bottom quartile; IGF-I, 0.98, 95% confidence interval (CI), 0.69-1.39; IGFBP-1, 0.95, 95% CI, 0.63-1.41; IGFBP-3, 1.10, 95% CI, 0.78-1.54; GH, 1.09, 95% CI, 0.82-1.46). These risks were similar for premenopausal women of age 45 years or less. Further adjustment for additional breast cancer risk factors did not change these estimates. In conclusion, circulating IGF-I, IGFBP-1, IGFBP-3, and GH levels appear to have no important association with breast cancer risk in a large cohort of premenopausal women.

Sesmilo G. et al. Effects of GH Administration on Homocysteine Levels in Men with GH Deficiency: A Randomized Controlled Trial. The Journal of Clinical Endocrinology & Metabolism Vol. 86, No. 4 1518-1524, 2001 GH deficiency is associated with increased cardiovascular mortality and early manifestations of atherosclerosis. Elevated serum homocysteine levels have been found to be associated with increased cardiovascular risk. The effect of GH replacement on homocysteine has not been investigated to date. We evaluated the effect of GH replacement on fasting homocysteinemia in a group of men with adult-onset GH deficiency in a randomized, single blind, placebo-controlled trial. Forty men with adult-onset GH deficiency were randomized to GH or placebo for 18 months, with dose adjustments made according to serum insulin-like growth factor I (IGF-I) levels. Fasting serum homocysteine, folate, vitamin B12, and total T (3) levels were determined at baseline and 6 and 18 months. Anthropometry, IGF-I levels; insulin, and glucose were measured at 1, 3, 6, 12, and 18 months. Nutritional assessment, body composition, total T(4), thyroid hormone binding index, and free T(4) index were assessed every 6 months. Homocysteine decreased in the GH-treated group compared with that in the placebo group (net difference, -1.2 +/- 0.6 micromol/L; confidence interval, -2.4, -0.02 micromol/L; P = 0.047). Homocysteine at baseline was negatively correlated with plasma levels of folate (r = -0.41; P = 0.0087). Total T (3) increased in the GH-treated group vs. that in the placebo group (net difference, 0.17 +/- 0.046 ng/dL; confidence interval, 0.071, 0.26 nmol/L; P = 0.0012). Folate and vitamin B12 levels did not significantly change between groups. Changes in homocysteine were negatively correlated with changes in IGF-I. For each 1 nmol/L increase in IGF-I, homocysteine decreased by 0.04 +/- 0.02 micromol/L (P = 0.029). In contrast, changes in homocysteine did not correlate with changes in folate, vitamin B12, total T(3), C-reactive protein, interleukin-6, or insulin levels. This study shows that GH replacement decreases fasting homocysteine levels compared with placebo. This may be one of the mechanisms involved in the putative modulation of atherosclerosis and cardiovascular risk by GH replacement.

Sesmilo G et al. Effects of growth hormone administration on inflammatory and other cardiovascular risk markers in men with growth hormone deficiency. A randomized, controlled clinical trial. Ann Intern Med 2000 Jul 18; 133(2):111-22. BACKGROUND: Growth hormone-deficient adults have increased cardiovascular mortality. Growth hormone replacement may affect cardiovascular risk. Inflammation plays an important role in atherosclerosis, and inflammatory markers are predictive of cardiovascular events. OBJECTIVE: To investigate the effect of growth hormone replacement on inflammatory and other cardiovascular risk factors. DESIGN: Randomized, single-blind, placebo-controlled trial. PATIENTS: 40 men with adult-onset growth hormone deficiency. INTERVENTION: Growth hormone or placebo given for 18 months at a dose adjusted for normal serum insulin-like growth factor I level. MEASUREMENTS: Anthropometric, hemoglobin A1c, and central fat values were assessed every 6 months. Levels of glucose, insulin, insulin-like growth factor I, and lipids were measured at 1, 3, 6, 12, and 18 months. C-reactive protein, serum amyloid polypeptide A, inteleukin-6, and lipoprotein (a) levels were determined at baseline and 6 and 18 months. RESULTS: C-reactive protein and inteleukin-6 levels decreased in growth hormone recipients compared with placebo recipients (differences between groups, -1.9 +/- 0.6 mg/L [P = 0.0027] and -1.3 +/- 0.5 ng/L [P =

0.013], respectively). Changes in serum amyloid polypeptide A levels between groups did not reach statistical significance (difference between groups, -2.4 +/- 1.2 mg/L; P = 0.056). Serum cholesterol levels, low-density lipoprotein cholesterol levels, and ratios of total cholesterol to high-density lipoprotein cholesterol decreased in growth hormone recipients in the first 3 months compared with placebo recipients (differences between groups, -0.86 +/- 0.17 mmol/L [-33.2 +/- 6.6 mg/dL] [P < 0.001], -0.63 +/- 0.20 mmol/L [-24.5 +/- 5.9 mg/dL] [P < 0.001], and -0.56 +/- 0.26 [P = 0.040], respectively), but the decrease was not maintained from month 6 to month 18. Lipoprotein (a) levels increased (difference between groups, 22.0 +/- 8.0 mg/L; P = 0.0096). Short-term increases occurred in glucose levels, insulin levels, and insulin-to-glucose ratios (differences between groups, 0.54 +/- 0.16 mmol/L [9.6 +/- 2.8 mg/dL] [P = 0.0018], 37.9 +/- 9.6 pmol/L [P < 0.001], and 6.0 +/- 1.8 [P = 0.0025], respectively), but only the increase in glucose level was maintained over the long term (difference between groups, 0.56 +/- 0.17 mmol/L [10.0 +/- 3.1 mg/dL]; P = 0.0026). Hemoglobin A1c values did not change. Truncal fat-to-total fat ratios decreased (difference between groups, -0.018 +/- 0.007; P = 0.0087). CONCLUSIONS: Long-term growth hormone replacement in men reduces levels of inflammatory cardiovascular risk markers, decreases central fat, and increases lipoprotein (a) and glucose levels without affecting lipid levels

Shalet SM, Brennan BM, Reddingius RE. Growth hormone therapy and malignancy. Horm Res 1997; 48 Suppl 4:29-32 The possibility that human growth hormone (GH) replacement therapy might either increase the risk of cancer recurrence in a child who has previously been treated for a brain tumour or leukaemia, or induce de novo cancer, has worried paediatricians for a number of years. Concern arises from animal experiments, the association of acromegaly with malignancy, and the Japanese experience of a cluster of de novo leukaemia cases in children treated with GH. It is reassuring that so far the results from single centre studies and from the pharmaceutical industry surveillance programmes have shown no evidence of an increased risk of malignancy, recurrent or de novo. The confidence intervals, however, are wide and the scientific nature of these studies is flawed as there has never been a prospective randomized study of GH replacement in children with radiation-induced GH deficiency. For clinical reasons, such a study is unlikely to be performed and therefore surveillance must be maintained at a very high level.

Slonim AE et al. A preliminary study of growth hormone therapy for Crohn's disease. N Engl J Med 2000 Jun 1; 342(22):1633-7 BACKGROUND: Crohn's disease is a chronic inflammatory disorder of the bowel. In a preliminary study, we evaluated whether the administration of growth hormone (somatropin) as well as a high-protein diet would ameliorate the symptoms of the disease. METHODS: We randomly assigned 37 adults with moderate-to-severe active Crohn's disease to four months of self-administered injections of growth hormone (loading dose, 5 mg per day subcutaneously for one week, followed by a maintenance dose of 1.5 mg per day) or placebo. We instructed all patients to increase their protein intake to at least 2 g per kilogram of body weight per day. Patients continued to be treated by their usual physicians and to receive other medications for Crohn's disease. The primary end point was the change in scores on the Crohn's Disease Activity Index from base line to month 4. Scores can range from 0 to 600, with higher scores indicating more disease activity. RESULTS: At base line, the mean (+/-SD) score on the Crohn's Disease Activity Index was somewhat higher among the 19 patients in the growth hormone group than among the 18 patients in the placebo group (287+/-134 vs. 213+/-120, P=0.09). Three patients in the placebo group withdrew before their first follow-up visit and were not included in the data analysis. At four months, the Crohn's Disease Activity Index score had decreased by a mean of 143+/-144 points in the growth hormone group, as compared with a decrease of 19+/-63 points in the placebo group (P=0.004). Side effects in the growth hormone group included edema (in 10 patients) and headache (in 5) and usually resolved within the first month of treatment. CONCLUSIONS: Our preliminary study suggests that growth hormone may be a beneficial treatment for patients with Crohn's disease.

Stochholm, K et al. Mortality and GH Deficiency a Nationwide Study. European Journal of Endocrinology. (2007)157 9-18 OBJECTIVE: To estimate the mortality in Denmark in patients suffering from GH deficiency (GHD).DESIGN: Mortality was analyzed in 1794 GHD patients and 8014 controls matched on age and gender. All records in GHD patients were studied and additional morbidity noted. Patients were divided into childhood onset (CO) and adult onset (AO), discriminated by an age cutoff below or above 18 years at onset of GHD.METHOD: Data on death were identified in national registries. Sex- and cause-specific mortalities were identified in CO and AO GHD when compared with controls.RESULTS: Mortality was increased in CO and AO GHD in both genders, when compared with controls. The hazard ratio (HR) for CO males was 8.3 (95% confidence interval (CI) 4.5-15.1) and for females 9.4 (CI 4.6-19.4). For AO males, HR was 1.9 (CI 1.7-2.2) and for females 3.4 (CI 2.9-4.0). We found a significantly higher HR in AO females versus AO males, both compared with controls (P < 0.001). In AO, mortality was increased due to cancer in all subgroups, due to circulatory diseases in all age groups for females and for males in the oldest age group. For CO, the increased mortality was due to cancer.CONCLUSIONS: We found a significantly increased mortality in GHD patients when compared with controls, possibly due to their hypopituitary status. Mortality was increased in AO female patients when compared with males. For CO and AO GHD, different causes of significantly increased mortality were identified.

Strassberger C et al. How robust are laboratory measures of growth hormone status? Hormone Research 2005; 64:1-5 Biochemical assessment of growth hormone (GH) status is required in both suspected GH deficiency and GH excess. GH secretion can either be measured through investigation of the pituitary or by monitoring markers that change as a consequence of GH action on its target tissues. The two most widely used and, to date, best validated biochemical parameters are immunoassay measurement of either human GH (hGH) or insulin-like growth factor (IGF)-I. The fundamental difference between measurement of hGH and IGF-I is that the first reflects GH secretion while the second reflects GH action. However, because GH secretion is pulsatile in nature, random blood sampling for determination of hGH levels is only minimally informative. Analytical methods for measuring GH and IGF-I show considerable between-method variability. Since these parameters are used in establishing diagnoses and in monitoring GH-related diseases, the endocrinologist should be aware of the specifications and limitations of the analytical methods available.

Sugimoto T et al. Effect of recombinant human growth hormone in elderly osteoporotic women. Clin Endocrinol (Oxf) 1999 Dec; 51(6):715-724 OBJECTIVE: Bone mineral density and growth hormone (GH) secretion rate both decline during normal human ageing. We evaluated the effects of recombinant human GH on markers of body composition and bone turnover in an open study in 8 elderly osteoporotic women aged 68-75 years (mean age 71 years). DESIGN: Subjects were treated with GH as a single daily subcutaneous injection (0.125 IU/kg/week for the first 4 weeks and subsequently 0.25 IU/kg/week) for 48 weeks. RESULTS: GH treatment caused a rapid (within 2 weeks) increase in serum levels of IGF-I and IGF-binding protein-3 (IGFBP-3) which was sustained throughout the study. Markers of bone formation and resorption were both gradually increased up to 24 weeks of GH treatment. The bone formation markers, osteocalcin (OC) and bone alkaline phosphatase remained high during GH treatment, while the bone resorption marker, deoxypyridinoline (D-Pyr), tended to return to baseline levels after 24 weeks of GH therapy. GH treatment for 48 weeks caused a significant increase in hand grip and a decrease in waist/hip ratio. The mean percentage changes in bone mineral density (BMD) of mid-radius and lumbar spine were + 2.1% and + 1.2%, respectively, although they were not statistically significant. GH treatment was well tolerated and no major side-effects except mild oedema and joint pain were found. Since GH treatment produced durable increases in bone formation markers, BMD continued to be monitored after discontinuation of GH treatment for another 48 weeks, during which significant increases in radial and lumbar BMD (8.1 +/- 2.1 and 3.8 +/- 1.4% above pre- treatment values, respectively) were recorded. CONCLUSION: These results indicate that GH attenuates the decrease in muscle strength and bone mass as well as the gain of abdominal fat with ageing in elderly women. The present data provide useful information about the application of GH treatment in elderly women.

Swerdlow A. et al. Growth Hormone Treatment of Children with Brain Tumors and Risk of Tumor Recurrence. The Journal of Clinical Endocrinology & Metabolism Vol. 85, No. 12, December 2000 GH is increasingly used for treatment of children and adults. It is mitogenic, however, and there is therefore concern about its safety, especially when used to treat cancer patients who have become GH deficient after cranial radiotherapy. We followed 180 children with brain tumors attending three large hospitals in the United Kingdom and treated with GH during 1965-1996, and 891 children with brain tumors at these hospitals who received radiotherapy but not GH. Thirty-five first recurrences occurred in the GH-treated children and 434 in the untreated children. The relative risk of first recurrence in GH-treated compared with untreated patients, adjusted for potentially confounding prognostic variables, was decreased (0. 6; 95% confidence interval, 0.4-0.9) as was the relative risk of mortality (0.5; 95% confidence interval, 0.3-0.8). There was no significant trend in relative risk of recurrence with cumulative time for which GH treatment had been given or with time elapsed since this treatment started. The relative risk of mortality increased significantly with time since first GH treatment. The results, based on much larger numbers than previous studies, suggest that GH does not increase the risk of recurrence of childhood brain tumors, although the rising trend in mortality relative risks with longer follow-up indicates the need for continued surveillance

Svensson J et al. Body composition and quality of life as markers of the efficacy of growth hormone replacement therapy in adults. Horm Res 2001;55 Suppl 2:55-60 Growth hormone (GH) replacement therapy in GH-deficient adults should be initiated with a low dose, independent of body weight or body surface area. Measurements of serum insulin-like growth factor I (IGF-I) concentrations, as well as clinical examinations aimed at detecting signs of fluid excess, are important as safety markers to avoid overtreatment with GH. At present, there is no optimal marker for the long-term efficacy of GH replacement therapy. The long-term maintenance dose of GH should, therefore, be titrated in each individual based on the clinical response, with the aim of normalizing body hydration, other measurements of body composition, quality of life and well-being, and biochemical indices such as serum IGF-I concentration.

Takala J et al. Increased mortality associated with GH treatment in critically ill adults. NEJM 1999; 341:785-92 BACKGROUND: The administration of growth hormone can attenuate the catabolic response to injury, surgery, and sepsis. However, the effect of high doses of growth hormone on the length of stay in intensive care and in the hospital, the duration of mechanical ventilation, and the outcome in critically ill adults who are hospitalized for long periods is not known. METHODS: We carried out two prospective, multicenter, double-blind, randomized, placebo-controlled trials in parallel involving 247 Finnish patients and 285 patients in other European countries who had been in an intensive care unit for 5 to 7 days and who were expected to require intensive care for at least 10 days. The patients had had cardiac surgery, abdominal surgery, multiple trauma, or acute respiratory failure. The patients received either growth hormone (mean [+/-SD] daily dose, 0.10 +/- 0.02 mg per kilogram of body weight) or placebo until discharge from intensive care or for a maximum of 21 days. RESULTS: The in-hospital mortality rate was higher in the patients who received growth hormone than in those who did not (P<0.001 for both studies). In the Finnish study, the mortality rate was 39 percent in the growth hormone group, as compared with 20 percent in the placebo group. The respective rates in the multinational study were 44 percent and 18 percent. The relative risk of death for patients receiving growth hormone was 1.9 (95 percent confidence interval, 1.3 to 2.9) in the Finnish study and 2.4 (95 percent confidence interval, 1.6 to 3.5) in the multinational study. Among the survivors, the length of stay in intensive care and in the hospital and the duration of mechanical ventilation were prolonged in the growth hormone group. CONCLUSIONS: In patients with prolonged critical illness, high doses of growth hormone are associated with increased morbidity and mortality.

Tivesten, A The Growth Hormone Secretagogue Hexarelin Improves Cardiac Function in Rats after Experimental Myocardial Infarction. Endocrinology, January 2000, p. 60-66 Vol. 141, No. 1 Several studies have shown that GH can enhance cardiac performance in rats after experimental myocardial infarction and in humans with congestive heart failure. In the present study, the hemodynamic effects of hexarelin (Hex), an analog of GH-releasing peptide-6 and a potent GH secretagogue, were compared with the effects of GH. Four weeks after ligation of the left coronary artery male rats were treated sc twice daily with hexarelin [10 microg/kg x day (Hex10) or 100 microg/kg x day (Hex100)], recombinant human GH (2.5 mg/kg x day), or 0.9% NaCl for 2 weeks. Transthoracic echocardiography was performed before and after the treatment period. GH, but not Hex, increased body weight gain. GH and Hex100 decreased total peripheral resistance ($P < 0.05$) and increased stroke volume ($P < 0.05$ and $P < 0.01$, respectively) and stroke volume index ($P = 0.06$ and $P < 0.01$, respectively) vs. NaCl. Cardiac output was increased by GH and Hex100 ($P < 0.05$), and cardiac index was increased by Hex100 with a borderline significance for GH ($P = 0.06$). In conclusion, Hex improves cardiac function and decreases peripheral resistance to a similar extent as exogenous GH in rat's postmyocardial infarction. The mechanisms of these effects are unclear; they could be mediated by GH or a direct effect of Hex on the cardiovascular system.

Toogood A. et al. Growth Hormone Replacement Therapy in the Elderly with Hypothalamic-Pituitary Disease: A Dose-Finding Study. J Clin Endocrinol Metab 84: 131–136, 1999 Adults over the age of 60 yr with organic disease of the hypothalamic-pituitary axis have a 90% reduction in GH secretion. This is distinct from the hyposomatotropism associated with increasing age and results in a significant reduction in serum insulin-like growth factor I (IGF-I), an increase in fat mass, abnormal bone turnover, and an adverse lipid profile compared with those in healthy subjects of the same age. These findings suggest that the elderly with organic GH deficiency might benefit from GH replacement therapy. However, the dose of GH required maintaining serum IGF-I levels in the normal range while minimizing side-effects in this group of patients is unknown. We have studied 12 patients with organic GH deficiency, aged 62.4-85.2 (median, 67.9 yr), each treated with three doses of GH (0.167, 0.33, and 0.5 mg/day). Each dose was administered for 12 weeks. The serum IGF-I level rose in a dose-related manner over the course of the study (P < 0.0001). From a baseline median (range) IGF-I concentration of 101 (49-148) microg/L to 149 (49-227) microg/L at 12 weeks (P = 0.003 vs. baseline), 200 (70-453) microg/L at 24 weeks (P = 0.002 vs. baseline; P = 0.04 vs. 12 weeks), and 239 (122-502) microg/L at 36 weeks (P = 0.002 vs. baseline; P = 0.07 vs. 24 weeks). The age-specific IGF-I SD score exceeded normal in two subjects taking 0.33 mg/day and in six subjects taking 0.5 mg/day. Serum IGF-binding protein-3 also rose over the course of the study (P < 0.001); however, the greatest increase occurred during the first 12 weeks, after which the IGFBP-3 level plateaued. Body composition changed significantly during the study, with a fall in fat mass (P = 0.0003) and an increase in lean body mass (P = 0.0001). GH was well tolerated in this elderly group, all of whom completed the study. Three patients developed side-effects while taking 0.5 mg/day; two developed headaches, and one developed arthralgia. This study has demonstrated that the GH replacement dose in elderly subjects is considerably lower than that required by younger adults with GH deficiency. In 50% of the subjects a dose of 0.5 mg/day was excessive, whereas 83% maintained their serum IGF-I within normal limits while taking 0.33 mg/day. No patient exhibited a supranormal IGF-I level on 0.17 mg/day.

Thum T et al. Growth hormone treatment improves markers of systemic nitric oxide bioavailability via insulin-like growth factor-1. J Clin Endocrinol Metab. 2007 Aug 28 CONTEXT AND OBJECTIVE: Impaired nitric oxide (NO) bioavailability and low levels of circulating endothelial progenitor cells (EPC) are correlated to an increased risk for development of cardiovascular diseases. We investigated whether improved systemic NO bioavailability and increased levels of EPC after GH treatment are related and mediated by the IGF-I. DESIGN, PATIENTS, AND RESULTS: Healthy middle-aged volunteers (n = 16) were treated for 10 d with recombinant human GH. Before and after GH treatment, we analyzed markers of NO bioavailability and EPC levels. GH treatment was responded by significant increases in plasma IGF-I levels. Urinary cGMP levels were increased and diastolic blood pressure reduced after GH treatment (P < 0.05). Likewise, plasma nitrate and nitrite levels were increased, whereas the NO synthase inhibitor asymmetric dimethylarginine was reduced. Correspondingly, IGF-I treatment increased expression of the asymmetric dimethylarginine-metabolizing enzyme dimethylarginie dimethylaminohydrolase-1 and dimethylarginie dimethylaminohydrolase-2 in cultured human endothelial cells. IGF-I levels correlated with cGMP concentrations (r = 0.51; P < 0.05). EPC numbers were increased after GH treatment and correlated with markers for NO bioavailability. These findings were also observed in mice treated with GH for 7 d. GH treatment additionally increased aortic endothelial NO synthase expression of mice. Importantly, blocking of the IGF-I receptor in vivo abolished the GH-mediated effects on markers of increased NO bioavailability.CONCLUSIONS: GH treatment induced markers of increased NO bioavailability and enhanced circulating EPC numbers in healthy volunteers. Animal data demonstrate increased NO availability to be mediated via an increase in IGF-I plasma levels. Thus, GH treatment enhances systemic NO bioavailability via IGF-I and may be beneficial in certain cardiovascular diseases.

Torella D et al. Cardiac stem cell and myocyte aging, heart failure, and insulin-like growth factor-1 overexpression. Circ Res. 2004 Mar 5;94(4):514-24 To determine whether cellular aging leads to a cardiomyopathy and heart failure, markers of cellular senescence, cell death, telomerase activity, telomere integrity, and cell regeneration were measured in myocytes of aging wild-type mice (WT). These parameters were similarly studied in insulin-like growth factor-1 (IGF-1) transgenic mice (TG) because IGF-1 promotes cell growth and survival and may delay cellular aging. Importantly, the consequences of aging on cardiac stem cell (CSC) growth and senescence were evaluated. Gene products implicated in growth arrest and senescence, such as p27Kip1, p53, p16INK4a, and p19ARF, were detected in myocytes of young WT mice, and their expression increased with age. IGF-1 attenuated the levels of these proteins at all ages. Telomerase activity decreased in aging WT myocytes but increased in TG, paralleling the changes in Akt phosphorylation. Reduction in nuclear phospho-Akt and telomerase resulted in telomere shortening and uncapping in WT myocytes. Senescence and death of CSCs increased with age in WT impairing the growth and turnover of cells in the heart. DNA damage and myocyte death exceeded cell formation in old WT, leading to a decreased number of myocytes and heart failure. This did not occur in TG in which CSC-mediated myocyte regeneration compensated for the extent of cell death preventing ventricular dysfunction. IGF-1 enhanced nuclear phospho-Akt and telomerase delaying cellular aging and death. The differential response of TG mice to chronological age may result from preservation of functional CSCs undergoing myocyte commitment. In conclusion, senescence of CSCs and myocytes conditions the development of an aging myopathy.

Valimaki MJ et alEffects of 42 months of GH treatment on bone mineral density and bone turnover in GH-deficient adults. Eur J Endocrinol 1999 Jun; 140(6):545-54 OBJECTIVE: To study the effects of GH treatment for up to 42 months on bone mineral density (BMD) and bone turnover. DESIGN AND METHODS: BMD with dual energy X-ray absorptiometry, serum type I procollagen carboxy-terminal propeptide (PICP), serum type I collagen carboxy-terminal telopeptide (ICTP) and serum IGF-I were assessed in 71 adults with GH deficiency. There were 44 men and 27 women, aged 20 to 59 (median 43) years. Thirty-two patients completed 36 months and 20 patients 42 months of treatment. RESULTS: The BMD increased for up to 30-36 months and plateaued thereafter. In the whole study group, the maximum increase of BMD was 5.0% in the lumbar spine (P<0. 001), 5.9% (P<0.01) in the femoral neck, 4.9% (NS, P>0.05) in the Ward's triangle and 8.2% (P<0.001) in the

324

trochanter area. The serum concentrations of PICP (202.6+/-11.5 vs 116.3+/-5.4 microg/l; mean+/-s.e.m.) and ICTP (10.5+/-0.6 vs 4.4+/-0.3 microg/l) doubled (P<0.001) during the first 6 months of GH treatment but returned to baseline by the end of the study (130.0+/-10.4 and 5.6+/-0.7 microg/l respectively), despite constantly elevated serum IGF-I levels (39. 6+/-4.1 nmol/l at 42 months vs 11.9+/-0.9 nmol/l at baseline; P<0.001). The responses to GH treatment of serum IGF-I, PICP, ICTP (P<0.001 for all; ANOVA) and of the BMD in the lumbar spine (P<0.05), in the femoral neck and the trochanter (P<0.001 for both) were more marked in men than in women. At the end of the study the BMD had increased at the four measurement sites by 5.7-10.6% (P<0.01-0.001) in patients with at least osteopenia at baseline and by 0.1-5.3% (NS P<0.05) in those with normal bone status (P<0.001 for differences between groups; ANOVA). Among patients who completed 36-42 months of treatment, the number of those with at least osteopenia was reduced to more than a half. The response of BMD to GH treatment was more marked in young than in old patients at three measurement sites (P<0. 05-<0.001; ANOVA). In the multiple regression analysis the gender and the pretreatment bone mass appeared to be independent predictors of three measurement sites, whereas the age independently determined only the vertebral BMD. CONCLUSIONS: GH treatment in GH-deficient adults increased BMD for up to 30-36 months, with a plateau thereafter. Concurrently with the plateau in BMD the bone turnover rate normalized. From the skeletal point of view GH-deficient patients exhibiting osteopenia or osteoporosis should be considered as candidates for GH supplementation of at least 3-4 years.

van Dam PS Somatropin therapy and cognitive function in adults with growth hormone deficiency: a critical review. Treat Endocrinol. 2006; 5(3):159-70. Both growth hormone (GH) and insulin-like growth factor (IGF)-I have receptors in the brain, in particular in areas that are involved in cognitive function. Therefore, it has been hypothesized that GH deficiency can lead to cognitive dysfunction, and that somatropin replacement therapy may have beneficial effects on cognitive function in GH-deficient patients. In this review, an overview is given regarding the possible effects of decreased activity of the GH/IGF-I axis and somatropin therapy in GH deficiency in relation to cognitive function. The available data regarding cognitive function in GH-deficient patients are limited, but suggest that this condition can lead to specific cognitive changes, in particular attentional deficits and altered processing speed. The underlying mechanisms and the effects of somatropin treatment on cognitive function in GH deficiency are still unclear. Similar studies to those performed in patients with GH deficiency have been performed regarding the cognitive changes in elderly patients with relatively low GH and/or IGF-I levels. Large controlled studies regarding the effects and safety of somatropin treatment in healthy elderly patients have not been performed.

Van Der Lely et al. Use of human GH in elderly patients with accidental hip fracture. Eur J Endocrinol 2000 Nov; 143(5):585-592 OBJECTIVE: To investigate whether early intervention with recombinant human growth hormone (hGH) after hip fracture improves functional recovery and long-term outcome. SUBJECTS AND METHODS: Functional recovery after hip fracture is often incomplete. The catabolic situation that develops after the hip fracture accident, and a state of malnutrition either pre-existing or developing after surgery, are main contributing factors for the poor clinical outcome. hGH has been used to promote anabolism in a variety of clinical catabolic situations. The study design was randomized, double-blind and placebo-controlled. A total of 111 patients older than 60 years with an accidental hip fracture (mean age 78.5+/-9.1 (s.d.) years) were randomized to receive either hGH (20 microg/kg per day) or placebo for a period of 6 weeks, starting within 24 h after the hip fracture accident. Thereafter patients were followed up for an additional period of 18 weeks. Efficacy was assessed by comparing the changes in the Barthel Index score of activities of daily living and in a patient's living situation between the hGH- and the placebo-treated subjects. RESULTS: Eighty-five (78.5%) patients completed the first 8 weeks of the study and 76 (68.5%) the entire study period of 24 weeks. When split according to age, a trend was found that for patients older than 75 years the changes in Barthel Index score from baseline were less in the hGH group than in the placebo group (-18.6+/-18 vs -28.1+/-26) at 6 weeks after surgery (P<0.075). There was an overall trend to a higher rate of return to the pre-fracture independent living situation in the hGH group than in the placebo group. Analysis by age revealed a significantly higher proportion of hGH- than placebo-treated patients returning to the pre-fracture living situation for subjects older than 75 years (93.8 vs 75.0%, P=0.034). hGH treatment increased IGF-I values to levels in the range of those of normal subjects of 50-60 years of age. CONCLUSIONS: A 6 week treatment with hGH (20 microg/kg per day) of otherwise healthy patients after an accidental hip fracture may be of benefit if given to subjects older than 75 years of age. The rate of return to the pre-fracture living situation in subjects of this age treated with hGH was significantly increased when compared with the placebo-treated group. The treatment intervention was well tolerated and no safety issues were recorded.

Wang P et al. The role of endotoxin, TNF-alpha, and IL-6 in inducing the state of growth hormone insensitivity. World J Gastroenterol 2002 Jun; 8(3):531-6 AIM: Critical illnesses such as sepsis, trauma, and burns cause a growth hormone insensitivity, which leads to an increased negative nitrogen balance. Endotoxin is generously released into blood under these conditions and stimulates the production of proinflammatory cytokines such as TNF-alpha, IL-6, and IL-1, which may play a very important role in inducing the growth hormone insensitivity. The objective of this current study was to investigate the role of endotoxin, TNF-alpha and IL-6 in inducing the growth hormone insensitivity at the receptor and post-receptor levels. METHODS: Spague-Dawley rats were injected with endotoxin, TNF-alpha, and IL-6, respectively and part of rats injected with endotoxin was treated with exogenous somatotropin simultaneously. All rats were killed at different time points. The expression of IGF-I, GHR, SOCS-3 and beta-actin mRNA in the liver was detected by RT-PCR and the GH levels were measured by radioimmunoassay, the levels of TNF-alpha and IL-6 were detected by ELISA. RESULTS: There was no significant difference in serous GH levels between experimental group and control rats after endotoxin injection, however, liver IGF-I mRNA expression had been obviously down-regulated in endotoxemic rats. Liver GHR mRNA expression also had a predominant down-regulation after endotoxin injection. The lowest regulation of liver IGF-I mRNA expression occurred at 12h after LPS injection, being decreased by 53% compared with control rats. For GHR mRNA expression, the lowest expression occurred at 8h and had a 81% decrease. Although SOCS-3 mRNA was weakly expressed in control rats, it was strongly up-regulated after LPS injection and had a 7.84 times increase compared with control rats. Exogenous GH could enhance IGF-I mRNA expression in control rats, but it did fail to prevent the decline in IGF-I mRNA expression in endotoxemic rats. Endotoxin stimulated the production of TNF-alpha and IL-6, and the elevated IL-6 levels was shown a positive correlation with increased SOCS-3 mRNA expression. The liver GHR mRNA expression was obviously down-regulated after TNF-alpha iv injection and had a 40% decrease at 8h, but the liver SOCS-3 mRNA expression was the 4.94 times up-regulation occurred at 40 min after IL-6 injection. CONCLUSION: The growth hormone insensitivity could be induced by LPS injection, which was associated with down-regulated GHR mRNA expression at receptor level and with up-regulated SOCS-3 mRNA expression at post-receptor level. The in vivo biological activities of LPS were mediated by TNF-alpha and IL-6 indirectly, and TNF-alpha and IL-6 may exert their effects on the receptor and post-receptor levels respectively.

Wren AM et al. The novel hypothalamic peptide ghrelin stimulates food intake and growth hormone secretion, Endocrinology 2000 Nov;141(11):4325-8 Ghrelin, a novel 28 amino acid peptide found in hypothalamus and stomach, was recently identified as the endogenous ligand for the growth hormone secretagogue receptor (GHS-R). We have now found that both intracerebroventricular (i.c.v.) and intraperitoneal (i.p.) administration of ghrelin in freely feeding rats stimulated food intake. The onset of increased feeding was rapid and after i.c.v. administration was sustained for 24 hours. Following i.c.v. administration of 3 nmol ghrelin, the duration and magnitude of the feeding stimulation was similar to that following 5 nmol neuropeptide Y (NPY). Plasma growth hormone (GH) concentration increased following both i.c.v. and i.p. administration of ghrelin. Release of adrenocorticotrophic hormone (ACTH) was stimulated and thyroid stimulating hormone (TSH) inhibited following i.c.v. administration of ghrelin. These data suggest a possible role for the newly identified endogenous hypothalamic peptide, ghrelin, in stimulation of feeding and growth hormone secretion.